Advance Praise for *Unprocessed*

"I love how Megan effortlessly intertwines her story with all that she learned about the food we eat and how it's processed. . . . A refreshingly simple approach on where to draw the line."

—Lisa Leake, #1 *New York Times* bestselling author of *100 Days of Real Food*

"Confused about why nutritionists like me advise eating relatively unprocessed foods? Megan Kimble spends a year taking a deep dive into the meaning of processing by trying to live an unprocessed life, and on a careful budget yet. Part memoir, *Unprocessed* takes us through Kimble's evolving understanding that we have real choices about the way we eat and that these choices greatly matter for our health, economics, and sense of community."

—Marion Nestle, professor of nutrition, food studies, and public health at New York University and author of *What to Eat*

"In Megan's thorough and lively search for a diet of real food, she delivers an important lesson in the processes that have led us away from our old nourishing ways. A meaningful and timely tale."

—Tamar Adler, author of *An Everlasting Meal: Cooking with Economy and Grace* and contributing writer for *The New York Times Magazine*

"Well-told story of a quest that has the power to change far more than the author's life. It's an important book for all of us who live and breathe and eat in America. I thought I knew this material, but I couldn't put the book down, and I came away from it recharged and better informed. . . . Fresh and smart, but also wise."

—Deborah Madison, author of *Vegetable Literacy* and *The New Vegetarian Cooking for Everyone*

"A very personal and honest report of her year-long effort . . . and many practical tips for improving our ways of eating without spending a fortune. An engaging read with valuable information."

—Andrew Weil, M.D., bestselling coauthor of
True Food: Seasonal, Sustainable, Simple, Pure

"Megan Kimble is the freshest voice in literary food writing since Dan Barber and Tamar Adler came on the scene. *Unprocessed* is a stunning debut by a perceptive observer of how our food systems actually work, but it also reveals the faces, processes, and values that are hidden in our food supply chains, written in disarmingly graceful prose that will stay in your memory for years to come."

—Gary Paul Nabhan, author of the award-winning
Growing Food in a Hotter, Drier Land and *Coming Home to Eat*

"*Unprocessed* should be required reading for every American eater. In this engrossing tale, Kimble lets us tag along as she processes our flawed food system and unprocesses her kitchen. Kimble's candor and can-do spirit empower and inspire."

—Jonathan Bloom, author of *American Wasteland*

UNPROCESSED

MY CITY-DWELLING YEAR OF
RECLAIMING REAL FOOD

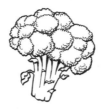

MEGAN KIMBLE

wm
WILLIAM MORROW
An Imprint of HarperCollins*Publishers*

HarperCollins books may be purchased for educational, business, or sales promotional use. For information please e-mail the Special Markets Department at SPsales@harpercollins.com.

FIRST EDITION

Designed by Diahann Sturge

Library of Congress Cataloging-in-Publication Data has been applied for.

ISBN 978-0-06-238246-7

15 16 17 18 19   ov/rrd   10 9 8 7 6 5 4 3 2 1

For my parents, Midge and Jeff Kimble.
Because of Katie, my best friend and faithful editor.

CONTENTS

Change is a process.

"Wait," Tyler says. "Isn't peanut butter processed?"

The peanut butter jar is in my left hand, spoon in my right; a banana, unpeeled, waits on the counter. I stick the spoon back in the jar and turn to face Tyler, my sister's husband, sitting at the kitchen table of my parents' house outside Los Angeles.

"No," I say. "It's just ground-up peanuts."

"Isn't that a kind of processing?"

"Well, yes. I mean, all foods are processed, at least to some degree."

"So then what's the difference between ground-up peanuts and, say, partially hydrogenated peanut oil?"

I sigh. I thought my sister had already explained the logic of my upcoming year to her husband, but evidently Tyler is feeling contrary this January morning so soon after the holidays. It's pestering like this that makes him feel more like a brother than a sister's husband, but I am nervous on the cusp of a year unprocessed and I don't want to argue semantics. "There are degrees of processing," I say, placing the peanut butter jar back on the counter. "I'm trying to find the line where a food becomes *too* processed." With the exception of, say, a raw, foraged mushroom—risky business—all food has undergone some processing before landing on our plates. By way of harvest or heat, all food is processed, and often it is the better for it.

But increasingly, it is not. Today, the word "processed" refers to adulterated foods—foods that have been shifted and shaped into packages that are *not* better, not for us or for the earth. All foods are processed, but if we understand the difference between an apple and a bag of Chex Mix—and we do—and if the space between the two matters for the health of our bodies and the environment—and it does—then the question of what makes a food too processed also matters.

I'd decided to see if I could go a year without eating a processed food. Or rather, a food I deemed "too processed." When I first hatched the project, around the time that Tyler was bugging me in my parents' kitchen, I thought that I should figure out precisely what made a food processed and *then* begin. But as it turned out, it would take me a year to figure out where to draw the line, to understand where our food system succeeds and fails in processing food from land. That figuring out is what you're holding in your hands.

I HEARD MICHAEL POLLAN INTERVIEWED on NPR's *Wait . . . Don't Tell Me* several years ago. The host of the show, Peter Sagal, introduced him as "the most well-known authority on food and food economics working today," a description that is as true now as it was then. The two chitchatted for a bit and then Sagal asked Pollan, "So, if you ever want to eat a cheeseburger, do you have to go hide somewhere?"

Pollan laughed. "Shortly after I got to Berkeley," he said, "I was in Berkeley Bowl . . . a local supermarket, which has wonderful fresh produce, grass-fed beef." What was Michael Pollan buying at the Berkeley Bowl? Fruity Pebbles—his son Isaac's Saturday-morning treat. "So I was reaching for a box of Fruity Pebbles," he said, "and somebody tapped on my shoulder. And it was this tall, bearded graduate student and he said [whispering], 'I'm watching Michael Pollan shop for groceries.'"

When you are ten years old, even if Michael Pollan is your father, Fruity Pebbles are fun to eat on Saturday mornings. When you are twenty-six, even if you know better, shrink-wrapped chocolate chip cookies are fun to eat on Saturday nights. With food, it's not just easy to look the other way, to ignore the ingredient label—it is, in fact, delicious to do so. On a Saturday morning, Michael Pollan is a father who'd rather relax than explain to a ten-year-old why the corn syrup in his processed cereal is causing his pancreas to overproduce insulin.

Although it is impossible to speak of food without discussing the dysfunction in how we now grow, prepare, and eat it, this is not a book focused on what's gone wrong. Michael Pollan, for one, has already led the charge of uncracking the truth of a food system gone astray. Since Pollan wrote *The Omnivore's Dilemma* and Gary Paul Nabhan wrote *Coming Home to Eat*—the epicenter of his 220-mile local food experiment was just south of Tucson, where I live and where my year unprocessed unfolded—and Barbara Kingsolver *left* Tucson to write *Animal Vegetable Miracle,* consumer consciousness has swelled. Awareness has shifted. Local, organic, sustainable—these are all words now in the public vernacular. But in early 2012, when I stopped eating processed food, farmers' markets accounted for only 1 percent of total food sales; organic foods represented only 2 percent of total grocery sales. If we knew what had gone wrong, why weren't we doing anything about it?

This is where I begin. You've likely heard the charge—Vote with Your Fork—but I wanted to test how feasible that advice really is. Today, many of us are stuck between knowing what we should do and feeling like we don't have enough time or money to do it. Eating unprocessed was my attempt to find another way in, unburdened by "should do," focused instead on "can do."

Change is hard. Small choices gain inertia and turn into habits, and we are all busy, broke, and stuck in our whirlwind cities. But if Suze Orman writes money books enlightening the *Young, Fabulous & Broke* about their financial futures, then this, I hope, is some small manifesto for the busy, urban, and broke about their edible futures.

IN THE SPRING OF MY SENIOR YEAR in college at the University of Denver, I saw Al Gore give the famous PowerPoint presentation that inspired the documentary *An Inconvenient Truth*. I had seen the film the previous Christmas with my sister and mom; those two hours sitting in a dark theater horrified us. The world was beautiful, it was whole, and we were breaking it apart. And then the credits rolled. The theater lights lifted and we walked, knob-kneed, out of the theater. Our fear dissipated into dinner plans.

The evening I went to see Al Gore in the flesh, I was on the precipice of all those decisions that come with college graduation. Riding the light rail downtown, I read a few pages in Ernesto Guevara's *Guerrilla Warfare*. I was taking a senior seminar about Che, and although I wasn't into the icon's militarism and ego, I was enthralled by his boldness, how he'd stuck his thumb into the spinning status quo and changed how one small part of the world worked. I was enthralled, but in my life, being this bold—Che bold—felt incompatible with an infrastructure already in place, one that included careerbuilder.com and an apartment lease. As commencement approached, we graduates were told again and again: Be bold. But I didn't really know *how*. I wondered: Does boldness exist only in military fatigues? Could it also wear a sundress and flip-flops?

Al Gore was, as I expected him to be, amiable and twangy. But unlike the movie experience, I was actively in my mind and body as I listened, fidgety and lacking the distance offered by film. The lights in the convention center never dimmed and so they didn't rise. I carried my terror with me all the way home. It was all happening now, chemicals in the air, a sweating world, it was nownownow—9 P.M. on a Tuesday. I called my dad, a quantum physics professor, arbitrator of big decisions.

"Right," he said. "It's scary stuff."

"But what do we do?" I asked. "What do *I* do?" I should change my major from English to astrophysics or environmental science, I could just stay in college for another year. I would learn the tools needed to fix this problem. Global warming was *my* generation's problem—this would be my life's big gesture.

"But, Megan," he said. "Do you like science?"

"I don't know. I could!"

"Big gestures are important," he said. "But big stuff starts at the day-to-day. You've got to like what you're doing on a Wednesday afternoon in order to solve the big problems."

Rather than figure out what should fill my Wednesday afternoons, I approached the professor who was teaching the class about Che Guevara and asked him for contacts in Latin America. I wanted to Make a Difference. I wanted to See the World and to Speak Spanish. My professor e-mailed a friend who owned a hotel in Nicaragua and needed a volunteer English teacher. So I finished my English degree and moved to Playa Gigante, a small fishing village of five hundred people, to work at the hotel and start a free English-language program for the town's residents.

I arrived in Playa Gigante expecting—well, I don't know what I was expecting. Fewer scorpions. More infrastructure. Less mud. More electricity. I lived in a bunk bed in the staff quarters, shared a bathroom with four surfers, and lived out of my backpack. Only after I arrived did I learn how closely Nicaragua had been tied to Che and Castro; how, inspired by the Cuban revolution, in 1979, a scrappy crew of guerrilla soldiers and untrained civilians overthrew a government backed by the biggest superpower in the world.

But my day-to-day life was simple, elemental. When I wasn't teaching my English class every morning, afternoon, and evening, I was reading, running on the beach, or drinking beer with Juan, the hotel's manager. Save for the quantity of beer I consumed—another?—I made very few choices. I ate what was given to me: scrambled eggs and *gallo pinto,* rice and beans, for breakfast; fried fish or fried chicken and *gallo pinto* for dinner. Playa Gigante had no grocery stores or markets, so if I wanted any food that wasn't stocked in the hotel's kitchen, I had to ask Juan to buy it for me when he drove the hour into Rivas, the closest city, to do our weekly shopping. (I'd lived in Playa Gigante for six months before I discovered that the town had a convenience store in the form of a man named Castro, who sold dried goods, eggs, and soda out of a back room in his house.)

When it rained, the electricity went out and my younger students didn't come to class. Rain or no rain, I went running in the afternoon, so I'd see them sitting on plastic chairs below corrugated zinc roofs or stirring *gallo pinto* over woodburning stoves. I'd wave at my adult students, fishermen, as they strung out their nets, tying knots and repairing lines. I ran around cows that stood like boulders, staring unblinkingly at the long-legged gringa; I darted around strutting wild turkeys and passed pigs burrowed into the cool mud.

My life was stark and I settled into its starkness. I settled in so much that I stayed in Nicaragua for a year instead of the three months I'd planned. And when I finally did come home, I was shocked—culture shocked, abundance shocked, choice shocked.

My first day back in Los Angeles, I went to a supermarket and wandered up and down the aisles, overwhelmed. Gloriously overwhelmed, it's true. There was peanut butter—so many kinds—and granola—so many flavors—and fresh vegetables—so many available at the same time. But as I marveled at the abundance, I also marveled that I'd ever assumed abundance was the only option. That I'd ever believed there would always be food, and that it would always be plentiful. For the first time in my life, I wondered: Why does anyone need the choice of nine kinds of peanut butter?

Of course, peanut butter seems to have nothing to do with global warming, with communism or capitalism, but the more I learned, the more I realized that everything is connected: consumption in the wealthy north and poverty in the developing south; a changing climate and a food system that exhales almost half of all greenhouse gases emitted in the United States; political unrest in Latin America and the policies we pursued at home.

The threads I tugged began to lead back to the same knot. And one way into the tangle of that knot was food. Food—at least, the way we now grow, process, and transport it—has changed the climate; ironically, now the changing climate will dictate how we can grow food in the future. Food leaves countries like Mexico, Peru, and Chile, and enters the markets in the United States—usually to the economic benefit of us eaters, instead of faraway producers. Food overwhelms us with cheap choice and we, in turn, overwhelm our bodies with too much of it.

I grew up a complacent eater and citizen, aware of issues but believing that my civic responsibility was to educate myself. To study hard and get a good job—patience, little girl—so that I could join the power brokers and finally turn my frustration with our broken system into a contribution, into some sort of solution.

Some challenges, like global warming, feel so insurmountable that it seems as though nothing can be done. But we live in a world full of insurmountable obstacles. And we do things. Without small specificity, without localness and precision of place, it is hard to ask and harder to answer: What do we want to change and how do we want to do it?

I pose this question to a friend in the parking lot of a hipster Tucson coffee shop, leaning on our bikes. It is time to go home, and John offers a concluding statement. "Our generation sucks," he says.

We have been talking about this all night—about 1970s counterculture, voter turnout, and the Occupy Wall Street movement, which was sweeping the nation at the time. If global warming is our generation's problem—if we are the people who will inherit a planet in spasm—why weren't we doing anything about it? We were doing *something,* sure—I worked in communications at the University of Arizona's Office of Sustainability; John was working on a Ph.D. in environmental anthropology—but it felt like we weren't doing *enough.*

In the fall of 2011, in a park in lower Manhattan, a small encampment protesting income inequality drew international attention. For a moment, a month or two, as the movement spread to cities across the world, it seemed like something might change, that Wall Street firms would finally be held accountable for bankrupting our future, and that we, the young people of America, would be the ones to hold them to it. But in practice, when my friend Sarah and I ventured to Tucson's Occupy encampment, we hovered, uncertain of what to do, how to participate. After scrawling messages in chalk on the pavement and participating in a group meeting, as dusk slanted toward dark, we talked about spending the night. "Then again, I have to be at work tomorrow morning," I said. "How does that work?"

I matriculated in the age of alarm, after world oil production peaked, when global climate change and economic instability were givens rather than what-ifs. I've never worked in an economy that wasn't unreliable or lived in a world that wasn't warming. Somehow, protesting in a park didn't seem like a sustainable solution to issues with such inertia.

So the question I again faced when I returned from Nicaragua was: *How?* How do we start to dig out from under this weight? How do we begin change—and how do we sustain it?

IT'S A SWELTERING WEDNESDAY NIGHT IN JUNE, midway through my year unprocessed, when I begin to figure out the answer to this question. I ride my bike to the Loft Cinema in Tucson to meet second-date Mark and arrive wearing Tucson's summer sash—that right-to-left line of soaked fabric that forms under my messenger bag like the "Indiana" ribbon of a Miss America contestant.

We're here for the Tucson premiere of *Heist: Who Stole the American Dream?*—a documentary about the 2008 financial collapse and corruption on Wall Street and in Washington. When Frances Causey, the film's director, and Kimber Lanning, the director of Local First Arizona, take the stage for a Q&A, an audience member asks the inevitable question: So, what can I do? What can any of us do, huddled by our air-conditioning units on this desert island, so far away from the traffic circles of Washington, DC?

Kimber ran a record store in Phoenix before she started Local First Arizona, a nonprofit organization that works to strengthen local economies in the state. Shaggy black hair hangs around her face; a brown dress wraps close to her curves; shiny heels tilt toward the audience and then lean back. She speaks without saying "um," without shifting her weight around her chair. Frances fidgets, rubbing the cord of the microphone up and down, but Kimber sits, composed and certain. Her answer is simple: Spend money better.

"The American consuming public is the elephant in the room," she says. "We forget that our individual buying power is the most power we have, any one of us, and we *give it away* without thinking."

Our dollars have the power to change the way things run, and yet we give them away with such *ease*. Money circulates, money travels, and money rushing through Wall Street does not simply appear out of the ether. I buy things and my dollars trickle toward the center. We treat money as an either/or—either we have money or we do not have money. But we often don't stop to consider what happens in the space between, how money flows through a community.

Kimber tells us this: If a community the size of Tucson shifted 10 percent of its spending to local businesses—a 10 percent *shift,* not an increase—within one year, we would create almost $140 million in new revenue for the city. What that also means, I realize, is that we would *withhold* that $140 million from the balance sheets of those corporations that then use our money to influence government policy, to grow unsustainable food, to waste energy—and to process and sell us foods that aren't good for us.

I want to grab my date, this man I barely know, and tell him—I've figured it out! Now I understand. But I hardly know him, so I sit quietly and buzz with this idea, this wonderful articulation of what I had felt about changing the way I bought food but couldn't quite say. My dollars reverberate, of course—the dollars I spend at Safeway or at a CSA. These dollars *matter*. So what if I spend my dollars in a different way? Distribute my small portion not to the center, to the bargain shops and industrial producers, but to the periphery—to the locally accountable corners of my country rather than the abstract black hole of its center?

I ride my bike home, chewing on this idea. It is precisely because I have so few dollars that I should treat them so preciously, should make sure that each and every one, vibrating out there in the world, is behaving itself. I love this idea because it is quiet, immediate, and personal.

MORE OFTEN THAN NOT, a dollar spent on a processed food is a dollar distributed to the center. Globally, processed and packaged foods constitute a $1.25 trillion market and ten companies control a quarter of that market. Ten companies, and we think that we have a choice in the foods we buy. The reason this consolidation matters, even if you are happy with the cheap-packaged tastiness it brings you, is that size engenders influence. The giants of our food system are also our political Goliaths. The American Farm Bureau Federation, Distilled Spirits Council, Cargill Inc., Mars Inc., the Grocery Manufacturers of America—again and again, the largest companies in any sector provide some of the largest campaign contributions in U.S. elections.

If a handful of companies controls a majority of our processed foods, and 70 percent of all food calories we eat are processed, then the logic is inescapable—most of our food dollars are spent supporting companies that may or may not serve our best interests.

The statement that almost three-fourths of food consumed across the world is processed comes from Carlos Monteiro, a prominent nutrition professor at the University of São Paulo in Brazil. Monteiro agrees with me—or, more likely, I agree with him: All food is processed. As found in nature, most plants and animals are inedible, toxic, or highly perishable; advancements in agriculture, preservation, and preparation over the past ten thousand years have offered huge gains for human nutrition. These gains have only begun to become undone in the past three decades, with the rapid rise in consumption of what Monteiro called "ultra-processed" foods—foods that have been manufactured to be "durable, accessible, convenient, attractive, ready-to-eat or ready-to-heat." This 70 percent figure, then, does not include pasteurized milk, frozen carrots, or canned tomatoes. "The most important factor now, when considering food, nutrition and public health, is not nutrients, and is not food, so much as what is done to foodstuffs and the nutrients originally contained in them, before they are purchased and consumed," he writes. "That is to say, the big issue is food processing—or, to be more precise, the nature, extent and purpose of processing, and what happens to food and to us as a result of processing."

I didn't know of Monteiro's research when I began my year and I didn't know what *exactly* made a food processed. But I had to start somewhere, so I began with the belief that a food was unprocessed if I could theoretically make it in my home kitchen. I could grind up wheat berries into flour, though I couldn't take that flour and sift out its endosperm and bleach it into fluffy whiteness. I could gather honey and grind nuts into butter, but I wouldn't refine sugar, stock up on chemicals, or mix emulsifiers. Whenever possible—whenever I could afford it—I'd buy organic and local, but I'd also be aware of when these modifiers fall short.

When I started my year unprocessed, I'd recently returned to eating meat after nearly a year of vegetarianism. I didn't eat much—maybe a serving a week. When I started my year, I decided meat would be unprocessed if it was locally raised and carefully slaughtered. When I ate out, I allowed myself the option to order meat if it seemed, based on some criteria I'd later determine, like a sustainable choice. So I ate the occasional carne asada taco or chicken salad, and although it was nice to be *able* to eat meat, mostly I didn't.

I did drink milk. I sometimes made yogurt, but mostly it arrived at my refrigerator packaged in gallon-size plastic tubs—unsweetened, without added flavoring or thickeners. Yogurt joined flash-frozen fruit in a blender for a morning smoothie. I filled my lunchtime Tupperware containers with home-cooked beans—pintos, chickpeas, lentils—and grains—barley, couscous, long-stemmed rice—with a generous helping of roasted or raw vegetables and a pour of extra-virgin olive oil. I made grilled cheeses on my George Forman from store-bought bread containing only some version of grain and water, and cheese grated from blocks, without de-caking agents or food coloring. I fried eggs with bright, gooey yolks—eggs that came from local farmers—and slid them atop jumbles of fresh vegetables, provisioned almost entirely by my Tucson Community Supported Agriculture share.

Basically, I ate everything that was obviously and intuitively food. Food defined, without chemical additions or processed subtractions.

In addition to the nature, extent, and purpose of processing, I wanted to consider its intent. Historically, we have processed food to make it safer and to preserve it, two advancements that significantly increased human health and longevity; today, the goal of processing has shifted to creating products that "are formulated to reduce microbial deterioration ('long shelf life'), to be transportable for long distances, to be extremely palatable ('high organoleptic quality') and often to be habit-forming," writes Monteiro. Add "cheap for the consumer but profitable for the corporation" and you've figured out the modern supermarket.

We are at a rare moment in history when the word "processed" might soon become meaningless. As GMOs, food additives, and pesticide-covered crops spread through our supermarket aisles, we may no longer even have the choice to eat unprocessed foods. Unless, that is, we do something differently.

When I started my year unprocessed, I was earning an annual salary of $16,780. I was a graduate student, taking four classes and working twenty-five hours a week on top of those classes. I was busy, broke, and I lived in a small one-bedroom apartment with a janky, understocked kitchen.

While there are challenges I can't grasp about living on the brink of hunger—challenges I address in the last chapter of this book—the fact of the matter is, most of us have several dollars a week that we could spend differently. The hypothesis of my year was that eating whole, unprocessed food would not cost significantly more than the ready-made subsistence I might gather from the industrial food chain. And, more important, it would not take significantly more time. Even though I eventually canned tomatoes, evaporated salt from the sea, and brewed mead, I didn't have the time or desire to turn food processing into a full-time dedication. I also ate out, went on dates, and tried to live my year unprocessed in the world and not away from it. I didn't expect to ditch my microwave; but I also hadn't bargained on processing meat, milking goats, or hoarding grocery receipts—for every single food item I bought. If the question of the year was how to unprocess my food, its experiment was how to afford it.

BACK IN THAT PARKING LOT WITH MY FRIEND, midway through my year unprocessed, as I consider John's statement that "our generation sucks," I realize how profoundly I disagree with this neat little summary. I disagree with a force that surprises me.

"What?" he says, seeing my expression.

"Well, saying that: That's sort of a showstopper, don't you think?"

He raises his eyebrows.

"What do we do with that? How do we un-suck ourselves?"

He shrugs, mounts his bike, and rolls away. As I pedal after him, I remember why, six months before, I had stopped eating processed foods. I was sick of talking about problems in coffee shops.

It may look like my generation is silently accepting what seems inevitable, but quietly, in the small corners of our country, we are working to untangle ourselves from the systems that reared us. Of course, I didn't start eating unprocessed for the politics—I did it for the food. Eating unprocessed wasn't just a way to opt out of a broken food system, it was also a way to opt *in*. To opt in to another way of eating, another way of being with food, flavor, and community. I wanted to spend money better, but I also wanted to eat better food. And conveniently, real food tastes better.

I am young, urban, and broke, and so it seems like I have little bargaining power. But I have my dollars. I decided to do something specific, something precise, and something very small; to protest the only way I knew how, against the problem I'd always believed I'd have to inherit. I stopped eating processed food. It was a beginning: a start in redirecting my precious dollars away from the center, away from fossil fuel food, stripped land, and unaccountable industries. Because in a world of seemingly insurmountable obstacles, there *has* to be something we can do—right?

1

SUPERMARKET

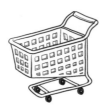

Processed sells.

The warmth of Safeway's fluorescent lights pulls me inside, pleasurably inevitable, and before I know it, I'm looking at a table stacked with brittle plastic boxes of pink-frosted sugar cookies. Behind the cookies, a refrigerated display case of MEALS TO GO and another of HOMEMADE GOODNESS stand tall. Because I am looking for the most tastily processed meal in the store, I stop to linger. I consider Safeway's Signature Café Broccoli Cheddar au Gratin entrée, packed neatly in a plastic dish and wrapped in image-splashed cardboard with a ticker-tape list of ingredients. A similarly packaged shepard's pie catches my eye, glistening with prideful peas and vivid carrots, almost outweighing the fact that I don't like shepard's pie.

I'm at Safeway because my year unprocessed begins tomorrow: Sunday, January 15. I've cleaned my cabinets of their accumulated processes—of low-fat cream cheese, hundred-calorie tortillas, and vanilla-flavored almond milk, all of which contain some refined version of sugar, wheat, or, in the case of the cream cheese, whatever it is that's used to make sorbic acid and guar gum. I've munched through the leftovers of my processed life—a bag of chocolate chips, two cans of Diet Coke, half a bag of pretzels—or given it away to hungry friends.

I am anxious for the year to start. Less than the actual logistics of eating processed, I'm nervous about the fact that soon, I will have to talk about it. Will have to explain my reasoning, my commitment to this schemed-up, hippie-sounding thing I've decided to call "unprocessed." When I told my sister Katie about my year's project, she asked a series of sensible questions, absorbed the constraints I'd established, and then promptly started e-mailing me recipes for unprocessed desserts. Tyler was skeptical; my mom, ever the midwesterner, said, "Well, that sure sounds like a challenge." I've told exactly two people in Tucson—Sarah and Hilary, my first and best friends in town, who both think it is a very Megan thing to believe so optimistically in the possibility of a year.

For now, it's just me in Safeway, here to buy my last processed meal.

On Sundays—every Sunday of my childhood—my mom, Katie, and I went to the grocery store, usually to the Vons supermarket in La Cañada. It was a ritual that anchored our Sundays week after week, year after year, as we moved from finicky five to surly sixteen. Although my vegetarian mother mostly filled our cart with vegetables and pasta, cheese and yogurt, the occasional cardboard-wrapped cookie or crinkly bag of chips was a concession to persistent pleadings.

Tonight, my indulgence is one of nostalgia as much as of process. Whatever I buy tonight will be my departure from the kind of place that has fed me for as long as I've known how to eat. I could, theoretically, keep shopping here this year; there are organic apples and free-range eggs, California-sourced kale and Arizona dates. But just as foods can be processed, so can commerce. If I wanted to keep my unruly dollars close at hand, then I had to forgo this kind of processed shopping experience, one where small dollars flow to a super-center. One problem—one reason for my nervousness—was that I wasn't yet sure where I might shop *instead*. I didn't think I could afford to provision my kitchen exclusively at the farmers' market, so Trader Joe's remained in my rotation, but skeptically so, as I learned how little the company shares about where they source their food. I had my eye on Tucson's food cooperative, a member-run operation, but hadn't yet scouted its aisles.

I tear myself away from the glistening shepard's pie and turn to the vastness of the store before me. One meal. I'm here for one meal. I don't want a plastic-textured entrée, but I don't know *what* I'm here to buy. In a supermarket, this is a very vulnerable way to be.

TODAY, THE LOS ANGELES CONVENTION CENTER SITS on the site of the first Safeway. In 1911, on the corner of Figueroa and Pico in downtown Los Angeles, Sam Seelig opened a modest store to "furnish to the public reliable merchandise, foodstuffs tested and valuable in health-giving as well as in economy," recalled a *Los Angeles Times* article in 1925. Until well past the turn of the century, grocery stores were outlets for dried goods stored in large, unmarked barrels; customers would present orders to clerks, who would then gather items from store shelves. (Indeed, until the Trademark Law passed in 1905, it was illegal for companies to brand or market food directly to customers.) But in 1916, when Clarence Saunders, a flamboyant force of a man—he would eventually build himself a pink palace—opened a grocery store in Memphis, Tennessee, he transformed the way food was bought and sold. At the Piggly Wiggly, Saunders established the fundamental tenet of modern supermarket shopping: Customers themselves would choose the food they buy. That we should serve ourselves at a supermarket seems so integral to the store's purpose as to be innate, but the fact is, had Saunders or another flamboyant grocer not decided that shoppers might actually want to select their own food, that they would enjoy the experience of wandering through long aisles, there would be no such Safeway for me to wander through today.

In *The Super Market: A Revolution in Distribution,* M. M. Zimmerman marveled at these intrepid customers—known then as "housewives"—willing to forgo the comforts of clerk-assisted shopping "in order to do her own choosing and to cart her own purchases." But comfort wasn't what the housewife wanted anymore. She wanted choice and she wanted it for cheap.

In 1929, an Irish immigrant named Michael Cullen proposed a new model for selling groceries: cheap food, and lots of it. He would sell three hundred items at cost and another two hundred at 5 percent below cost. He would "lead the public out of the high priced houses of bondage into the low prices of the house of the promised land." Cullen rented a six-thousand-square-foot warehouse on Long Island, stocked it full of wholesale and discount goods, and called it King Kullen Grocery Co. King Kullen would be the "World's Greatest Price Wrecker," and so it was; to King Kullen the masses flocked. By 1936, there were seventeen outlets in New York doing $6 million worth of business. King Kullen, it is said, was the country's first supermarket.

BEFORE I CAN REACH A ROW OF REFRIGERATORS labeled PURE & WHOLESOME, I am pulled into an aisle full of yogurts, cheeses, and puddings—the pull is unexplainable but explicit—so I follow this urge up DAIRY CHOICES and swing a left at the end. Before I turn into FROZEN CHOICES, I survey the end-aisle display facing me. It holds a disparate assortment of frozen foods: Green Giant baby brussels sprouts with butter, White Castle frozen cheeseburgers, and DiGiorno Rising Crust Pizza. Though it appears like someone with a very particular set of munchies stocked this freezer, these are high-profit, highly advertised items, likely to be bought "off list"—on impulse. These items are not bought; rather, they are *sold*.

With the "revolution in distribution" offered by the first supermarkets, no longer could grocers be depended on to guide customers to specific brands. Today, aggressive food marketing is all but assumed, but in 1957, Vance Packard's revelations in *The Hidden Persuaders* were scandalous: "Buying psychologists have teamed up with merchandising experts to persuade the wife to buy products she may not particularly need or even want." After surveying more than five thousand shoppers, a study cited by Packard found that "today's shopper in the supermarket is more and more guided by the buying philosophy—'If somehow your product catches my eye—and for some reason it looks especially good—I WANT IT.'"

In the years following *The Hidden Persuaders,* as food manufacturers and retailers jostled to be first in the receiving line for this impulse, these hidden persuasions gradually became more overt. By the 1980s, retailers had built an intricate framework of slotting fees—"rent" that food manufacturers pay to secure shelf space—and trade allowances—advertisements those manufacturers promise to run to generate interest—to help shoppers buy exactly what retailers want them to buy. Those two hundred items King Kullen promised to sell below cost are now known as "loss leaders," discounted specials that get you in the door to buy more expensive items.

MY SISTER KATIE once pulled her pants down in the middle of a supermarket. I wasn't there—Katie was four, so I was a stay-at-home two—but the story is a Kimble family staple. Katie had a halo of ridiculously curly blond hair and bright blue eyes; she was adorable and temperamental and she wanted ice cream. My mom refused. Katie demanded. I can just see her there, in the middle of the Pasadena Ralph's, fuming, glaring up at my mom, fists clenching in frustration. She had already stomped her feet and still my mom had given her a gentle but firm no. What recourse did a four-year-old have? With a defiant shove, Katie yanked her elastic-waist pants and cotton underpants down to her ankles and stood back up, hands on her hips. She looked my mom in the eye, daring her to ignore *this* spectacle.

The ice cream was not bought.

I'm midway through the second FROZEN CHOICES aisle, past the ice cream and somewhere under the domain of breakfast, deep within the Eggo Waffles, Jimmy Dean Sausages, and Eating Right Frozen Oatmeal—I pause to wonder how re-heating cooked-then-frozen oats is easier than microwaving raw oats—when I spot a rectangular blue cardboard box, covered in beige flying disks, shooting yellow stars, and the bubble words: KRUSTEAZ MINI PANCAKES.

Once Katie and I had passed tantrum age, when all threats of public nudity had passed, we were essentially set loose in the grocery store. My family rarely went out to eat and Katie and I packed our lunches every day, so the grocery store was the domain in which we were allowed to exercise the freedom of choice—within reason. My mom cooked us vegetarian dinners every night—stir-fries and pastas, baked potatoes and veggie enchiladas—and so, she figured, a few Doritos here and there wouldn't hurt. Even as my mom fought to get healthy foods in our bodies, she struggled to find foods we'd willingly consume. So Katie and I roamed, tossing our choices exuberantly into the cart. Lunchable Snacks and Cheddar Blast Doritos—and, for me, Krusteaz Mini Pancakes.

A mini pancake is a golfball-size pancake—a flattened golfball, uniformly toasted, round and smooth. Every morning, I'd arrange eighteen of these disks in piles of three; after a minute and a half, staring eagerly at the whirring microwave, I'd pop the door open to flip each stack of mini pancakes from top to bottom, ensuring no pancake endured too much sog. "Why don't you just heat them in one layer?" my sister demanded, always the know-it-all. But I ate my mini pancakes in stacks of three because sinking my teeth into a thick stack of pancakes, cupping this little stack between sticky thumb and forefinger, dipping each bite's edge into a spill of syrup, running my tongue in the grooves between each disk's edge—this was so much more satisfying than folding one floppy pancake into my mouth. I remember the feel of a stack of mini pancakes in my hand more than almost any other food from my childhood—the billow of sweet pancake steam when I opened the microwave, the spongy chewiness of each bite, the sticky fingers to be licked clean of maple syrup when the little stacks had disappeared.

After we had finished our shopping, after we loaded the groceries into the car and pushed the cart back to the hold, we each pulled one snack out of the trunk as a treat for the two-mile drive home. I would snag a heel of the fresh French baguette peeking out from a long paper bag; Katie would take the end of a sourdough baguette, her favorite. We would peer across the expanse of trunk, searching for the flagpoles of bread. A four-inch tear, and then we scampered back into the backseat to gnaw on our bread in smiling silence.

ALTHOUGH I HAD RESOLVED to journey down every aisle, I cannot muster the energy to confront HOME CARE, BABY CARE, or PARTY, PRINT & PAPER. Steering into an aisle is a commitment, and purposefully so. Although doctoral students in the sociology of shopping or the psychology of food continue to write dissertations about supermarket layout and design, about aisle width, length, and "profit maximization consistent with customer convenience," the fundamentals haven't changed in decades. Supermarket design resides in the delicate balance of exposing you to as many products as possible without aggravating you so much that you throw your oranges in the air and run screaming from the store. The basic premise of food merchandising is exposure, as studies by those same doctoral students have proven again and again—the more you see, the more you buy.

Hence, long aisles. A long aisle forces customers to look at all the products within that aisle, even if they've already grabbed the one they need. Unfortunately, long aisles tend to stress customers out, which makes them buy less;

midaisle "escape hatches" are one solution to this stress problem (but not a favorite one, as customers usually opt to escape); another solution is to put everything you need at the back of the store, so that to grab a carton of milk, you must first cross an aisle of cereal.

I wander up an aisle called SNACK TIME, passing bags of Frito-Lay Potato Chips and boxes of Wheat Thins, stopping only in front of a row of exuberantly orange cheddar-flavored Chex Mix. My hand floats forward—I'll just have a handful, a processed aperitif to the last processed meal. But once I am holding it, I remember that no one eats just a handful of cheddar Chex Mix, not when it is so crunchy and orange, so rhythmically hand-mouth, hand-mouth.

In *The End of Overeating,* David Kessler, a pediatrician, lawyer, and the former commissioner of the Food and Drug Administration, interviewed numerous food industry insiders in an attempt to figure out why it is that some foods are so irrationally irresistible. Why do our bodies keep eating some foods even when our minds say *stop*?

Although there are exceptions, most manufactured food products have been carefully designed and tested by a team of food engineers and focus groups to ensure that they "optimize palatability to ensure profitability." According to Kessler, one brand of orange juice went through sixty-five product prototypes before it was ready for supermarket shelves. Maxwell House coffee went through eighty-seven variations before it "tasted right."

"If you can find that optimal point in a set of ingredients," one consultant told Kessler, "you may be well on your way to converting that array of chemicals and physical substrates into a successful product." A successful product is one that we buy again and again, one we consume independent of hunger or health. And, often, that success can be traced to just three ingredients: sugar, fat, and salt. Foods that combine sugar, fat, and salt pull our evolutionary triggers in ways that make us eat more, regardless of hunger—a reaction that remains from the days, thousands of years ago, when sugar, fat, and salt were hard to find, much less in combination. Sugar, fat, and salt, combined in intriguing ways, create foods that are "high in hedonic value, which gives us pleasure," writes Kessler. When he asks a consultant if he designs foods specifically to be highly hedonic, the consultant replies: "Yes, absolutely."

THE IDEA THAT THE FOODS WE EAT might be designed rather than simply harvested is still a relatively new one. We've processed foods for thousands of years, but usually for one of two reasons: to make the food more digestible, its nutrients more available to our bodies, or to preserve it—to preserve summer for winter, for example, or an acre's crops for a village's meals. Today, the primary reason we process food is to sell it. Processing improves texture, augments appearance, enhances taste, and makes better "mouthfeel." We process food to preserve it not just seasonally, but indefinitely. Without context—without advertising—an outsider might guess that today, the purpose of processing is to make foods *less* nutritious.

Until the 1950s, the history of food processing in the United States more or less mirrored the rise of urbanization. If you lived on a farm, as most Americans did until the turn of the twentieth century, you grew your own food or you traded for it with your neighbors. Move to a city, as most of us did, and suddenly it was up to someone else to harvest and transport that food to you. With industrialization came industrialized food—mass-marketed, factory-processed, and necessarily preserved to endure greater distances between producers and eaters.

Entrepreneurs bounded into this new market, producing product after product to fulfill the demand for foods that "kept infinitely without spoiling," as James Kraft wrote in the patent for his new processed cheese in 1916. Consumers loved this "pasteurized loaf cheese" because it was dependable. It looked, tasted, and felt the same every time you used it—and, before widespread refrigeration, it stayed good tucked inside little tins stacked in your kitchen cabinet.

Over the first half of the century, processed foods gradually permeated American supermarkets—Oreos were introduced in 1915, Wonder Bread in 1921, Spam in 1937—but it wasn't until the 1950s that process hit its heyday. After two world wars and a great depression, processed foods promised convenience, stability, and anytime access, and so Americans opened their kitchens and cabinets to the constancy of industrial processing with exuberance. In 1952, the first frozen fish sticks were sold; in 1953, Kraft Cheese Whiz hit supermarket shelves; in 1954, C. A. Swanson & Sons sold the first microwavable TV dinner for ninety-eight cents. In that same decade, National Starch started making modified starches—made from corn, tapioca, and potatoes—which gave those frozen TV dinners the shape, moisture, and texture they needed to stay palatable (and stay ninety-eight cents). The 1950s were the decade in which chemical fertilizers took over our fields, when artificial additives began flowing from factories, and new highways connected ever-distant markets.

In 1958, the FDA updated the 1938 Federal Food, Drug, and Cosmetic Act with a Food Additive Amendment. The amendment sensibly defined food additives as any substance intentionally added to foods. These substances, it declared, would be subject to premarket approval by the FDA "unless the use of the substance is generally recognized as safe." The "generally recognized as safe" clause—now referred to as GRAS—was intended to protect obviously safe foods like salt and yeast from being subjected to a long food-additive approval process. What happened instead is that food companies realized that they, too, didn't want to wait while sodium nitrate or guanosine monophosphate trudged through this long approval process—so they started submitting new additives as GRAS based on their own (often in-house) expert testimony. Unlike food additives, GRAS ingredients don't need to be approved by the FDA before they can be used. According to a 2010 study by the Pew Health

Group, more than ten thousand chemicals are added to the array of foods available for human consumption—the vast majority of which haven't been formally reviewed by the FDA. Today, most food additives are innocent until proven guilty.

I TURN DOWN A VAGUELY NAMED AISLE—if this is LUNCH & DINNER, what is the rest of the store?—and press on, past boxes of garlic-seasoned instant potatoes and cans of Campbell's creamed corn. There are tins of tuna and a can of red sockeye salmon and then finally the aisle is over, but I nearly run into a round table of individual Kraft Mac 'N Cheese cups stacked in concentric circles like a fountain of champagne glasses. I pull into a rare negative space behind a cardboard case of Doritos and take stock of my surroundings.

A young woman in tight jeans and a soft sweater stretches her neck forward to read a label on a bottle of salad dressing. Two guys in sweatpants roll past. They pause and one pulls a can of something from a shelf and gestures to his friend; the friend doesn't even look at it before he nods in agreement. My eyes are blurry after so much brightness, and I realize, now that I have focused on something besides boxes and labels, I'm not the only one who seems bleary-eyed. No one makes eye contact—no one even looks at each other.

In 1957, motivational analyst James Vicary described this as the supermarket's "hypnoidal trance." To better understand impulse purchases, Vicary set up hidden cameras and followed women as they entered a supermarket, analyzing their eyeblink rate, an indicator of internal stress. The women's eyeblink rate began at an average of thirty-two blinks per minute; rather than increasing in frequency as they wandered around the store, which would have implied an increase in tension, the women instead began to blink at an average of fourteen blinks per minute, indicating they'd gone into a kind of "light trance . . . that is the first stage of hypnosis," wrote Vance Packard in *The Hidden Persuaders*. "Mr. Vicary has decided that the main cause of the trance is that the supermarket is packed with products that in former years would have been items that only kings and queens could afford, and here in this fairyland they were available."

At the turn of the century, corner stores were stocked with dozens of items; in the 1960s, the "thousands of items offered" made national headlines. By 2007, the average supermarket stocked an average of forty thousand food and beverage products.

I stand behind the Doritos, wanting everything, and so wanting nothing. My senses have been so confounded by this shouting match of a supermarket, this explosion of food and things-like-food, that my desire to eat one dish, to experience one flavor, has been sent skittering. While I sympathize with the turn-of-the-century housewives who rankled at their lack of autonomy at the grocery, we have swung too far in the opposite direction. There are too many choices; there is too much of what seems like freedom, too many packages parading as abundance.

For me, grocery shopping is as much about making food as it is about making identity. Although my eyes blur and my stomach growls, I am reluctant to leave this bright place, to commit to one product over another and thus commit to my own departure from this supercharged place of nostalgia and culture—both the culture of my family and friends and a larger one, the culture of American eating. I have wandered through supermarkets to distract myself from loneliness or to assert independence; I have bickered over baguettes with my sister and gossiped over cookies with my best friend. We come to the grocery to stock our kitchen cabinets but leave having made some statement not just about who we are, but who we want to be. Who we *could* be, once we go home, unload our paper bags, and begin to create something.

My head spins, eyes blur, and my blood sugar dips, so an hour and seventeen aisles later, I remember the DiGiorno pizza I saw, justifying the salary of an advertising executive in an office somewhere. I steer around floating Safeway shoppers as I hustle back to the freezer aisle. My eyes blur again as I scan the array: diet pizza, restaurant pizza, organic pizza, deep-dish pizza, celebrity chef pizza, breadsticks & pizza, until finally, I spot a DiGiorno Rising Crust Supreme Pizza. The image on the cover of the cold cardboard box is outlandishly flawless, the picture of pizza perfection. The colors on the vegetables glisten, impossibly bright; the crust swells with unfeasible pride. When I swing back through the bakery, I spot a single serving of thickly frosted carrot cake, so again I fold to the demands of the hidden persuaders. I navigate around displays to the front of the store, speed through the self-checkout, and flee, finally, to the safety of my car.

My frozen pizza, after it is no longer frozen but piping hot, is salty, cheesy, and saucy, crunchy on the underside of the crust and gooey on top. It is all the things that a pizza should be. I eat two slices while watching an episode of *Mad Men* on Netflix—Donald Draper sells the allure of cigarettes to the 1950s—and then during a second episode, I eat one more. This represents half the pizza, but I'm not particularly full. Actually no. I'm still hungry, so I have one more piece. When I head into the kitchen to clean up, I realize that there is no cleanup. The cardboard box goes into the recycling bin and my grease-spackled paper towel sinks into the garbage. I slide a silver fork out of the dish rack and eat the carrot cake straight out of the plastic container. It's decadent; marvelously addicting. Half an inch of white frosting peers over the side of the cake like a roof's overhang. After I leave three thick fork trails in the sticky cake, after I fold a bite in my mouth, a stream of rich sweetness sprawls through my mouth. I can imagine, written in the notes of a Safeway food chemist, "excellent mouthful, good viscosity." The cake is moist—"superb water retention"—and consistently sweet, bite after bite—"high sucrose stabilization."

Unprocess Yourself: Grocery Shopping

No matter where you shop for food, read the ingredient label on every item you buy. The simple act of turning a package or carton over to peer at its underbelly might be enough to change your mind about buying it. Of course, the best and easiest way to shop unprocessed is to buy foods *without* ingredient labels—bananas, avocados, oranges. The second best is to buy packages containing just one ingredient—rolled oats, milk, honey. Beyond that, look for ingredient labels with words that you understand. If you don't recognize an item on an ingredient label, figure out what it is. Before I owned a smartphone, I used to call my sister in the middle of the day to Google me through ingredient list conundrums. Now, I consult my Chemical Cuisine app, published by the Center for Science in the Public Interest—download it for free on Android or iPhone. (They also publish a print guide.) Enter an ingredient and you'll find out what it's made of, where it comes from, and what it's used for.

Set up your processed parameters *before* you go to the supermarket. Make a shopping list and try to stick to it—an endeavor that'll be easier if you shop at markets that are trying to sell you reasonable foods instead of cheap, high-profit edible items.

Surprises happen. If you discover an unexpected and unwelcome ingredient in a food you just *have* to buy—if something stubborn inside you kicks and says, *I am* not *going to give* this *up*—then don't. Yet. Go home, think it over, and plan an unprocessed alternative.

2

WHEAT

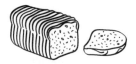

Grain is unprocessed if it is whole.

My year unprocessed starts with a stomachache. After consuming 2,400 calories in a single evening—the slice of carrot cake alone contributed 870—I wake up with what feels like a brick in my belly. I shuffle around my kitchen and pour water into the coffeepot; it groans to life as I peer into the fridge. I pull out a container of plain Greek yogurt, douse it in mesquite honey, and slice a banana over the creamy mixture. After my stomach unclenches and my body awakens, I set to my day's task: shifting Sunday's anchor from supermarket to kitchen. On my first morning of unprocessed, on the inaugural Sunday of a year of Sundays, I bake bread.

My first loaf of bread begins with a bag of Trader Joe's 100% Whole Wheat Flour. I believe that whole-grain flour, as opposed to refined white flour, is unprocessed because I believe I could mash up a bunch of wheat berries in my kitchen and make something grittily like flour. This is yet a theoretical belief on the fifteenth day of January; today, on this first day of unprocessed eating, all I have is a crumpled paper sack holding two pounds of whole-wheat flour and a hazy belief in its integrity.

I have never baked whole-wheat bread before—I've never baked *any* kind of bread that required kneading rather than stirring together sweet batter. While I am in my apartment baking bread, Hilary is in hers, overseeing chicken in a pot that will become chicken in a soup. Sarah is assembling ingredients to toss together in a salad; later tonight we will all converge for the first unprocessed potluck.

The philosophy that guides my cooking and my kitchen is this: Don't let the perfect be the enemy of the good. In cooking, as in life, even as we strive for flawlessness, most often what we achieve is good enough. If one's oven knob is so old it no longer displays temperature settings, 350-ish is good enough. If one does not own a one-eighth-teaspoon measuring device, a pinch will do. This philosophy generally serves me well, as I cook with confidence rather than compliance. My sautés and scrambles generally benefit from this sense of adventure, and I have a fair enough understanding of ratios that my baked goods rarely suffer from inexactitude. So when I try my hand at whole-wheat bread, I approach the task with the same sort of shoulder shrug. Wheat, water, yeast, honey, and oil. How hard could it be?

According to my recipe, I should dissolve yeast in one-quarter cup of warm water (110 degrees) and allow it to proof for three to five minutes.

I don't pause to consider the relative hotness of 110-degree water. One hundred and ten degrees sounds hot to me, so I release a stream of tap water into a stove pot and set it to boil, reasoning that I'll let it cool down to 110 degrees postboiling while I work on the other components of my bread. I measure out six cups of whole-wheat flour, a teaspoon of sea salt, a third of a cup of honey, and a fourth of a cup of olive oil. The final ingredient, apart from the proofed yeast, is the water, so I return to my steaming pot on the stove. I dunk my finger in, and indeed, it is hot. I measure out two cups for my flour mixture and a fourth of a cup to whisk with my yeast.

The yeast plunks into the water. One tablespoon, two; they plop into the water and then promptly sink in two fists of beige, decidedly not forming, as the recipe says they should, a creamy foam on the surface. The yeast huddles on the bottom of the glass, hugs the sides, sticks together as I attempt to whisk it about. I persevere. Yeast-water meets flour-oil-honey. I knead, I wait, I knead again. After six hours, the dough seems like it has risen a little—it certainly has not *doubled* as the recipe suggests that it will, but it seems a little lifted, a bit cheerier. The supper hour fast approaches, so I mold the dough on a pan to take to Hilary's. Maybe something magical will happen in the heat of the oven. Maybe the oven will transform this sad log of dough into something more, will bestow upon its heaviness five loaves and two fishes.

I hold the loaf pan aloft as I descend the narrow cement stairs into Hilary's basement-floor apartment. Sarah is already there. "Megan!" she cries, opening the door with wide eyes and cheerful yellow pants. I give her short frame a tight hug as I duck into the warm apartment. It smells like soup, a cozy complement to the flickering candles and stacked bookshelves. After a night in Safeway and a day in my kitchen, I am thrilled to be among friends instead of food. As Hilary emerges from her tiny kitchen, I pull back my dish towel to reveal my day's project.

"Damn, it shrunk on the way over," I say when I see that the small accumulation of cheer has wilted into concavity. "Cowardly bread, why won't you rise!"

"It looks lovely," Sarah says.

Hilary nods in agreement. "Yay unprocessed!"

"Are you nervous? Ready?" Sarah asks.

"Yup to both. I think it'll be good to just *start*. I ate most of a DiGiorno pizza last night. Might need the full year to recover."

"Well, I'm excited," Hilary says. To help me ease into new habits, or perhaps ease herself out of her bad ones, Hilary has decided to join me in unprocessed eating for the first two weeks of my year. Though she'd decided friendly relations with her on-again off-again boyfriend required that pizza still be allowed, her unexpected enthusiasm allows my new and nervous commitment to begin among company rather than in confinement. If I'd feared that a year unprocessed would confine me to my kitchen—that by unraveling my food's source, I would similarly unravel my social life—then this meal with Hilary and Sarah proves that even if the food changes, the dinner can still be the same.

"I brought wine!" Sarah exclaims, and then pauses, horror-struck. "Wait. Is wine unprocessed?" Hilary stops her stirring and looks up at me with a gaze that says, plainly: *It sure better be.*

"Yeah, really," I say, agreeing with Hilary's look. "I'm going to try to make it at some point this year, but until then, I'm operating under the assumption that I could theoretically ferment a bunch of grapes at home."

Sarah and Hilary shoot each other a glance, relieved.

After fifty minutes in Hilary's oven, the spread of dough doesn't budge. It emerges breadlike, something less like a loaf and more like biscotti, more like a cutting board, like a wheat Frisbee. But it's warm and it tastes like wheat. It's Minute Maid bread, cooked from concentrate. "I like dense bread!" Hilary insists. Both Sarah and Hilary are low-maintenance dinner companions, so we eat it. We break the bread, slather it with honey, and the year of unprocessed begins.

I BEGIN WITH BREAD because bread began us. Bread is born from wheat, wheat bred from land. If civilization began with agriculture, then agriculture began with grain. We hunted, we gathered, and when we ran out of sustenance, we moved on. But then, ten thousand years ago, in the Fertile Crescent of the Nile River Valley—in China, in Mesoamerica—something shifted. As gradually as soft silt accumulated on the floodplain of the Nile—or maybe it was as sudden as a flash flood rumbling across a plain—we realized that the foods we were gathering could be planted and grown closer to home. However it happened, it happened because a human, porous and soft-skinned, began to see a stalk of wheat differently. We began to process our landscapes.

We harvested seeds from wild emmer and einkorn wheat—archaeologists have dated emmer cultivation in the Fertile Crescent to at least 8800 BC—and we clustered together while we waited for the seeds to germinate. We cared for the shaggy stalks that soon emerged, harvested and stored the kernels of energy. More of us survived the winter, so more of us planted, harvested, stored; we learned discipline and patience as we tended our crops.

I cannot imagine a world where this idea, caring for crops, was ever *new*. The world that shaped my imagination is a world where agriculture is as inevitable as gravity. Straight highways cross Texas, the state where I was born, highways that lean into curving rows of cotton and corn, green and beige, seamless and ceaseless.

But wheat was revolutionary. Wheat was the first sign that the raw materials of a fertile world could be molded to fit our desires. Bread and its early manifestation, porridge, was one of the first foods human hands prepared with intention, one that freed us from the uncertain search for sustenance in the wild.

What is the difference between a stalk of wheat in the field, inedible and unapproachable, and the soft dust that floats through our kitchens and settles on our eyebrows? How did they do it, those early humans: How did they wrestle wheat from the field and into a loaf?

A STALK OF WHEAT looks like a matted feather duster, like a skinny girl hanging upside down on a jungle gym. Nestled at the scalp of this wild splay of hair are wheat berries, the seed of the stalk, the source of our food. When our ancestors began eating wheat, they shucked these stalks by hand. They gathered wheat berries, ground them into meal, and mixed this meal with water. First there was flatbread and porridge, grain paste and gruel. Leave a bowl of wet gruel sitting in a warm spot for a few days and the wild yeast spores of the air, then as now, will burrow down into the paste; will munch through sugar and begin to ferment. Dough will rise.

Today not only do we rarely rely on the wild yeasts of chance to leaven our bread, we also rarely harvest wheat by hand. Across the world's breadbaskets, wheat berries emerge from a field through the help of a combine. A combine harvester gets its name from its function; as it passes over a field, it reaps, winnows, and threshes, combining the three steps of harvest into one. In the rotating hull of a combine, grain, chaff, and straw go their separate ways; the grain passes through two sets of "fingers" (sieves, basically) that clean the kernels of their thin paper coats; the kernels shuffle out a spout in the back and fall into the bed of a truck. What emerges from a combine is a wheat berry. Grind these wheat berries into flour—between a rock and a hard place or in the grinding gears of a grain mill—and you have whole-grain flour.

Refined white flour emerged in the 1800s when we started tinkering with the innards of these wheat berries. Wheat bran is the rough outer coating of the berry, the source of the seed's fiber and nutrients. Peel away the wheat bran and you've got the wheat germ, the part that sprouts when wheat kernels are planted. Wheat germ contains lots of fiber and also most of the grain's oils, which means that it spoils easily. The germ and bran, once removed, leave behind the endosperm: a fluffy sack of concentrated starch—that is, sugar— meant to feed a growing plant. The reason white flour—the flour stripped of bran and germ—lasts so much longer in our cabinets than whole-grain flour is that white flour has so many fewer nutrients to offer the pests that compete with us for its calories. White flour has so much less protein, fiber, calcium, vitamin B, iron, and folic acid than whole-wheat flour that, beginning in the

1940s, U.S. law required millers to add back these last four vitamins and minerals, producing the deceptively named "enriched flour."

So why do we eat white flour? Simply put, we like it better. It makes fluffier cakes and pastries; its bland flavor is well suited for four-year-olds or bologna; and it spoils slower in our cabinets. Whiteness confers purity; this is not a modern phenomenon. Even the ancient Greeks sought refinement through refining. Archestratus, a contemporary of Aristotle, was aflutter when he tasted refined barley bread from Lesbos, "a bread so white that it outdoes the ethereal snow in purity."

Today, the reason white flour is so white is that it's been bleached to cover the natural yellowing that occurs as it ages; the reason cake flour is so fluffy is that it's been treated with chlorine dioxide or chlorine gas, which causes the starch granules to absorb water and swell, producing a stronger "starch gel." Although no one has yet proven that the chlorine that accumulates in our fat molecules causes us harm, chlorinated flour is illegal in the European Union. In the United States, Betty Crocker still serves it with a smile.

IT'S ANOTHER MONTH before I attempt to bake bread again, using the same paper-wrapped bag of Trader Joe's 100% Whole Wheat Flour. Having come to my senses and remembered that water boils at 212 degrees Fahrenheit, nearly double the tepid temperature required to activate yeast, I do not boil warm water this time. I force myself to stick to the recipe, step-by-110-degree-step, even when my dough becomes a bit sticky, even when it congeals to my fingers, stretching between my hands like Elmer's Glue, crying for another half cup of flour. No, I tell it. We are not the ones calling the shots here; we are players in someone else's game. After the dough rises, falls, and rises again, I pat the sticky mess into a log shape and slide it into the oven. I'm sitting on my couch reading, feet away from my clanging oven, when the yeast begins to metabolize. One molecule of sugar yields two molecules of alcohol plus two molecules of carbon dioxide, but what this article on yeast metabolism does not say is what this smells like. It's warm—the smell itself is warm. Sweet and sourdough, fermenting honey. It smells like Sunday, or rather like something primal that existed before Sundays ever did.

Fifty minutes later, I don my oven mitt and pull the baking sheet out from the oven. On top of the baking sheet is a loaf of bread. Tall, perched, overseeing the expanse of dirty metal with an unmoving gaze: It is a proper loaf of bread. I set the pan down, remove the oversize oven mitt, and pick up the loaf with my bare hand. It is piping hot, but it's a hotness I can't help but touch, can't help but examine. I made this—from flour floating in water, I made this thing, this package of discrete, portable *food*. I don't wait for the loaf to cool; I cut a slice from the end and fold a spongy hunk into my mouth. It tastes and feels and *is* bread.

The problem with baking bread at home is that now my home smells like bread. A serrated knife crunches across the loaf. I pull a jar of honey from the cabinet and slather it on this second hunk of bread. The plan, an hour before this smell took over my home, was to make a sandwich for lunch with this fresh bread and leftover collard greens. But now the bread is baked and the smell is in me. After I sample a slice slathered in butter, I wrap the rest of the loaf in a dish towel and continue about my reading, my e-mailing and note-taking. But still the bread holds sway. As I continue about my afternoon, the loaf in the back of my mind, it occurs to me that across ten thousand years, across continents and technology, perhaps the primary characteristic that distinguishes me from those distant humans who first planted wheat is that I have struggled with my weight—that I have struggled with *too much* weight.

Please stop asking me, stranger on the street and man in the grocery store, but: I'm six-foot-one (yes, I played basketball). I've gotten this question weekly since I was fourteen years old, since I sprouted early and had to learn how to inhabit and handle such a roomy body. When I was fifteen, my body stopped expanding upward and turned to a roominess that went outward. The spring after I turned sixteen—a junior in high school, center on the varsity basketball team—I hit 190 pounds. So my mom—five ten and 180 herself—made us an appointment with a Pasadena nutritionist.

"You're vegetarian?" Dr. Lisa asked my mom. "What do you normally cook?"

Um, pasta. Corn on the cob, sautéed veggies, and lots of rice, sometimes tofu. We ate cereal for breakfast, sandwiches for lunch, and veggie lasagna for dinner.

"Too many carbohydrates," said Dr. Lisa. "Too little protein."

So I turned to egg whites and away from chocolate-covered pretzels, and twenty pounds slid off easily given my young metabolism. That twenty came and went throughout college. On during freshman year, along with half my dorm; off sophomore as I replaced my morning croissant with cereal and yogurt; on again in my junior year when I studied abroad in steak-and-potato Argentina.

And then I graduated from college. I moved to Nicaragua, to the five-hundred-person town of Playa Gigante. Rob, the owner of the four-room Hotel Brio, offered me a spot in one of two volunteer bunks and two meals a day in exchange for the three daily English classes I would teach to the town's residents. I spent my mornings in the kitchen with Isolina, the hotel's cook, helping her make *gallo pinto* and flour tortillas. An oil-filled frying pan sizzled while she diced onions and sweet green peppers, hissed when she scooped them into the pan, crackled as they drowned in oil and Isolina instructed me on the proper way to fold in black beans and then rice. Isolina told me about her daughters, eleven and sixteen years old, while we made flour tortillas. To-gether we would pat the soft dough into a circle, born of white flour, lard, and water, kneading it gently with the tips of our fingers, sifting the circle around and around, flatter and flatter, before casting it into the iron pan hot on the stovetop. I ate every morsel Isolina gave to me, and as I spent more time with her in the kitchen, she began piling my plates higher. When life consisted of two meals a day, the bigger the meal, the better. Nicaraguan food is delicious, but it is country food, high in calories by intention, fuel for the fishermen and farmers who populate small towns like Playa Gigante throughout the country. Unlike these fishermen and farmers, I was standing in front of a whiteboard all day; I was eating fuel but burning only words. The pounds piled back on.

I came home. I ate salad and not fried chicken. I waited and exercised, but still the pounds clung, stubborn and homesick for the tropics. So, after two months of frustration, I turned to Weight Watchers, as so many of my friends, my mom included, had done in the past.

Weight Watchers parses food into points. Foods acquire points according to their calories, fat, and, inversely, fiber. When I ventured to Weight Watchers, my six one, 190-pound frame exercised regularly, so I got to eat twenty-eight points a day. Vegetables have zero points, a cup of butter has fifty-one, and an eight-ounce potato has three. The idea is to fill up on low-point foods—fruit or nonfat yogurt—and sprinkle in a few high-point foods—cheese or chocolate. Meals became the sums of their parts, ingredients the measure of their calorie-fat-fiber components. I had forgotten about Dr. Lisa's carbohydrate rule—that is, to avoid—until Weight Watchers helpfully reminded me that bread, especially white bread, is a points black hole, full of calories but not fill-you-up fiber or essential nutrients. If bread is about calories and losing weight is about losing calories, then it seems that losing weight meant losing bread.

Back in 2009, I wasn't the only one thinking this way. Control Your Carbs! cried the mainstream media. Lose Your Wheat Belly! Food companies perked up, recognizing an opportunity for a new food product: a carbohydrate that didn't contain carbohydrates. The way to achieve a low-carb carbohydrate is to replace the wheat's gluten, the glue that holds bread together, that which makes it springy and cohesive, with an artificial binding agent. Like, say, guar gum—the ground endosperm of guar beans, also used to manufacture paper—or sodium stearoyl lactylate—a "dough conditioner" that emulsifies bread and improves its ability to "resist abuse." What I didn't realize at the time was that this bread, made from additives and conditioned by chemicals, was adulterated bread, a diminishment of wheat. At the time, it simply meant fewer points for more food.

When I began my year unprocessed, I was still tempted by the hundred-calorie tortillas and low-carb flatbreads sold in the Safeway bakery. The promise of diet dessert still coaxed me into believing I could have both my cake and skinny jeans. I knew better, but still I bought them, conditioned by my past. But when my year of unprocessed began, low-carb carbs finally fell off the table. Bread would simply be bread, carby and starched. Even while my Weight Watchers–trained, Dr. Lisa–driven eating self gave a twitch, the rule was simple enough. There would be no chemicals in my diet—no diet in my bread.

THE FIRST LEAVENED LOAF of whole-wheat bread pulled from my oven doesn't make it through its first night. A warm third of it disappears straightaway under a cover of melted butter. The next third disappears in two thick slices at dinner, when I finally make my sandwich; the bread hugs grilled red onions, goat cheese, and sautéed collard greens. And the last third? The last third of the loaf disappears around the dangerous midnight hour. It is pulled apart in hunks, great tears of bread that accept honey dripping from a spoon like a thirsty plant soaks up water.

I have made delicious bread and from whole ingredients. Success. But as I brush the crumbs from my butcher block, wipe down my counters, and scrub my baking sheet, I feel like I've failed myself. A loaf of bread in less than twelve hours. I have a hard time getting myself to bed, and when I finally do, I lie on my back, staring up. A hard ache in my stomach reminds me of my psyche's failure.

As much as I believe this project is about something bigger than me, something political or social, environmental or generational, I realize as I lie there, blinking at the ceiling with a fist in my stomach, that this year is also about teaching myself how to eat. How to eat real food in moderate amounts, to avoid the compulsion that emerges after so much bottled restraint. I want to learn how to eat without the anxiety I acquired when I was just sixteen years old, when I was so newly formed, so raw and awkward. It makes me sad to think of my sixteen-year-old self, so sure that everyone was looking at the expanding rear end of her stretchy pants, the tight waist of her jeans. I sprouted so quickly, and my mom saw the pain I felt inhabiting such a big body when I still felt so small. I love that she tried to fix it, that she turned to nutrition as a cure for low confidence. But still, I wish that this sixteen-year-old could have lingered, just a bit longer, in a world where food was fuel and glee instead of guilt and restriction.

A mind is a terrible thing to spend on a body. I don't want to live the rest of my twenties, my thirties and forties, devoting so much energy to that boom-bust cycle of weight gain and loss. What are we supposed to eat? What do we eat to keep us healthy, strong, and supple? We are handed confusion, offered the uncertainty that theorizing science has served to nutrition. New diets are scrawled on chalkboards like the day's specials and we take them. We shuffle down the lunch line with our plastic trays, and we have little choice but to acquiesce to this confusion.

I did Weight Watchers for three months and I lost weight. I lost weight by losing carbs, by erasing fat, by faking sugar, but finally I lost weight by gaining control—control over everything I put into my mouth. Bread, in all its manifestations, crusty and springy, sweet and baked, is what Weight Watchers calls a "trigger food," one that "sets off a course of overeating where control is lost and excessive amounts are consumed." Control is lost—the passive voice indicating the kind of out-of-mind experience that occurs when your body continues to eat even when your mind actively wants it to stop. Everyone succumbs to different triggers, but the most common contain some components of the fat-salt-sugar trifecta that evolved over a millennium of humans searching for quick, dense food in the wild.

I cannot forget that there is a fresh loaf of bread in my apartment. Fresh bread occupies the corners of my mind like a waiting task. A bill that needs to be paid, a load of laundry to be washed. Bread is to be eaten—there can be no leftover bread.

If whole-grain flour is like burlap, white flour is a wispy cotton ball. When these soft bundles hit our digestive system, they dissolve like cotton disappears in a gust of strong Texas wind. A loaf of whole-grain bread, on the other hand, sticks around and sinks in. It hurts to eat this much bread. This pain is precisely because it is so unprocessed. My stomach must now do the work of breaking down its fibers and its oils, its grist and germ, its starches and sugars, and so my stomach gnaws throughout the night, focusing its energy on breaking down the onslaught I've thrown at it, on unraveling the dense proteins wound within each granule of grain.

IF AN UNPROCESSED GRAIN is a grain that's been passed whole through history, most grains I eat today fail this test. Ancient grains are categorically different from modern varieties, Model Ts to today's Hummers. Different varieties of the wheat plant are classified according to their level of gluten, which is a protein found in all grain species. Hard wheat has a lot of the stuff, which provides solid architecture for bread; soft wheat has less and so combines easily with foods like sugar or eggs. Gluten is the "muscle of bread." It's gluten that gives wheat its elasticity—the reason why bread springs and cakes sponge.

I'm learning about the chromosome count in wheat in an article published in *Scientific American* in 1953, nearly sixty years before gluten wiggled its way into the mainstream vernacular. In the 1930s, Russian geneticist and botanist

Nikolai Vavilov collected thirty-one thousand samples of wheat from across the world and classified them according to the number of chromosomes contained in each nucleus. Wild einkorn, said to be agriculture's founder crop, has seven chromosomes. When einkorn hybridized with an unknown wild grass, it produced a fourteen-chromosome offspring, the oldest of which is wild emmer wheat, once the most widely grown crop of the ancient world. Thousands of years later, farmers hoping for greater yields began crossing fourteen-chromosome with seven-chromosome varieties, producing today's standard grain, the twenty-one-chromosome "common wheat."

Just as it takes more energy to get a Hummer moving than it did a small Model T, it requires more energy and effort from our bodies to break down seeds with more chromosomes, to access the nutrients bound tightly within these protein coils. Too much effort, in fact. Today, studies suggest that all this work leads the villi, the lining of the small intestine, to become truncated, unable to accept or digest the nutrients bound within wheat, initiating what's known as celiac disease.

My best friend Kara has struggled with her health since I met her ten years ago. We met in college; when we lived in the same apartment building our senior year, Sundays were grocery day. We'd troll the aisles, filling our carts with semisensible choices—bagged lettuce, frozen chicken breast, bags of presliced bread. We tried to choose healthy foods, but for Kara, what constituted "healthy" became a shifting, slippery object. No matter what she ate, her stomach seemed to reject it. Throughout college, she went to doctor after doctor, was tested for malady after malady. Her health swung up and down, and by the time we graduated, the best indicator of her well-being was not the answer to the question "How are you?" but to the question "How's your stomach?" I watched as Kara wrestled with the confusion and anxiety of such a simple question: What should she eat? What could she eat that would offer her the energy needed to dash to class but wouldn't cause her to double over in agony? I remember a rough few months when Kara wondered if she was just allergic to *food*. Some days, all she ate was popcorn and carrots, not because she was trying to lose weight but because she couldn't lose another day to pain.

Finally she learned what it was that her body couldn't tolerate—those springy proteins that bind wheat and other cereal grains together. She wasn't the only one figuring this out. In the past decade, the gluten-intolerant has become a new cohort of consumers buying food across the country. Gluten-free is the new modifier of choice on food packages ranging from crackers to salsa. ("Of course salsa is gluten free!" Kara yelps when she sees this new labeling. "Why on *earth* would there be wheat in *salsa*?") Although gluten intolerance—which for some is associated with celiac disease—seems like the basis of a new fad diet, it's rather a symptom of a diet gone astray.

In 2009, a cohort of gastroenterologists analyzed stored blood samples from a group of nine thousand healthy young men who had been stationed at Warren Air Force Base between 1948 and 1954, and compared their results with a group of twelve thousand age-matched men stationed in Olmsted County, Minnesota. Within this sixty-year span, within these analogous groups of people, they found that instances of celiac disease had increased fourfold—that is, that the number of people who can't digest gluten had increased by 400 percent.

"Reasons for the increased prevalence of celiac disease over time are unknown," the study reports in a scientifically underwhelmed tone. However, "the most likely explanation may be environmental, such as a change in quantity, quality, or processing of cereal. Several major changes in wheat genetics and bread processing . . . as a result of industry food processing have occurred in the past forty years."

In 1953, a *Scientific American* writer counted the chromosomes in our wheat; in 2009, a group of gastroenterologists counted the number of us who can no longer eat that wheat. Nine thousand years ago, a wheat berry transformed human nutrition; today, it's transforming it all over again.

AFTER BREAD FAILS ME and then I fail it, I take a break from the carboloading. I drive to Nogales, Arizona, for a three-day conference about foodsheds along the U.S.-Mexico border. The word "foodshed" was popularized in 1996 by sociologist Jack Kloppenburg, who wrote, "While a [food] system can be anywhere, the foodshed is a continuous reminder that we are standing in a particular place; not anywhere, but here." Like a watershed, a foodshed describes the way that food flows through a particular place—it begins in geography, traverses markets, and ends in culture, consumed through cuisine.

I volunteer to be a driver for Sunday's Farming in the Borderlands tour to get free entry into the conference on Monday and Tuesday, but as I maneuver a heavy fifteen-passenger van over rutted roads and up muddy hills, I wonder if I shouldn't have just paid the registration fee. As I spin my attention into guiding this heavy van around the sharp turns of backcountry roads, the man in the front seat next to me doesn't stop talking. On the way to Avalon Organic Gardens, he tells me about "restorative agriculture," which is different from sustainable agriculture because it *restores* the land. On the way to the Native Seeds/SEARCH farm, he tells me about hitchhiking through Mexico, suggests that I take a shortcut along River Road, and then harrumphs when I decide to stay in line with the six-car caravan carrying a hundred farmers, ranchers, and foodies who are here, a dozen miles north of the Mexican border, to learn how it is that one grows food on parched land.

On the way home from Dos Cabezas Wineworks back to El Esplendor Resort, as the sun creeps down the front windshield, Kyle, the loquacious farmer, stops talking. He turns his back to me to look out the open window, the white hair of his ponytail billowing in the hard breeze, his stonewashed T-shirt fluttering around wiry arms. He looks back at me.

"What was your favorite part of the day, Megan?"

I glance back at him. I'm exhausted—out late, up early, clenched hands all day—so I frown, thinking. "Oh!" I say, the wheels of my brain finally creaking forward as the van slides off the dirt road and onto the cement highway. "I loved seeing the White Sonora wheat growing at Native Seeds/SEARCH." It had been why I signed up for this excursion in the first place—to learn more about this heritage breed of wheat growing in the desert for the first time in half a century.

The Native Seeds/SEARCH farm is the heart of a seed-saving nonprofit based in Tucson. The farm cultivates native crops of the desert Southwest and northern parts of Mexico and saves these desert-adapted seeds to sell and distribute to local farmers. If agriculture began with wheat, then it survived because farmers saved seeds. Plant a field of corn, say, and you save enough kernels from the cobs of your harvest to plant another field next year. Save seeds from the healthiest plants, and after enough years, you'll have selected for better crops. Depending on the plants you select, you might end up with better yields, better flavor, or better adaptation to the intricacies of a place, to its soil, weather, and culture.

That all changed in the 1950s, when Norman Borlaug developed his hybrid dwarf wheat and activated the Green Revolution, which prioritized yield above all else. Since then, seed has become commercialized and homogenized, selected for the lowest common denominator that will yield successful crops—and sold to farmers, rather than distributed to community seed banks. Today, ten companies control 73 percent of the world's seed stocks. Rather than relying on the natural capital inherent in saved seeds, farmers now have to pony up the cash before they can plant another harvest. For some farmers, this is a good deal—they know the seeds they get will produce better yields and eventually earn them more money. But for others, it simply means they must rely on corporations instead of their own harvest.

For us eaters, the homogenization of seed stocks means that the foods we're eating have been grown for quantity instead of quality, yield over taste or nutrition.

I tell Kyle about my unprocessed project, how I'm wondering about wheat's journey from farm to kitchen, from past to present.

He nods and looks out the window again. He remarks, "You know, I grew up on a wheat farm in central Kansas. My great-great-grandparents were wheat farmers in Russia who immigrated to the U.S."

The sun has dipped below the Santa Rita Mountains, the light dashes after it, my passengers nod off in the four rows behind me, and *now* I find out that I've been talking to a fourth-generation wheat farmer for the past eight hours. I am a horrible journalist.

"Oh?" I say. "Do you still grow wheat?"

"Nope. I'm gluten-intolerant."

"Really?"

"I think it's because I grew up eating so much of that refined stuff," he says. "I can see it in the difference between me and my older brothers. When I was only five or six, we moved into the city, but on the farm, when my brothers were growing up, we milled our wheat right at home. That's what everyone did. Or they brought bags over to the community mill, ground enough wheat to keep them for a couple of weeks."

The decline of small mills across the United States reflects a similar decline in small anything—farms, butchers, grocers. In 1873, there were 23,000 mills in the United States; by 1998, that number had dropped to 201, with four companies accounting for 70 percent of all the wheat milled in the country. While this number is startling, it's information I haven't been able to do anything with except file it away in the "bummer, man" folder that contains many tidbits I learn about industrial food production.

As I focus on controlling the fifteen-passenger van hurtling north along 1-19 back to Nogales, I'm suddenly grateful that Kyle is such a self-propelled conversationalist.

"You know," he says lightly, "all the flour you buy in the store is rancid."

I steal a glance sideways. "How so?"

"As soon as you break apart a kernel of wheat, the components begin to oxidize. The oils break down. It's why raw flour tastes bitter. The fats have turned," he says. "Not only that, the minerals in the germ interact with the air. You lose magnesium, calcium, zinc . . . all these diminish as the flour oxidizes. The nutrient profile just plummets."

"Wait. Seriously? How have I never heard about this?" I read books about food for *fun*; if anyone's to know about rancid flour, it's me.

"Well, it doesn't immediately harm you, not like when dairy or meat turns. But there are subtle, long-term effects on the body."

"Such as?"

"Have you ever heard of phytates?

I have not.

"They're nutrient blockers. Phytic acid occurs naturally in the bran of all grains. If you don't treat phytic acid, if you don't ferment the grain or soak it, the phytic acid will combine with minerals in the intestinal tract and block their absorption. That's why humans ate fermented grains for so long—why all bread used to be sourdough."

"Wait, so this is *all* flour?"

He nods. "The flour they sell at bulk food stores is the *worst*." He packs his frustration into this last word, imagining the bins of innocent flour subjected to fresh waves of oxidation every time someone flaps up the lid and lets in a whoosh of air. Every time *I* flap up the lid and let in a whoosh of air. I'm flummoxed. How is this *not known*?

"So what do we do?"

"Well, for one, we've got to get back to local processing. And eat sprouted or fermented grains."

Our conversation pauses as I exit the freeway at Rio Rico Drive and swing the van up to El Esplendor Resort. Thirteen sleepy heads nod good-bye as their bodies unfold out of the cramped car. I still have to drive this heavy van, property of the University of Arizona, back to Tucson, but I can't, not yet.

"Do you have a minute?" I ask Kyle. "Rancid, and wheat processing . . . the mills."

He nods and leans against the door of the van. "Once wheat berries are sucked up in the big hopper of a combine, they're poured through a big spout into the back of a semi and trucked to a granary where they're stored in these twenty-story silos for God knows how long. When the price of wheat hits a sweet spot, they're trucked off and traded on the Chicago commodities exchange. Most of the wheat is shipped to China—I don't know, maybe half of the grain we produce—but some is bought by big flour companies, shipped to Philadelphia or Minneapolis," he says. "These companies grind it up, stick it in a bag, and then truck it back across the country, where it sits in a warehouse, sits in a storeroom, sits on a shelf." Oxidizing, oxidizing all the while. "Until finally you buy it."

"Wow."

"And the whole-grain flour you buy in the store . . . You know it doesn't really come from the same grain, right?"

I shake my head.

"It's just like anything else these days. Millers specialize. We make so much white flour in this country that most millers sieve apart the bran, germ, and endosperm, and sell them as component parts. Whole grain could be made with bran from this warehouse, germ from another, doesn't matter from where. When you buy whole-grain flour at the store, you're often not buying parts from the same piece of grain."

By the time I'm driving back to Tucson, my exhaustion has melted into a wide-eyed sort of mania. I will eat rancid flour no longer. I will no longer buy flour cobbled together from granaries across the country, will no longer eat Humpty-Dumpty wheat—the food that has fallen apart and cannot be fixed. I go online and find a surprisingly robust and varied community of home grain grinders. I flail around awhile, attempting to ascertain where I fall on the "stone vs. burr grinder controversy" and decide how much a reasonable person might spend on a home grain grinder—fifteen dollars or five hundred. I read articles and reviews. Finally, around midnight, as this day clicks toward the next, I commit. The Victorio Hand Operated Grain Mill sets me back sixty dollars but it gets four out of five stars on BePrepared.com. (Incidentally, a subset of the home-milling population includes survivalists preparing for the apocalypse.) Although I can't really afford this grain mill, I am wide-eyed and manic about all the flours I can mill at home, all the bulk bins full of rancid flour I can now avoid. With Victorio, "there's a simple way to replace overly processed, vitamin deficient foods with the fresh, natural goodness of home-ground products." Although the foodie-slash-survivalist blogosphere insists that this grain mill will both save me money and keep me fed after our food system collapses, owning a hand-operated grain mill feels less about financial and food security than about putting Humpty-Dumpty back together again.

WHEN I WAKE UP MONDAY MORNING, I wonder how far off the unprocessed deep end I've gone. I just bought a hand-operated grain mill because a skinny, gray-haired farmer told me industrial wheat is rancid. The question that kicked in when Kyle revealed the truth about rancid grains—how is this not known?—continues to rattle around my head, and so I turn to the establishment for verification.

As it turns out, the establishment doesn't have much to say about this particular issue; there are so many interests invested in maintaining the reputation of industrial flour that academic studies don't go near it. (Because, after all, it is the system, Archer Daniels Midland and General Mills, that funds much of nutrition research in the first place.)

Finally, I give up on mainstream verification—isn't it the mainstream that I'm protesting in the first place?—and buy a book that I should have bought long ago: Sally Fallon's *Nourishing Traditions: The Cookbook That Challenges Politically Correct Nutrition and the Diet Dictocrats*. It had been recommended to me before, by a diverse set of foodie friends, but I had resisted it for the same reason, I now realize, that I am resisting Kyle: It is dressed in hippie attire, its cover clothed in a sketch of a smiling sun, the title displayed in handwritten type.

Nourishing Traditions is based on the research of Weston C. Price, a dentist who traveled around the world in the 1930s documenting the health and diet of a variety of indigenous cultures. In *Nutrition and Physical Degeneration,* a wandering 524-page tome published in 1939, Price documented teeth as a microcosm for the whole body; in more than fifteen thousand photos, he showed how transitioning from a traditional diet, no matter the kind, to a modern "Western" diet—defined by refined grains, sugar, and processed fats—resulted in tooth decay and general malnutrition. Although in 1950, a scientific journal dubbed Price "the Charles Darwin of nutrition," his work remained largely unknown until Fallon came across it in the 1990s and, with the help of nutritionist Mary Enig, digested Price's dense research into the readable *Nourishing Traditions.*

"All grains contain phytic acid," writes Fallon. "Untreated phytic acid can combine with calcium, magnesium, copper, iron, and especially zinc in the intestinal tract and block their absorption." You can treat phytic acid either by fermenting grain into sourdough—by incorporating wild yeast into your dough, usually by way of a sourdough starter—or by soaking and sprouting it. A grain is, of course, a seed, so a sprout is its attempt to form a new plant, which breaks down long starch molecules and growth inhibitors, making the grain easier for your body to digest. "[Untreated grains] may lead to irritable bowel syndrome, and . . . serious mineral deficiencies and bone loss," writes Fallon. And finally: "If you buy grains that have been rolled or cracked"—which includes any grain with an oily germ, like corn, oats, or rice—"they should be in packages and not taken from bins, where they have a tendency to go rancid."

EVEN IF FARMERS DID SAVE THEIR OWN SEEDS, or sourced them from seed-saving groups like Native Seeds/SEARCH—even if they did successfully re-introduce heritage crops, like White Sonora wheat, into their fields—they still need someone to *buy* them. And most customers, like chefs and bakers, don't want hard wheat berries. They want fluffy flour.

When I finally meet Jeff Zimmerman, the owner of Hayden Flour Mills, he is covered in it. His black jeans are dusted in so much whiteness that they appear stonewashed; his glasses are coated in a layer of dust like fogged-up windows. "Megan!" he says. "Great! Awesome!"

I'd been nervous to meet Jeff. If four companies process most of the wheat we consume, Jeff is one of the remaining two hundred working to bring milling back to the community. The headquarters of Hayden Flour Mills is located in the back room of Pane Bianco, a Phoenix pizzeria and bakery owned by Chris Bianco (once dubbed the best pizza chef in the United States by both the *New York Times* and *Bon Appétit*) and managed by his brother, Marco Bianco. I'd felt intimidated peering into this room behind the kitchen. The beautiful hulk of an Austrian mill, built of impeccable blond wood and gritty gray stone, dominates the room. But there is something about the current of wheat flour wafting through the small room, the dust smeared haphazardly on Jeff's lanky arms, elbows, and knees, and the way he says, "Megan!"—I am cheered into comfort.

"So what's up?" he says. "What do you wanna know?"

He cleans off his workstation while he talks, moves a table scale into a cabinet, brushes fallen wheat berries into an empty hundred-pound sack, dusts swaths of flour with a bristled brush. I had expected to have to explain myself to him, to justify my interest, my project, my bona fides, but I realize, as he pauses in his work to look at me, my curiosity is qualification enough. So I ask how he started—why he began milling wheat.

"I was eating a tomato," he says, and then stops and looks at me to make sure I'm paying attention.

"Mm-hmm."

"I was eating this tomato, one of those heirloom varieties, and it occurred to me: Was there ever an heirloom wheat? We've got heirloom chickens and veggies, but I couldn't find any heirloom grains."

I nod.

"It was a sort of comedy of errors, how it all happened. I found Marco Bianco here, who agreed to let me use this amazing space! And then I found Gary Nabhan, the famous Gary Nabhan, who was trying to grow the White Sonora seed. At the same time, can you believe it! I don't know, somehow we wrangled something together."

Jeff watches me scribble on my notepad, a small smile on his face. "You're tall. I've got a tall family, too. My daughter hates when people ask her, but I'll ask you anyways . . ." He comes over to me and measures himself against my stature.

I can't help but laugh. "I'm six one."

"Cool," he says. "Okay, so we're going to grind up some wheat here. Do you know the story of the White Sonora?"

White Sonora wheat is one of the oldest varieties cultivated on the American continent. Unlike corn, wheat never grew wild in the Americas; White Sonora was first grown in its namesake desert around 1650. From there, the wheat traveled in the saddlebags of Padre Eusebio Francisco Kino north into Arizona and soon spilled into fields across the Southwest. During the Civil War, the central valleys of California and Arizona, not the Great Plains of Kansas or Oklahoma, were the country's bread basket, as the region produced millions of pounds of White Sonora wheat flour for Yankee and Rebel troops.

In 1874, Charles Trumbull Hayden, a man generally credited as the founder of Tempe, opened the first mill in Arizona to process the bushels of White Sonora pouring out of the state's fields. Hayden Flour Mills thrived on the banks of the Salt River, passing through three generations of the Hayden family. But by the 1930s, thirsty populations had siphoned Colorado River water away from the Gila and Salt Rivers flowing through Arizona, the rivers the Pima Indians—the region's primary producers of White Sonora—depended on to irrigate their wheat fields, and the Pimas' expanding wheat economy began to contract. In 1998, the Bay Milling Company, which had since taken over operations, abandoned the mill, and the once-rolling fields of Sonora wheat crumbled back into the desert.

That is, until Jeff Zimmerman came along. Zimmerman grew up on a small farm in North Dakota—the kind of farm that might just have grown grain to send to a community mill. After he graduated from Arizona State University, he worked for Intel's plant in Chandler until, after getting laid off, he decided to do something different. Not long after his tomato epiphany, he met Marco and Chris Bianco, who agreed to house the mill in the back of their famous pizzeria.

Zimmerman registered the trademark for Hayden Flour Mills, bought a 1,600-pound stone mill, and started looking for grain to grind. This search led him to Gary Nabhan, an internationally recognized ethnobotanist who had acquired White Sonora seeds from Tohono O'odham farmers and planted the seeds at the Native Seeds/SEARCH farm. Nabhan connected Zimmerman to

Anson Mills's Glenn Roberts, based in South Carolina, who donated two tons of White Sonora seed to the project, seed that was planted in fields around the state with the help of a USDA grant.

Jeff hands me a step stool—"even though you could probably just dunk 'em in, right?"—and I pour a bucket of wheat berries into the mill's hopper. I flip the switch to on. Slowly, grumbling with the heft of inertia, the stone starts spinning. As it picks up speed, a subtle smell of sweet flour fills the warm air.

"Now we've got to set the distance between the bed stone and spinning stone," he says, and so I release a wood gear and ease the spinning stone down. "Not too far," Jeff cautions when a sharp grinding pierces the slow whir; he comes over and raises the stone a bit. "You don't want them to grind too close; they'll get hot and kill the enzymes in the wheat." I nod. "Okay, you ready?" he asks. "Let 'em loose."

I pull a lever and a stream of berries crowds into the spout, shimmies into the damsel, the amazingly named device that feeds the grains into the millstone, and then, moments later, flour wafts out of the mill spout.

Jeff cups his hand and gathers the flour. "Feel it," he says.

I pluck some out between my thumb and forefinger and rub it around. "It's pretty coarse."

"I'll put it back through the mill again," he says. "But what you did, just there—you know how we say 'a rule of thumb'? Some people say that's where the expression came from. Or maybe that's just why millers started using it. They would test the fineness of their grain by rubbing it just like that."

"That's so cool!" I exclaim.

Jeff beams, as excited as I am. He shuts off the mill, grabs a bucket full of flour, and scoops three heaps into a one-pound plastic bag. He seals it up and presents it to me. "Go forth and bake. Let me know how it goes."

FINALLY, MY MINIMILL ARRIVES IN THE MAIL. It's a heavy, narrow device, smaller than a wine bottle, bigger than a ruler. I mount it on the edge of my coffee table, the only counter in my apartment with a lip wide enough to support the two-inch base. I wind the flat-top screw snug to the wood and give the rectangular metal canister a shake to make sure it's snug. It extends only six or seven inches above the coffee table; the housing that will hold whole berries before they crowd into the grinder is smaller than a fist.

Although I now have a sack of Jeff's freshly ground flour in my kitchen cabinet, any lingering doubts and morning-after regret that may have surfaced when I woke up on Monday and remembered I'd bought a hand-operated grain mill dissolved on Tuesday when I opened my weekly e-newsletter from the Tucson CSA. Along with okra and corn, green beans and chilies, for the first time since I joined the CSA, we will also receive a half pound of Paloma White Winter Wheat berries harvested at Crooked Sky Farms, just south of Phoenix. Clearly, the world wants me to mill wheat.

But not yet. The mill is mounted and I crouch before it, ready to grind, until I realize that I forgot to wash my berries. Reluctantly, I accept that washing my wheat—rinsing off the bits of straw and dirt that were carried off the field—is a necessary step, so I pour the baggy into a mesh sieve and stick it under the faucet. I spread the berries across a baking sheet to dry and call my parents, as I do on most Sundays. Zoey the dog barks when my mom puts me on speakerphone. My dad shouts hello and we have one of those speakerphone conversations, nice because it's like being back at the dinner table but also vaguely stressful because everyone must slowly shout to be heard.

When I tell them I'm about to bake bread, my dad says, "Your mom used to make bread almost every Sunday. The whole house would smell. Remember that, Midge?"

"With that silly bread machine," she says, her voice increasing in volume as she leans in to the phone. "I wonder where it's ended up."

I interject. "Hey, Mom, thanks for the gift card. You really didn't need to do that." Last week, I'd collected my mail to find a card signed *For unprocessed,* with a hundred-dollar Trader Joe's gift card folded between the flaps.

"I know. I just wanted to," she says. "I worry about your money. Do you have enough?"

"Yup," I say. I don't actually know if I have enough. I had been both relieved and reluctant to receive the gift card. Reluctant because I wanted to eat unprocessed on my own terms—and within my own budget—but relieved for the support. I've just started a new job, working as a part-time marketing coordinator for the University of Arizona's Office of Sustainability, but have yet to receive my first paycheck. With January's rent out the door, my unprocessed grocery tab had been accumulating on my credit card. I knew I'd have enough money soon, but knowing is more stressful than having, and so I am grateful for the help.

Twenty minutes later, when I hang up the phone, water continues to cling in the berries' crevices. I remember farmer Kyle telling me that one of the biggest costs of industrial wheat production is the energy required to run the drying machines that keep a twenty-story granary at 14 percent humidity, so I wander into my bathroom and grab my hair dryer. Five minutes with a Revlon Ionic Ceramic and the berries are ready to rumble. Corralled into a cup, poured into the mill's housing, I press on the crank, unconvinced that anything's going to happen. It's not going to move—this won't work. Sixty dollars will not buy me the ability to mill wheat in my own home—I am already planning my e-mail to Kyle, to the Victorio company. But then the crank shifts forward, the berries dive inward, and out of the milling cone spills a fine dust of speckled beige flour. Flour! I keep grinding and the flour keeps spilling, melting from the turning crank of the milling cone. Flour, whole from a berry; flour, whole from a field.

As I watch the wheat berries crowd together over the slowly rotating mill, as I grind the crank and the wheat tumbles out the other end, transformed into the soft Spackle of flour, the process becomes so much less mysterious. Stalk to berry to flour, soil to seed to energy: I get it, just a little bit, how it was that someone ever imagined food from the earth.

It takes seven or eight minutes of continual motion to crank through two cups of wheat berries, and by the end, my right bicep burns. I kneel over my coffee table and run my fingers through the bowl of flecked flour. It's *warm*, surprisingly so. It's not hot, not burning, but certainly warmer than the air. (Warm like 110 degrees?) And so I don't wait; I bake bread. I bake bread now, with my warm flour. Yeast dissolves, oil whisks, honey floats in swarmy bubbles, and my freshly ground whole wheat crumbles and dissolves into a humid mess. Two cups of wheat berries produce four cups of flour, but my recipe calls for six, so I pull from my cabinet the bag of Sonora wheat flour that Jeff gave me.

Kyle's bitter words echo in my mind, so I lick my pointer finger and stick it into the bag and then lick the fine dust that sticks to my skin. It tastes like . . . nothing, really. It textures more than tastes, smooth like chalk dust as I rub it around my tongue. I grab another taste, and this time it tastes sort of mineral-sweet. I grab the bag of Trader Joe's Whole Wheat Flour, the same flour that formed my first loaf of bread, and remove the clothespin clasping it shut. I've never, before this moment, tasted raw flour, but in goes my finger and out goes my tongue. It's grittier than the Sonora wheat. It's gritty and bitter. I squish the flour between my tongue and the top of my mouth and the granules release a stream of sour flavor. I cannot believe that I've never noticed this flavor before—I cannot help but roll my eyes at this bag of flour, so unequivocally earning its own demise.

Again I bake bread. Throughout the day, the dough rises and falls with my kneading. It rises, falls, rises, and then arranges itself into loaves of dough. "The word *dough* comes from an Indo-European root that meant 'to form, to build,' and that also gave us the words figure, fiction, and paradise (a walled garden)," writes Harold McGee in *On Food and Cooking: The Science and Lore of the Kitchen*. "This derivation suggests the importance to early peoples of dough's malleability, its clay-like capacity to be shaped by the human hand."

My human hands shape this hybrid bread, built of the grains of the Sonora wheat and the flecks of my little grain mill, still perched on my coffee table.

Forty minutes later, my hybrid loaf of heirloom wheat and fresh flour doesn't emerge from the oven as high as I expect. It's a roomy bread, sprawled across the baking sheet. But, as one must do when confronted with bread fresh from the oven, I slice off a broad slab from one end. It requires no honey, asks for no butter. I grab the opposing crusts and watch as the dough stretches apart between the two sides, the air bubbles popped apart by warm yeast now yawning open, expanding wide, until finally they split.

The bread rolls through my mouth with yeast-wheat-honey warmth as I chew through its fibers. It's so much better than my first loaf, both because my baking skills have improved and because I can feel the flakes of wheat rubbing through my mouth, because I can imagine them whole.

I could eat the whole loaf. The smell is everywhere, in my hair, my throat, on my clothes. But this particular loaf of bread doesn't trigger me. I want to eat more, but I don't want the stomachache, don't want the rush of insulin as my body wrestles with its starches. Instead, I slice it up. I slice it up, put it away, and on Monday morning, when I am dashing out the door to work, I toss a tomato between two slabs and slather on some goat cheese. Six hours later, the inside of the bread has gone soggy, but the outside crust continues to crunch, sweet like oranges, dense like nuts. It's a carby lunch, this thick bread. It's a fatty one, too, this rich cheese. But it fills me up, satisfies me, and although it takes less than ten minutes to consume, the memory of it lingers throughout the afternoon, sticks to the inside of my stomach and the back of my tongue.

There are so many competing narratives weaving the story of what to eat. How do we know whose to read, what story to enact in our own lives? Why should I buy into Kyle's story of food, this wire-framed, gray-haired man who happened to climb in my front seat? It is complicated, wheat is, and so there isn't an easy answer. In the nine thousand years since human hands began cultivating bearded stalks of grain, our diet has become increasingly reliant upon their fruits. Even as I delight in the grinding crunch of my minimill, I realize that I will have to venture away from it at some point; that I will have to eat the faux-whole grains out in the world, pieced together like Humpty-Dumpty. So I return, again, to the philosophy of my kitchen: Don't let the perfect be the enemy of the good. Even if I continue to buy wheat berries to grind into flour, there will be compromise bread. Later in the week, after my hybrid bread has disappeared and I need a quick lunch, I will pull from my freezer two slices of Ezekiel Sprouted 100% Whole Grain Bread—made of the same primary ingredients but sold presliced in a plastic bag—and it will be good enough.

The way I eat wheat will be different from how Kara does, or Kyle, or all those whose bodies have rejected the onslaught of grains foisted upon them. But what I learn from my hand-operated grain mill is that it's worthwhile to wrestle with our own stories. And as I mill my own wheat, I feel like finally, after ten years of confusion, I am reclaiming bread for myself.

Unprocess Yourself: Wheat

Any food store with a bulk section sells wheat berries; you can grind them into flour if you feel like adding a grain mill to your kitchen machinery. You can also boil wheat berries and add them to salad or sautés. Many farmers' markets sell freshly ground flours; if someone's gone to the trouble of milling flour, it's likely because they're growing an heirloom variety of wheat. If you aren't going to use your flour within a few weeks, seal it and put it in the freezer.

To make a basic loaf of whole-wheat bread, you'll need whole-grain flour, warm water, active dry yeast, and salt. Honey and oil are good additions, but not necessary. You want roughly a three-to-one ratio of flour to water, with about two tablespoons each of yeast and oil, a teaspoon or so of salt, and about a fourth of a cup of honey—but a precise recipe will help immeasurably the first few times you make bread. To proof your yeast—which is simply "proving" that it's still active—add yeast to about a cup of warm water along with a spoonful of honey (for the yeast to munch on). The water should foam—that's the yeast doing its thing. Mix the remaining liquids and combine with flour. Knead until the dough forms a smooth mass. Leave the dough to rise—I usually cover it with a warm, wet cloth to help the yeast propagate—and come back in an hour or two to knead it again. After it rises again, shape the dough into a loaf, score the top, and bake on a baking sheet for about forty-five minutes, or until the crust turns golden brown.

I like making bread, but usually it comes into my kitchen presliced and in a crinkly plastic package. When buying bread, I always look for

3

SWEET

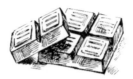

Sugar is processed if it is made.

When I lived in Nicaragua, the world stopped at 6 P.M. Or, rather, our days did. We pulled chairs to the patio, cracked open beers, and watched *la puesta del sol,* the putting of the sun. So close to the equator, the sun set at six year-round. We might lose ten minutes in the winter and gain ten in the summer, but it didn't matter. Time *was* the sunset. Bug spray evaporated on skin, loose clothes tickled in the breeze, and the sun hung inches over the ocean. It'd dip a toe in, testing, wavering, and then shimmy its fat belly into the water, bobbing for another minute before finally melting into blue. It was always then, watching the sunset with Juan on the hotel's breezy patio—after I'd finished my beer, before we retreated inside at the behest of the mosquitoes—that I wanted chocolate. Just a nibble. Just a bite, a chunk, a small, melting mouthful.

"A day without chocolate is a day wasted," my grandmother always said.

"Megan, chocolate isn't good for you," said Juan. "Here, have a tortilla." Juan was the manager of Hotel Brio and my best friend in Playa Gigante. I babysat products made from sprouted grains. Food For Life—also sold under the name Ezekiel—sells breads, tortillas, and cereals made from whole, sprouted grains. The generic brand of most natural food stores will have a version of sprouted, whole-grain bread. At the Tucson Co-op, a loaf of Ezekiel 4:9 Sprouted Grain Bread costs $4.49—roughly the same price as any whole-grain bread stocked at the supermarket.

Ingredient label fun! That same loaf of Ezekiel bread contains: sprouted wheat, filtered water, sprouted barley, sprouted millet, malted barley, sprouted lentils, sprouted soybeans, sprouted spelt, fresh yeast, wheat gluten, sea salt. Basically, bread—and any grain-based product, like pasta or flour tortillas—should contain grain, salt, yeast, and water. Maybe oil. That's it.

I'm on the unprocessed fence about wheat gluten, which is basically ground-up wheat protein, added to give bread lift and structure. Many at-home bread recipes call for it, although the process of making wheat gluten requires grinding up whole grains after they've been vigorously washed to remove the starch—not exactly on my kitchen to-do list, but then again, neither was grinding whole grains. Your call.

Anything else—like sulfur dioxide, anything ending in "glyceride," calcium propionate, or calcium sulfate—are usually added as preservatives. Your bread *should* mold after a few days on the counter. I freeze mine and defrost by way of a toaster. (Spread that toast with a generous heap of almond butter and slice a banana on top and you've got breakfast.)

Keep in mind that bread is effectively sugar tied up by fiber—starches are just long chains of glucose units—so it doesn't keep you full for very long. I'm all about feeling full, so I don't eat a ton of grain products. (Also, see: bread, trigger food.)

Juan's daughters when his wife came to visit from their home in Masaya, a town an hour away; I scavenged the beach with curious Malinda and braided baby Leslie's hair. Life was good in the tropics, so I hushed my chocolate cravings with crumbly chocolate-flavored cookies and honey-filled tortillas. But finally, after five months of chocolate-free days, Kara came to visit. She didn't bring me chocolate, but we had bigger plans. We ventured into the open-air market in Rivas, through chaotic stalls, around water in the gutters, and found a woman who sold raw, unshelled cacao beans for five dollars a pound. In Hotel Brio's hot kitchen, we roasted the cacao beans in a frying pan and then passed an hour and two beers laboriously peeling away papery outer shells to reveal the shiny, smooth cacao nibs within. A food processor's spinning blade whirred the nibs into clumpy dirt; into the spinning darkness, we dumped a spoonful of butter and a stream of granulated white sugar, and peered, rapt, as the blade spun the dirt into mud. The noise of the food processor brought Juan and Isolina back into the kitchen and they, too, peered into the spinning food processor. Juan exclaimed, surprised: "It looks like chocolate!"

It looked like it, but it wasn't quite *it*. The smoothness of the spinning belied the grit within. The paste crunched around our mouths with an effect that, taken cumulatively, was chocolate-y. But the sugar hadn't incorporated into the cacao, the butter into the sugar, so although our concoction was chocolate-like, it was not *chocolate*.

For most of its early history—for at least the last three thousand years— chocolate was consumed in liquid form, usually prepared by brewing ground cacao in hot water, much like coffee is today. It was a bitter brew, one drunk to invigorate rather than indulge. Indeed, the Aztec king Montezuma II reportedly drank a daily fifty golden goblets of *xocolatl,* or "bitter water," made of unsweetened cacao ground up with spices. (Montezuma evidently believed *xocolatl* was an aphrodisiac; if ever there was a man who needed *xocolatl,* it was the emperor of fifty wives.)

Xocolatl became chocolate—cacao became cocoa—about five hundred years ago, when the bitter bean finally found sugar. Montezuma offered Spanish conquistador Hernán Cortés a sip of the frothy liquid in 1519; after the first commercial shipment of chocolate landed in Sevilla in 1585, cosmopolitan cafés throughout Europe started concocting hot beverages made with sugar and chocolate.

The process of chocolate begins when a heavy, football-size pod—christened *Theobroma cacao,* "the food of the gods," by Swedish botanist Carolus Linnaeus—is cracked open to reveal thick columns of fiber woven with slimy white seeds. After fermenting in this sweet mucus for a week or so, the seeds are cleaned, roasted, and deshelled, producing the nibs of cacao most of us recognize. It wasn't until 1828 that a Dutch chocolatier developed a screw press to separate cacao butter from the solid; in 1847, a British bloke figured out how to combine chocolate liquor—the liquid form of cacao—and sugar in the right quantities, at the right heat, to create the world's first portable chocolate bar. Chocolatiers speak of "conching" and "tempering"—grinding the chocolate nibs finer and finer; applying heat to evenly crystallize fat with solid—but essentially, chocolate is some combination of cacao butter, cacao solid, and sugar.

Sugar defines chocolate like heat defines summer, like lightness signifies day. Sugar and chocolate are the original dynamic duo. Just as good couples bring out the best in each other, cacao's complexity marries sugar's straightforward sweet with such delightful ease it seems impossible that one ever existed without the other.

For my year unprocessed, would I have to go so long without chocolate? I'd made it through a year in Nicaragua without chocolate because my days had been filled with other delights—early morning ocean swims, tropical rainstorms, mangoes fresh off the tree. Although my Tucson days are happy ones, they are filled with fewer of these dense moments that had made life in the tropics so sweet. If sweetness is a taste, it is also an experience; it is the crystallization of desire.

A MONTH INTO UNPROCESSED, I feel constantly stressed out. I am on overdrive, hypervigilant about reading ingredient labels and querying menus. Out in the world, unprocessed follows me around like elevator music. At the Office of Sustainability, my new boss asks me, bemused or simply amused, what's in the Tupperware containers I bring for lunch every day. (CSA veggies and wheat berries; leftover whole-grain pasta; grilled winter squash and garbanzo beans.) Another coworker, a gruff facilities management guy, shakes his head, incredulous, when I pull out a mason jar full of bright orange carrot soup and sit down for lunch. "What is *that*?" he asks. I try to be nonchalant about unprocessed, but as my friends and coworkers hear about my endeavor, they ask questions. Their questions aren't posed as challenges, but I am still standing on unsteady legs, and so I stumble; I become defensive. "No, there *is* a difference between kinds of process!" I insist, defending the hummus spread across my whole-grain toast. When my office mate turns thirty, we gather in the kitchen to sing "Happy Birthday"; after we sing, as everyone else digs into the cake, I feel awkward, leaning against the wall with nothing to do with my hands, so I return too quickly to my desk. I feel like I am traveling around Tucson with a giant *U* hung around my neck.

Katie continues to e-mail me recipes for desserts sweetened with dates or honey, and dutifully, I attempt to make many of them—unprocessed pumpkin pie, with a date and coconut crust; unprocessed frozen yogurt, with bananas and almond butter; unprocessed apple cobbler, with rolled oats and honey.

But when I get home from work or class, long past sunset, after I eat dinner and do the dishes, I don't really want homemade cobbler. I want, instead, a bite of ready-made, dark, melting sweetness. I want chocolate. But if refined sugar is processed, then chocolate is, too.

While different cultures prefer different combinations of bitter, sour, and salty foods, according to anthropologists, an affinity for sweetness appears in almost every society across human history. Before sugarcane spread across the globe, there were dates, figs, and honey in the Mediterranean; oranges and berries in Asia. Apples in the Garden of Eden. In the *Oxford English Dictionary,* something that is sweet "affords enjoyment or gratifies desire." It is "pleasure, delight, the pleasant part of something." It is the best part.

WHEN KATIE AND I WERE KIDS, my mom instituted a rule called One Sweet a Day. "Can I have a Coke?" I'd ask, and the answer was yes only if I hadn't had a sweet before, with the understanding that I wouldn't ask for another one after. My mom seems to have manufactured the dictum out of desperation, as a way to rein in the voracity of her skinny daughters' sweet munchings. (The ravenousness that led Katie to pull down her pants in the name of ice cream had only intensified when I became a partner-in-crime for her sugary scheming.) Katie and I began to treat the idea of "one serving" with such abandon—plucking a bowl-size latte mug from the back of the cabinet to hold our ice cream; cupping our hands together to get the most mileage out of a "handful" of jelly beans— that my mom resorted to micromanaging our sugar. "Thirty jelly beans, Katie!" she'd call from her desk as Katie tiptoed into the pantry. "Only thirty!"

My mom trusted us to report back on our activities outside the home, to tell her whether or not we spent thirty cents of our lunch money on an orange-swirl Popsicle, and perhaps because One Sweet a Day seemed as inviolable a rule as Do Your Homework (or because the Popsicles stained the corners of our lips a telltale red), we always told. When Katie and I got to high school, One Sweet a Day became of secondary concern to 11 P.M. Curfew and No Texting at Dinner, but the rule stuck with us. Katie and I would pass each other at school, one or the other clutching a chocolate chip muffin, and grin with the glee of breaking a neglected rule.

On our yearly visits to see our Grandma Kimble in her home in Floydada, Texas, we arrived with a box of dark chocolate truffles from See's Candies. She was in her mideighties at that point, skinny and wearing too-big skin, alert and trapped in an unresponsive body. Grandma Kimble reigned over her days from the perch of an overstuffed electric chair that lifted and lowered her with interminable slowness. "Going down!" she'd cry, leaning back into the upright chair, poking the down button with her crooked fingers. She'd hold on to the button ten, fifteen, twenty seconds while we waited for her to regain her rightful place in the small living room.

"Milk chocolate is for wussies," she'd declare, peering at the box through the spectacles that magnified her bright blue eyes into sparkling orbs. She'd hem and haw over the paper-wrapped truffles—her frail shoulders folding around the box like a curved curtain—before finally plucking one out and passing the box down to Katie and me.

Even Grandma abided, in her own way, by One Sweet a Day. She'd savor the truffle, clasping it between arthritic fingers to savor each bite of rich, smooth chocolate. She might pluck out another truffle after her first, but only if it was a special day, and she never ate more than two. I was seven, eight, nine, and I didn't understand why not. Why not splurge for another? She was, after all, so *old*. I tried to ask her once, as polite as I knew how, why she didn't eat more truffles now, you now, just in case.

"Be*cause,* darlin'," she'd say, folding into the drawl she'd acquired after living in West Texas her whole adult life. "Now I've got something to look forward to tomorrow."

Though in adulthood, there is no longer a need to rebel by illicit muffin or extra truffle, I still feel the power of One Sweet a Day. And usually I follow it. But now One Sweet a Day is not a restriction but an allowance. A command that I shall have one sweet a day, every day. A dictum that says a day without sugar is a day deprived.

WHAT IS SUGAR? The word contains duplicity—sugar is itself duplicitous, enticing us into highs and then casting us off into lows. Sugar is "hey baby, how *you* doin'?"—it is syrup to salt's sultry. Sweetness is bliss, saccharine is smothering. We "sugarcoat" that which we want to evade. Sucrose is chemistry, insulin its moderator. Sugar flourishes in the tropics but lives in the liver.

There is cane sugar: white, brown, crystallized, or powdered. Cane sugar is organic or vegan, cooked or raw, turbinado, Demerara, or muscovado, all the glistening hue of pale dust. There is coconut sugar and date sugar, palm and maple. There is calorie-free sugar—stevia, Truvia, SweetLeaf—sold in impossibly weightless plastic sacks; there are narrow plastic cylinders of white crystals called simply fructose. There are bottles, jars, and canisters of liquid sugar: blackstrap molasses, barley malt, brown rice syrup, maple syrup, agave nectar, and honey. Desert honey, mesquite honey, raw honey; pumpkin-, ginger-, or prickly-pear-flavored honey. There is, of course, fiber-bound sugar, a bite of a bright Pink Lady apple. Crunchy flares of juice, apple skin in teeth, sweetness that trickles, slowly, into the bloodstream.

All sugars are some combination of three simple molecules: glucose, a building block for plant growth and animal energy; fructose, found mostly, as the name would suggest, in fruit; and galactose, which is found only in milk. Fructose is about twice as sweet as glucose, so it's the presence of fructose that defines a sensation of "sweetness"—fructose is the difference between a potato and a pear. Sucrose, which occurs naturally in sugarcane and sugar beets, is half glucose, half fructose. Usually, when we're talking about sugar, we're talking about sucrose.

When we encounter these sugar molecules, they are wound into complex chains of carbohydrates and starches; digestion unwinds these molecules, turning food into glucose, the body's primary unit of energy. Glucose—or *glukus,* which means "sweet" in Greek—is a chain of carbon, hydrogen, and oxygen. When our bodies break down these chains, they become carbon dioxide and water, which, in turn, yield adenosine triphosphate, or ATP, the "molecular unit of currency" for energy transfer within cells. In other words, sugar becomes glucose becomes ATP, becomes a neuron firing and an arm swinging.

Compared to a potato or a carrot, both of which must be broken down by stomach acids and pushed through the small intestine before their energy is incorporated into the bloodstream, a process that can take upward of two hours, it takes minutes for sugar in the mouth to become glucose in the blood. Because our bodies digest all chains of sugar molecules, starches and sucrose alike, the same way, it's essentially irrelevant at the molecular level where this glucose comes from. The only chemical difference, for example, between table sugar and high-fructose corn syrup is a slightly higher ratio of fructose to glucose in the latter: a 55 to 45 percent ratio instead of 50–50 in sucrose, a small enough difference to be essentially irrelevant. What is more important is how—in what—the sugar is packaged.

THE FIRST TIME I GNAWED ON A HUSK OF SUGARCANE, after it had been hacked from the ground by a swinging machete, I was surprised at how sweet it wasn't. In the space between my post-Nicaragua life in Los Angeles and a move to Tucson, I'd found an adventure in Brazil. I'd been there a month when a friend invited me on a weekend trip to her grandfather's farm. We arrived to a flurry of aunts, uncles, and kisses, and soon we were bumping in the back of a truck as the eighty-eight-year-old Senhor Tabosa, his small, sinewy frame blazing with energy, barreled up a winding dirt road that swung through a deep green mountainside. When we paused to collect açai berries scattered beneath a tall roadside palm, Senhor Tabosa slid a machete from the floor of his truck, bounded over a barbed-wire fence, and toppled a long skinny cane with a quick, quiet crack. *"Açúcar!"* he exclaimed, shedding the sugarcane's husk with a few deft strokes of the machete, and handed me a foot-long section of beige fibers, huddled together like a tamale. It was a crunchy first bite, thick and full of juice sliding down my chin. The juice was warm from the Brazilian sun and the fibers were sweet but not sticky-sweet, not cloying or bursting or smooth. The sweetness didn't dissolve, but crunched and chewed its way across my mouth, into my gums, down the back of my throat, thick like an accidental mouthful of seawater. The sweetness was subtle, almost vegetable.

By quantity, sugarcane is the world's most cultivated crop—an estimated 23.8 million acres planted around the world produce an annual harvest of 1.7 billion tons of sugar—and Brazil is the world's largest producer. Sugarcane's sweetness is not incidental, like that of a fruit or flower, in which sweetness serves the seed. The whole *point* of sugarcane is sweetness.

For several thousand years after humans discovered that the knobby reed contained sweetness inside its awkward exterior—sometime around 8000 BC, likely in New Guinea—the sugar in sugarcane remained largely untapped. In 6000 BC, after the Persians stumbled across the "reeds that produce honey without bees" on the banks of the Indus River, sugarcane sprawled to southern China, spread across Southeast Asia, and finally arrived to India, which is where granulated sugar was likely invented. A fellow named Dioscorides visiting India from the Mediterranean first documented this new substance, "a sort of crystallized honey . . . not unlike salt in its texture, and it can be crunched in between the teeth like salt."

As least, Dioscorides is thus quoted in the book *Food in the Ancient World from A–Z,* which I find deep in the stacks of the University of Arizona library when I turn from the supermarket to the annals of historic wisdom in my quest to find unprocessed sugar.

"You go, girl!" exclaims the librarian, a middle-aged man wearing an oxford button-down and sporting long dreadlocks, when I ask him why this book is being rejected at the electronic kiosk. "You're the first person to check this book out." He slides a bar code on the front. "Ever!"

Sugar remained on the periphery of European culture until about AD 1100, when the Crusaders, deployed by the Catholic Church to counter Muslim expansion, encountered people in the fields of Tripoli "sucking enthusiastically on a honey reed they call *Zuchra* . . . delighting themselves with [its] beneficial juices." In what might be a prescient commentary on our modern relationship to sugar, this ancient scribe reported people who "seemed unable to sate themselves with this pleasure in spite of [its] sweetness."

Until well into the seventeenth century, granulated sugar was a rarity in European households—imported from India, the sweet granules were so expensive and used so sparingly that they were classified as a spice or, occasionally, as medicine. Thomas Aquinas officially permitted the consumption of sugar during religious fasts, as "though they are nutritious themselves, sugared spices are nonetheless not eaten with the end in mind of nourishment, but rather for ease in digestion; accordingly, they do not break the fast any more than the taking of any other medicine." So useful was sugar as medicine that, for centuries, the expression "like an apothecary without sugar" meant a state of desperation or helplessness.

But it was in the Americas, after Christopher Columbus colonized his conquered soils with the hardy, adaptable reed, that sugar finally came of age. "Sugar—or rather the commodity market which arose demanding it— has been one of the massive demographic forces in world history," writes anthropologist Sidney Mintz in *Sweetness and Power: The Place of Sugar in Modern History*. Indeed, as soon as soil in Spanish Santo Domingo sprouted sugarcane, ships departed from the coast of Africa filled with thousands— eventually millions—of slaves to harvest and process the quick-growing cane. As sugarcane production in the colonies rose, the price dropped in Europe and sugar spread to the masses. Sugar was a rarity in 1600, a luxury in 1700, and by 1800, when Europeans were consuming five hundred million pounds a year, it was a necessity.

BACK WHEN A SATURDAY'S SWEET might be spent on a bowl of Frosted Flakes or, if we were lucky, cinnamon rolls, Katie and I watched *Mister Rogers*. I remember the knotted beige carpet that filled our family room, how I would gnaw at it with my fingernails, trying to reinvigorate its fluff, and I remember something that Mister Rogers used to say. Maybe he only said it once, or maybe it was a refrain, but as he stood there in his funny cardigan, explaining how to make crayons or sneakers or fortune cookies, he said: There is a difference between things people make and things that are made.

There is a difference between foods people can make with their hands and foods that are made by machines. People can make sweet corn into a corn tortilla; people can't really make high-fructose corn syrup, not without access to a laboratory and an advanced degree in chemistry. If there is a difference in sugar that is processed and sugar that is not processed, it is the difference between sweetness fabricated and sweetness found.

Making sugar from sugarcane is essentially a liquid-to-solid operation. Extract juice from cane. Boil juice to evaporate water. Concentrate extract into syrup. Apply more heat. Crystallize syrup into granulated sugar. Refine.

That last word is the loaded one, the step when things start happening in the passive voice. Once sugarcane juice crystallizes into something solid, the crystals are spun through a centrifuge to further dry the sugar solids and remove any impurities. Molasses is the stuff that gets sucked out of the centrifuge, and by "the stuff," I mean all the nutrients, which is why blackstrap molasses is considered one of the world's most nutritious foods while white sugar is deemed one of the most nutrient-poor. What's known as raw sugar is sugar here, the crystallized cane with molasses removed. But truly raw sugar can contain mold, fibers, or other contaminants, so often the raw sugar that appears on supermarket shelves has been purified, either chemically, in the case of Demerara sugar, or steam-cleaned, in the case of turbinado sugar. Much like Humpty-Dumpty "whole grains," standard-issue brown sugar is usually refined white sugar that's been mixed with molasses.

To make refined white sugar, the "raw" crystals tumbling out of the centrifuge are dissolved and purified with phosphoric acid and then filtered through a bed of activated carbon or, more commonly, bone char. According to the Vegetarian Resource Group, hundreds of years ago, "sugar refiners discovered that bone char from cattle worked well as a whitening filter, and this practice is now the industry standard." This is why Whole Foods sells a vegan version of sugar—because of the bone char.

Initially, the incentive to process sugar as much as possible was a fairly obvious one. The purer the sugar, the more easily it combined with other foods. Refined sugar is also an excellent preservative, and back when sugar was getting going, keeping fruits fresh and vegetables edible wasn't so easy as sticking them in the freezer. (Hence, jam.)

"The history of sugar making and refining has been one of irregular improvement of the level of chemical purity," writes Mintz in *Sweetness and Power*. Sugarcane is a plant full of sucrose; the story of sugar's processing is simply that over the years, we've figured out more efficient ways to package that water-bound sucrose into portable crystals. And then, inevitably, to slide it into all of our favorite foods.

THE ANSWER TO THE DINNER-PARTY UNPROCESSED QUESTION—"Wow, is that hard?"—is sugar. Sugar is in *everything* and if you decide refined white sugar is processed, most everything sold at the supermarket becomes off-limits. Of course sugar shows up in chocolate bars, vanilla yogurt, and fruit preserves. Less obvious is why the *first* ingredient listed in Jack Daniel's Honey Dijon Mustard is high-fructose corn syrup; why sugar appears in Prego Traditional Marinara Sauce, in Kraft Balsamic Vinaigrette Salad Dressing, in Progresso Light Chicken Noodle Soup and 100% Natural Whole Wheat Bread.

If added sugar is "defined as any sweetener containing the molecule fructose that is added to food in its processing," writes nutrition scientist Robert Lustig in the journal *Nature,* then logic dictates that a food containing added sugar was processed.

I don't want sugar in my salad dressing or mustard; I don't need it in my bread or tortillas. Over the past fifty years, sugar consumption has tripled worldwide and it is no wonder. If sweetness is desire, why wouldn't we pack more and more of it into our foods? The problem with this logic is in its accumulation. In the United States, we consume an average of six hundred calories a day just from added sugar. We are hooked on sweetness and our bodies are taking a beating because of it. "Sugar dampens the suppression of the hormone ghrelin, which signals hunger to the brain. It also interferes with the normal transport and signaling of the hormone leptin, which helps to produce the feeling of satiety," writes Lustig. "And it reduces dopamine signaling in the brain's reward center, thereby decreasing the pleasure derived from food and compelling the individual to consume more."

If sweetness is the best part of something—a day, a sunset—then it should be overtly enjoyed rather than hidden in processed packaging. Sweetness should be savored as a delight rather than consumed by compulsion. My issue with sugar is less its processing than its ubiquity.

Although a chain of glucose is a chain of glucose, how your body responds to sugar depends on quantity and speed—how much sugar you eat and how fast you eat it. The quicker the sugar hits your system, the more pressure it exerts on your body to respond quickly. When you eat sucrose, the fructose goes straight to your liver while the rest of the body—including your brain— pitches in to use glucose. Too much sugar consumed too quickly overloads the liver. Though they both contain the same kind of sugar, if you eat an apple or drink a cup of its juice, your body responds differently. In the apple, sucrose is bound up by fiber and cellulose—sticky duct tape that takes time and effort to unwind and rip open. A cup of apple juice, on the other hand, is cyber in its immediacy. There is no packaging that slows the arrival of sucrose and that all-at-once arrival stresses out your body. With sugar, as with e-mail, the ease of the sender becomes the burden of the receiver. If an apple is a neatly wrapped package, then refined sugar is e-mail spam.

If sweetness is the best part, it is only so because it was once precious and scarce, not assumed and available. "If the stars should appear one night in a thousand years, how would men believe and adore; and preserve for many generations the remembrance of the city of God which had been shown!" wrote Ralph Waldo Emerson. "But every night come out these envoys of beauty, and light the universe with their admonishing smile." And so it is of sugar today, the assumption of omnipresence diminishing the power of its sweetness.

It is not sugar itself that I'm opposed to, not sweetness or desire. It is simply its presumption, its conquering gene that has lingered since Columbus colonized a new world's soils with the sweet fibers cultivated by slave labor. The issue is not sugarcane, of course—it is rather the assumption that to have sweetness in our lives, our lives must be filled with sugar.

"THE BEES ARE CRANKY TODAY," says Jaime de Zubeldia when I arrive at ReZoNation Farm. "They're always cranky in early spring."

"Why?" I ask. I've just arrived and the thought of cranky bees makes me want to climb right back in my car and return to Tucson. I was already driving north through Saguaro National Park, winding west toward Avra Valley, when I remembered that the last time I was stung by a bee, my leg acquired a swollen, balloon-size protrusion that had throbbed for days.

But my hunger for honey has driven me this far without attention to allergy, so I follow Jaime through the gate and into the house he shares with his wife. As it turns out, the bees are cranky because they, too, are hungry. In early spring, there's not much blooming in the desert, so "they're spending their resources on laying eggs and raising bees," says Jaime—on growing the hive rather than gathering nectar to make honey. "It's like you have a lot of mouths to feed and not enough in the refrigerator. Stresses them out."

Before cane sugar swept through the Mediterranean world, honey was the sweetener ancient civilizations depended on. My trusty *Food in the Ancient World from A–Z*—I now feel like it is mine, or at least that its existence depends on my reading of it—informs me that beekeeping was first documented in Egypt around 2500 BC, but that humans were likely collecting honey long before that. Seven-thousand-year-old clay pots have been found in the republic of Georgia, still containing trace residues of honey, evidence of the ancient custom of sending a departed into the afterlife armed with a jar full of sweet syrup. Three thousand years before that, a rock painting in a cave in Spain shows two people raiding a wild beehive, evidence that we've gone out of our way to find honey for at least ten thousand years.

Bees do most of the work in the processing of honey from nature. They venture out into the world and suck up flower nectar, which they then regurgitate into hives, into the empty spaces of wax honeycombs. Nectar accumulates in the honeycombs as bees flap their wings, drying the water-based nectar into sweet syrup.

Scattered across ReZoNation's two and a half acres are fifty hives that, over the course of a year, yield Jaime roughly fifty pounds of honey. "The job of a beekeeper is just to provide the bees with space and entice them to stay," Jaime says. That space is in fact called "bee space," a term coined by beekeeping pioneer Lorenzo Langstroth in 1851. Langstroth's discovery that bees build better hives when given a finite, defined space—three-eighths of an inch between removable frames—revolutionized the beekeeping industry. Before Langstroth hives, which allowed the beekeeper to remove frames and inspect the health of the hive, beekeeping had been a hobby sport, racked by risk and infection.

The introduction of the movable frame hive, the wax comb foundation, the centrifugal honey extractor, and the bellows smoker, all of which appeared between 1851 and 1873, "transform[ed] beekeeping from a sideline interest to an industry," writes Tammy Horn in *Bees in America.*

After we each don a wide-brimmed beekeeping hat, faces swathed in mesh, Jaime loads a small smoker with scrap paper and slowly pumps a thick, sweet smoke. The smoke distracts the bees and lowers their defenses, allowing him to reach two glove-adorned hands around either end of a top bar and slide it, heavy with honey, swarming with bees, into the light. He peers at it, muttering, to himself or to the bees. The bees clump and climb, cluster and canoodle. They preen and wag, burrow and mosey. More brown than yellow, more collective than individual.

Most of Jaime's hives are top-bar hives, basically U-shaped bee boxes covered by rows of rectangular wood beams. The box becomes a hive when Jaime fills the space with young bees. The bees scurry into the world, collect nectar, and return to their bee space, where they begin knitting wax combs along the bottom of these bars. When the landscape is in bloom, hardworking bees can weave a hive of pentagon-shaped wax combs from empty space in a matter of days. It's only then, when the hive is built, that the bees turn their energy to the task of filling these holes with honey.

As Jaime slides the first frame back into the bee box and pulls out another, I ask, "What are you looking for?"

"Just looking," he says. He extends a finger in among the bees, brushing them gently one way and another. "Trying to see if I can find the queen." The bees don't seem to be doing much except bumping into each other, but as Jaime progresses through the frames, left to right, moving closer to the center of the box, the dark interiors of the wax-crusted combs begin to glisten with honey. If he were going to harvest this honey today, Jaime would brush the bees away, break the comb into a bucket, and carry that bucket to his kitchen table. He'd place this bucket, the one with centimeter-wide holes scattered across its base, atop another plastic bucket fitted with a plastic valve. Jaime's special smashing stick—a repurposed top bar from one of his hives—would crush honey and comb together, and gravity would pull that honey through the holes, toward a valve siphoning honey into a jar.

Most honey today is extracted via centrifuge. Beekeepers slide combs into the slots of a centrifuge; as it spins, honey seeps out of the combs and accumulates in the bottom of the barrel, where it can be siphoned into a jar and then later spooned into tea. As Jaime hands me a steaming mug, I ask, "Why don't you use a centrifuge?"

He grabs a beekeeping supply catalog from the top of a cluttered coffee table and shows me their selection—a twelve-frame spinner sells for $2,000, a go-big or go-home eighty-four-frame spinner for $6,200. "The up-front cost is limiting," he says, deadpan. "I sometimes borrow one from the Community Food Bank, where I used to work."

"Can you taste a difference?" I ask. "In honey that's extracted in a centrifuge?"

"I don't think it tastes quite as complex," Jaime says. "When I crush the combs, you get some comb in the honey, which offers nutrients and texture."

While many small-scale beekeepers spin honey out of hives with a centrifuge and call it a day—I don't notice a difference when Jaime offers a taste test of spun versus crushed—many more use heat to clarify the semisolid grainy sweetness into something more like syrup. Some industrial-scale honey processors go one leap further, refining the syrup to remove all traces of pollen. Which is a problem, because according to the FDA, honey without pollen isn't honey. In 2011, according to *Food Safety News,* three-fourths of the honey sold in U.S. grocery stores wasn't actually honey, meaning it had been ultrafiltered to remove any identifying qualities. (Organic honey fared slightly better.) Ultrafiltering involves heating honey, watering it down, and then high-pressure blasting it through very small filters to remove any lingering pollen. You want your honey to have pollen not only because it's more nutritious but also because it's safer. Some Chinese honey—which accounts for almost half the honey consumed in the United States—has been shown to be contaminated with chloramphenicol and other potentially dangerous antibiotics. But without pollen, that honey isn't traceable to its source.

Jaime's honey—rather, the honey from his bees—is, on first encounter, crunchy. Opaque, both in the jar and on the end of a spoon. Granulated and crystallized, solid against my tongue until the creaminess liquefies, rolls, and expands. A honey's flavor depends on the flower the bees drink their nectar from—bees gorging on orange blossoms produce sweet, citrus-tinged honey, while clover-bombarded bees create the common cinnamon-hinted honey. Jaime's honey is mesquite honey, made by desert-adapted bees sourcing their sugar from the blooms of this enduring desert tree, and it's smoky and thick, strong and sweetly lingering.

I HADN'T ATTEMPTED another chocolate-making adventure since I returned stateside—chocolate was everywhere, wrapped in bars and shaped in kisses, ready for the nibbling. But I have yet to find even the most eco-friendly chocolate made with any sweetener except cane sugar, so when my sister comes to visit at the end of February, when I am reunited with my sweet-seeking partner-in-crime, it is time to try again. When Katie comes to visit, her husband, Tyler, stays at home in Seattle. When I pick Katie up from the tiny Tucson airport and she exclaims, "Old people really *do* flock to the desert in the winter!" I realize how long it's been since it was just the two of us, scheming and silly together.

Katie is in the last year of her Ph.D. program in environmental economics, a short dissertation away from becoming not Dr. Kimble, as I had for so long assumed she would be, but instead Dr. Grooms. Tyler and Katie got married the summer before I moved to Tucson, and I was still adjusting to the new nomenclature. A boyfriend becomes a husband and a name disappears, this last name that had joined us, announcing our relation, codifying strange moments of self-recognition in another being. But when Katie arrives to Tucson, I remember that even if we are different people on paper, we are still as united as we have always been, inescapably joined by genes and knobby limbs that sprawl like sugarcane.

Katie wants to go to Trader Joe's for our chocolate-making provisions, but I've started to feel uncomfortable about my reliance on the market's mysteriously sourced wares, so I insist we drive the extra mile to Sunflower Farmers Market.

"You know the Trader Joe's brand?" I ask as we drive along Speedway Boulevard. "They actually buy most of that food from big food companies at bulk rates and put it in their own packaging."

"Oh, I don't know about that," she says, dismissive. "They have a lot of organics."

Katie doesn't want to hear about Trader Joe's ills—and really, neither did I. We are eaters of the Trader Joe's demographic, devotees addicted to artisan wares at big-box prices. Trader Joe's is successful in large part because of people like us, who want good food that is not only sustainably sourced but also agreeably, impossibly affordable. It is true that Trader Joe's stocks a stunning array of organic food, which makes it easy to ignore the fact that the company is deliberately silent on its sourcing. (In 2010, *Fortune* reported that the Trader Joe's brand pita chips come from Stacy's, a division of Frito-Lay and that Trader Joe's yogurt comes from Danon's Stonyfield Farms. Want more information? Good luck.) The neighborhood corner-store vibe that's consciously cultivated also makes it easy to forget, if you ever knew it in the first place, that although the company headquarters are in Monrovia, California, Trader Joe's is owned by a wealthy German family.

As we pull into the parking lot of Sunflower Farmers Market, which is of course not a farmers' market, but rather a chain of natural food stores, Katie says, acutely, "Well then, who owns Sunflower?"

"I don't know," I admit. "I think it started in Arizona. But I guess it's all over the Southwest now."

In addition to ingredients for our dinner—whole-wheat pasta, fresh mozzarella, tomatoes, and basil—we buy cacao powder, a stick of butter, and honey. "Can I buy a bar of chocolate for myself, in case it doesn't work out?" Katie asks as we're standing at the register.

"No!" I exclaim, offended. "There *will* be chocolate." This time, we will buy preground cacao; we will heat the butter, the honey will bind, and there will be chocolate.

While the intricacy of Jaime's honey had satisfied me for weeks, deliciously complex and surprisingly filling, honey is not, at the end of the day, chocolate. It is the fat, salt, sugar conundrum all over again—good in isolation, but transformative in combination.

When we get home, we unload the groceries and stand in my tiny kitchen, towering over my tiny stove. Together, we watch as a stick of butter melts into a creamy pool. I measure out a cup of unsweetened cacao powder; Katie folds in half a cup of honey. I whisk; Katie watches.

"Looks like chocolate syrup!" she says, hopeful.

She pulls a fork from my sticky drawer, pokes it in the molten liquid, and blows on it until it cools. I follow her lead. She takes a lick. I take a lick. We look at each other and shrug. "It tastes chocolate-y," she says, encouraging.

I pour the butter-honey-cacao syrup into a square glass Tupperware and slide it into the fridge. A couple of hours later, after we cook and eat dinner, I turn the mold over. The maybe-chocolate solid doesn't budge. Katie slides a knife along its edges and offers the Tupperware another vigorous, upside-down shake. The chocolate doesn't quite fall; it lingers and sticks, dithers and waits.

Finally, the mass lumbers toward the table and lands on a plate with a soft thud. Katie slices the mushy solid into neat little squares. Two pairs of fingers, pinched like fleshy tweezers, pluck two cubes of gooey sweetness. Katie and I look at each other, eyes wide, waiting for the pile on our tongues to dissolve, to claim its identity either as chocolate or not-chocolate. Within seconds, the cube becomes a stream of thick sweetness running around the corners of my mouth. It melts so quickly, so liquidly. It is delicious. But it is not chocolate. Rather, as I pluck another square off the table and examine the shiny film left behind on my fingers, I realize—we have made chocolate-flavored butter.

"Don't worry, Megs," Katie says, digging into a bag of popcorn. "You'll get it next time."

"Easy for you to say," I snap, with unwarranted crankiness. Soon Katie will return to Seattle, to a husband and chocolate truffles sold on every corner, and I will remain in my self-imposed year without chocolate.

My disappointment in yet another chocolate failure is not merely a physical one, not just a craving left unsatisfied. Rather, it is a failure to find comfort. For Montezuma and his fifty golden goblets, chocolate was about longing, lust, or immortality. For Grandma Kimble, her daily dose of chocolate was in some way about the opposite, about mortality. Small moments of delayed gratification that, once fulfilled, swelled into forward movement, a reason for the next day. In my life, small moments of anticipated pause carry me through hectic days, and giving up chocolate for a year meant giving up one of those small moments of comfort and calm—and their delicious anticipation—which accumulated into something like a day or a week lived happily. I teeter, I realize, on the self-indulgent edge of a woman in a Dove Chocolate commercial who unfolds a square of foil in a sunny apartment, closing her eyes and smiling as she eases into "her moment." But what is happiness if not "your moment"? What else is family besides leaning on your grandmother as she bends over a box of paper-wrapped truffles, plucking one thing from everything? What is sisterhood if not snuggling on a couch and snapping apart thick, dark squares? Giving up chocolate meant giving up this comfort, depriving myself of something that was bigger than the food itself, more intimate and softly human.

CHOCOLATE, REAL CHOCOLATE, is made by reincorporating cacao powder—the dust that results when the oil is pressed from cacao nibs, which are then pulverized—with its original fats. I'd been attempting to make chocolate with butter made from milk, and when Katie leaves, I finally realize the glaringly obvious: Real chocolate is not made with cow's butter. It is made with cacao butter.

I turn to the Internet and find Vivapura: Pure Superfoods for Life, a company based in Patagonia, a town thirty miles south of Tucson, that sells only Raw, Organic, and Ethical Superfoods, which include Bee Pollen, Spirulina Crunches, and Raw Cacao Butter. The Vivapura website directs me to my nearest distributor of these raw superfoods, so I get in my car and drive ten minutes along Speedway Boulevard until I hit Country Club Road—an indicator of what's to come—and turn into the parking lot of Whole Foods. After wandering the aisles, contemplating the vastness of sugar's variety, I spend an outrageous amount of my paycheck, an embarrassing twenty-eight dollars, on a pound, a *War and Peace*–size slab, of raw cacao butter. ("No," says a Whole Foods employee, "I have no idea how long cacao butter keeps in the refrigerator.")

On the Vivapura blog, I find a recipe for "The Best Chocolate Ever." Or rather, it is a fourteen-minute YouTube narrated by Susan, a very pretty British woman who has long hair and silver rings around both nostrils and says things like, "This will take a while, so don't worry about leaving the hob on."

The first thing to do, Susan tells me, is melt my cacao butter in a bowl placed over some hot water, so I dump a quarter cup of the grated cacao butter, which has a consistency rather like soap, into a metal bowl balanced over a saucepan filled with boiling water. The melting of the cacao butter should take quite some time—"You can go watch some YouTubes," Susan says with an ironic chuckle—but mine melts almost as soon as it hits the metal, so I hurry to stir in a half cup of cacao powder, three tablespoons of honey, and a dash of salt.

"Tempering is bringing the cacao into a place where it's really, really happy," says Susan. "Allowing it to click into place." Tempering is controlling temperature; by heating and cooling the chocolate, I allow the triglycerides of the cacao butter to lock into place with the solids of the cacao powder and the glucose molecules in the sugar. When the chocolate hits 120 degrees, measured by the cheap meat thermometer I purchased for this endeavor, I remove my bowl from the pot of water and set it on the counter to cool.

While I wait for the shiny liquid to hit ninety degrees, Kara calls me from Denver. It's 10 P.M. on a Saturday night, and she is walking home from a bar, crying. She broke up with a serious boyfriend a week ago and it is one of those terrible breakups that happens not because anything is wrong but because it's not right. I had gone through nearly the same breakup a year before, and I tell her that it will get better; that I, too, stood in a corner of a bar after I'd forced myself to go out with friends, stood there so paralyzed by sadness that my friends had told me to go home and so I, too, had walked home from the bar crying, had eaten pizza, peanut butter, and chocolate until my stomach seized in the same agony as my mind. I talk to her until she gets back to her apartment, until she promises to go to bed and call me in the morning. As I go back to stirring my chocolate, reheating it over the simmering saucepan, I remember another reason for chocolate—not simply as a pause to look forward, but as comfort for looking back.

I pour the shiny chocolate into a rectangular mold and slide it into the fridge to set—and set myself to the couch to wait. Two hours later, when I bend into the cold fluorescence of my fridge, I find a bar of chocolate. A proper bar of chocolate. I flip the mold over and the bar falls right out, crisp and quiet.

The bottom of the bar is shiny, and when I pick it up and break it apart, the bar snaps. Susan has said shine and snap are the mark of a good tempering and my bar *snaps*! I cannot believe it, so I keep snapping the bar into little chunks, snap after crisp, quiet snap, until I am left with a mound of shiny chocolate chunks. Finally, I settle down from the snapping and taste one of the pieces. It tastes like chocolate and it feels like chocolate; the cacao butter melts in my mouth slowly, releasing cacao and honey in an even stream of bitter sweetness. There is no doubt. It is chocolate.

WEEKS LATER, as my Saturdays stretch in mild March warmth, I buy wax paper and blue ribbon. I've ordered a chocolate bar mold online—a hard sheet of clear plastic shaped like the tomb of a Hershey bar—and bought another slab of Vivapura Cacao Butter (as it turns out, the limiting factor to how long a bar of cacao butter will stay in your refrigerator is not how well it keeps). I'd first heard about the Tucson Food Swap from a friend of a friend but I am nervous about actually going with my own wares. Wares that I will barter with others, as my chocolate will function as the currency of my participation. The premise of a food swap is to cut money from the middle, to step off the merry-go-round of dollars earned to be spent, and *this* seems like the point of my year unprocessed.

The night before the swap, I putter around my kitchen, nervous not only because I'm venturing into this unknown world, but also because, for the first time this year, I will offer the products of my fledgling culinary skills for a stranger's appraisal. If bread did not prove it, then the long road to chocolate surely has—in the kitchen, I have more enthusiasm than skill. While this gusto gives me the confidence to tackle ambitious projects, it also translates into less-than-discerning judgment about that which I create. I am nervous that what I think of as delicious bars of real, snappy chocolate will be deemed as juvenile attempts at homemade sweetness.

But I have been practicing the art of chocolate making for a month now, and it keeps getting better. Today will be the first day I use my homemade vanilla extract—I've been soaking a Madagascar vanilla pod in a glass vial full of vodka since December; been watching over the months as the flavors of the pod soak into the alcohol, infusing it into a deep amber. (Most commercially available vanilla extract is made precisely this way, but at a scale writ large and with ethyl alcohol, so the reasons to make your own are that it's fun, cheaper, and tastes better.) Along with extract, my cabinet contains a jar of grainy raw honey and a canister of raw cacao powder. On Saturday evening, it all sits in a row on my countertop, expectant. I stand before it, apprehensive, and think: *G-ma, this one's for you.*

I melt a hunk of cacao butter, mix in a scoop of cacao powder, whisk, and wait. I apply heat and honey, whisk, wait, and pour the liquid into the mold. Again and again, batch after batch, as soon as the bar hardens enough for me to pop it out of the mold, I pour in another round of sweet, shiny liquid. I work in the kitchen until well after it gets dark. As twelve shiny bars await snappily in the freezer, I line twelve squares of wax paper along my counter. The bars get wrapped like taffies, their sides tied with perky blue bows.

On Sunday, I take my bars of chocolate to La Cocina, a colorful restaurant with a broad patio of cast-iron tables and chairs scattered below strings of twinkle lights. When I meet Lori, the organizer of the swap, and ask her where I should I set my chocolate, she exclaims, "Chocolate! Oh, you'll be able to swap that for *anything.*"

I wander through the food swap, sampling wares and awkwardly introducing myself to new faces. One man harvests olives from neighborhood trees and cures them in herb-filled brines in his basement; one woman bakes cookies using locally harvested mesquite flour; a college student collects small, spotted eggs from the quail that live in her backyard. The swap works like a silent auction—at each station is a piece of paper where you can write your offer.

"Megan/Chocolate for Enchilada Sauce"—a whole homemade jar of it—or "Megan/Chocolate for Dill Pickles." No one has to accept my chocolate as a swap, just as I don't have to accept pecan pie or zucchini bread.

I'd set out small snaps of chocolate on a plate as samples and Bianca of the enchilada sauce comes up to me as I wander about. "You're Megan, right?" she says, peering at my name tag. "That chocolate—it is just amazing." Lori comes up to ask, "How did you *do* it?" and Sara, another swap participant, says, "Yeah, we really needed a chocolate swapper in the mix."

My chocolate bars are not perfect—they lose their snap as the morning progresses, sharp edges melting into smushed fuzziness—but no one turns them down. I don't try the zucchini bread—filled with flour and sugar, as is the pecan pie—but it looks like a tasty loaf of homemade zucchini bread, nothing more, nothing less. The salsas are delicious, certainly better than anything I might buy in a store, but they are just salsa. There is no money involved, only our time, so perfection is not expected. After an hour of wandering and chatting, sampling and offering—after turning down several swaps as my supply dwindles—my chocolate buys me a jar of enchilada sauce, a dozen quail eggs, two homemade beers, a bag of mesquite flour, three jars of salsa, a canister of mole powder, and a jar full of olives.

When I get home, I have no Pacific sunset to watch. There is no breeze, no Spanish, no Juan. Instead, I sit on my hot porch, stare up at a saguaro, and treat myself to the swig, kiss, and pucker of my glass bottle of homebrewed beer. I watch the desert colors fade to pastel, and I bite into a small snap of cold chocolate.

Unprocess Yourself: Sugar

If you're going to eat something sweet, make it count. The fact that sugar is really not good for us will not make me stop eating it—life is too short to live without sweetness. Rather, knowing this makes me much more careful about how and when I let sweetness into my life.

Check savory foods like mustard or marinara sauce to make sure they don't have added sugars. Don't buy presweetened foods, like honey-flavored yogurt or maple-cinnamon oatmeal. Instead, buy plain or unflavored foods and add the sweetness in yourself. You will, I promise, add less than what would have been added for you (and skip a bunch of other artificial ingredients). Marinara sauces and salad dressings often contain added sugars—whole-wheat bread is another common culprit, as is, unbelievably, deli meat. I've seen breakfast cereals filled with as many as five kinds of sugar—if you want a little sweetness to start your morning, add it yourself. Food for Life sells unsweetened granola; so do most natural food stores.

For sweet treats, look for foods that have been sweetened with natural sweeteners like honey, maple syrup, molasses, or dates, all of which come packed with good nutrients and are often used in much smaller quantities. Lärabars are my favorite sweet snack, made with some variation of dates, dried fruit, and nuts. You can make homemade Lärabars with a food processor and the same ingredients, although I love the portability of a prepackaged bar when I find myself hungry in a processed-only place.

When faced with the many varieties of sugar—both granulated and liquid, added and in bulk—remember: Sugar is sugar. There are important differences between types of sugar, but what's more important than the specifics of each kind is quantity. Less sugar is better sugar.

To make chocolate, you'll need: cacao powder or paste and cacao butter; a sweetener, like agave or honey; and salt and vanilla extract. Measure two units of cacao powder or paste for every one of cacao butter. Cut the cacao butter into small pieces, which will help it melt evenly. The best way to melt the cacao butter is in a double boiler; if you don't have one, you can balance a glass or aluminum bowl on top of a saucepot of hot (not boiling) water. The butter will melt pretty quickly; as soon as it becomes liquid, add the powder and whisk until smooth—the mixture should have the consistency of chocolate sauce. Take the bowl off the heat and let the chocolate sauce cool for about half an hour, or until it reaches room temperature. Reheat the water and warm the liquid chocolate while stirring; add a tablespoon or two of honey, a pinch of salt, and a dash of vanilla extract. After a minute or two—while the liquid is still shiny—remove from heat and pour into a mold; leave it in the refrigerator for at least an hour to set.

4

PRODUCE

A million melons are processed.

In April, when the indecisive desert swings between winter nights and spring days, Sarah and I plant a garden. When I heard that a student group at the University of Arizona was planning to break ground on a campus community garden, I'd immediately called Sarah. Sarah lives with her boyfriend in a single-story two-bedroom apartment tucked into a sprawling single-story complex full of identical two-bedroom apartments. When I go over to her place, the only way I don't knock on the wrong door is by seeking the porch haloed by sunflowers, the steps tiered by lanky tomato plants.

So when I had asked, "Hey, do you want to share a garden?" she said, without missing a beat, "Yes."

"The dues are sixty dollars for six months," I said. "Do we want to claim a whole plot?"

"Hmm, maybe just half?" Sarah said. "Twenty-one feet seems like a lot of feet."

On a warm Saturday morning, we plant watermelon starts, bell peppers, and cucumbers; we transplant a beefy-leaf zucchini plant, the shrugging petals of a hopeful sunflower-to-be, and faint outlines of future tomatoes. After a morning of work, as we stretch our backs and survey our effort, our attempt seems so small, so fractional compared to all the land that could be planted—but it also seems wildly optimistic, this attempt by two novice gardeners to transform desert soils into something fertile and fresh.

ON A HURRIED MONDAY EVENING after a long day of deadlines, I rush across town and arrive late to a lecture about localizing Tucson's food system. The room is packed, so I find a seat on the floor and lean against the back wall. Three men rise in turn from their chairs on the stage to discuss how we might build a more secure, just, and sustainable foodshed in southern Arizona. Localize production, invest in slow money, build community, encourage innovation. It is interesting, really it is, but two hours into the evening, twenty slides into the second lecture, approaching a hungry and exhausted eight o'clock, this thought flashes through my mind: If I see another image of a smiling farmer handing a heavy bag of red tomatoes to a sundress-adorned woman carrying a sun-hat-adorned child at a sun-dappled farmers' market, I will run screaming out of the room.

The last time I went to a farmers' market in Tucson, it was ninety-five degrees at 9 A.M. Sweat dripped down my back and hair stuck to my neck. Dehydrated and sans sunglasses, I squinted through hard brightness at the exhausted farmer who squinted back at me. He tried to be friendly but he was exhausted—he'd gotten up at five to load a truck to drive an hour; he'd been standing in this heat since seven. Was I going to buy his carefully tended tomatoes or simply squeeze them and move on?

To be fair, I don't often make it to the numerous farmers' markets scattered throughout Tucson because I'm a member of the Tucson Community

Supported Agriculture program, which furnishes me with a weekly supply of locally grown, organic produce for twenty dollars. Even though this is a spectacular bargain for a week's worth of vegetarian meals, often, on Wednesday afternoons when I swing by the Historic Y Courtyard to pick up my share, I am in a hurry. I have not finished everything I was supposed to do in a day and I am tired and maybe cranky because, let's be honest, who *really* is in a good mood at 5 P.M. on a Wednesday?

I just want to grab my food and run. I want to rush anonymously through the courtyard, just as we rush anonymously through Safeway or Target. I queue up in line and close my eyes rather than glare at the woman who is picking up every goddamn eggplant from the black crate that says 2 EGGPLANTS before she finally puts one in her canvas tote and begins the process anew.

But I am not anonymous. After two years of weekly visits, Sara, a CSA volunteer, recognizes me. She says, "Hey, Megan!" and checks "Kimble" off her clipboard list. In the summer, she reminds me, "You have sprouts!" I have fresh bean sprouts waiting in the cheese fridge, a perk I've added to my share for an extra two dollars a week. I can't help myself, exclaiming, "I *know!*" and then, "They're *so* good." I grab a copy of the weekly newsletter to scan the recipe page, and again, I cannot help myself and I tell Sara, "I tried that okra jambalaya recipe last week and it was great. I would never have thought to use okra like that."

Try as I might, I cannot be cranky. Grudgingly, I act chipper. Impatience is taboo here, so impatiently, I act patient. And so, week after week, I am more chipper. I *am* patient. I laugh and joke, and always, without fail, after ten minutes, I leave laden with two heavy bags of fresh produce and a mood transformed.

THE FOOD THAT CATALYZES THIS TRANSFORMATION comes from Crooked Sky Farms, so called because Frank Martin, the farm's owner, once got lost in the borderlands south of Tucson and found himself on Crooked Sky Road, where the big desert sky curved along a jagged mountain range.

When I visit Crooked Sky's Phoenix fields, my Civic ducks under the freeway overpass, clicks right onto the Frontage Road, and there it is. A farm. A long expanse of checkered fields, green rows of the spring's last greens lined up in tufts like perky ponytails, dirt furrowed under encroaching vines; fresh off the freeway, it announces itself so emphatically, so obviously. *Farm!*

I follow three hand-painted green arrows around three thick fields to arrive at the farm's offices. I park and walk through a dusty clearing crowded with John Deere carts, a large washtub, and rusted steel machinery—a hand-crank wheat cleaner and an old-fashioned corn shucker, I later learn—and climb three soft stairs into a small trailer. At the invitation of the office manager, I perch in a chair in front of one of the three cluttered workstations, stacks of papers spreading in the space between computers like spilled water. A cartoon painting of a rooster tacked to the wall declares, *What happens in the barn, stays in the barn.* Another poster features a retro-looking alien crouching under a spaceship with a cursive caption: *Alien Invasion—I only came for the chilies!*

"You're in my seat," Frank says as soon as he clambers through the door.

I stand up.

"I'm just kiddin'," he says. "Wanted to see if you could take a joke."

I laugh, to demonstrate that I am of good humor.

Frank coughs, a thick, reverberating cough. "I have allergies," he says, easing into the chair I have just vacated. Frank looks like a farmer. He's wide and sturdy, with bristled cheeks, thick skin, and matted gray hair. He wears the farmer's uniform: a checkered oxford button-down and faded blue jeans.

"Oh?" I say.

"You're a member of the Tucson CSA, right?" Frank asks. "How do you like it?"

"Yeah. I love it. It's such a great community," I say, aware of how trite the words sound. "The produce is just wonderful. I mean," I stutter, "*your* produce!"

"Good," Frank says, satisfied. "Let's go look at the farm."

We climb into a John Deere cart, Frank coughing as he shifts into drive. Frank coughs as he tells me how he grew up trailing his parents through the West, following the migration of farmwork from Oregon to California, Nevada to New Mexico, and finally, to Arizona, "which is where the truck broke down." Frank started working on a commercial cotton farm when he was nine at a time when workers weren't allowed to leave the fields while crop dusters blew over with thick, pesticide exhalations.

"We'd just put our sleeves over our mouths," Frank says. "That started all the problems I have today. I'm all cut up inside."

Frank farmed cotton as long as he had to—"we were dirt-poor"—and then enrolled in the University of Arizona's master gardeners program. "What they said then was, 'There are two ways to start a farm: marry or inherit.' Neither of those was going to work for me. I just started small."

The first time Frank sold produce he'd grown himself was the first day the Prescott Farmers' Market opened for business. He was thrilled to make sixty dollars. "But farmers' markets are either really good or really bad," he says. "Either you're long or you're short, and if you've harvested too much, you gotta come home and feed all that food you didn't sell to the chickens." He first heard of the Community Supported Agriculture model in 1999, when two students at Prescott College approached him and asked if he might grow five different things for six weeks to distribute to a fixed set of people. "I thought people might get sick of beets, week after week, so I planted a bunch of different stuff. By the third week, they were sure glad that I had."

As a member of the Tucson CSA, I technically own a very small, very temporary fraction of this farm. My farm share—$120 every six weeks—helps Frank invest in operating costs up front; the investment of a thousand members across eight different CSA programs helps diminish the risks inherent in growing food. Collectively, we pay the salaries for his twenty-three employees; we pay for fuel for his carts, tractors, and delivery trucks; for water, rent, and taxes. Collectively, we receive dividends in the form of eggplant and arugula; we reap our investment in the assurance of a weekly delivery of organic, heirloom fruits and vegetables that cost us, on average, 40 percent less than if we bought that same food in the supermarket. Frank drives me through a field of spindly artichokes-to-be, past a flowering profusion of squash, and maneuvers the cart into a dirt row that cuts through a field dense with greens.

"Why do you farm?" I ask him. As Sarah and I struggle to care for seven feet of soil, the fact that one person might be responsible for so much land seems both optimistic and totally incomprehensible. Surrounded by fields of food that Frank has grown, I feel the same sort of worry I feel when I call an electrician to fix my air-conditioning unit or when I bring my car to a mechanic—when I realize that I don't understand so many of the mechanisms that sustain me. It sometimes amazes me that anyone does.

"I grew up so poor. Without electricity," he says, "and I'm not *that* old." Again, he stops the cart and shifts his weight so he can look me in the eye. "The fact that I could take such a small seed and grow so much food, it was a miracle. It seemed like magic to me." He looks back to his left, over his fields. "Shoot, it still is magic."

With rare exceptions, most people who farm do so because they like it—because growing fields full of food from slight seeds is a miracle, one of the few miracles that remain visible in a world that runs on nanochips.

But this story skirts a bizarre fact, one that has become true only within my lifetime. Today, many farmers in industrialized countries do not grow food from seeds. Today, farmers grow commodities from patented products. Farmers grow wheat to feed the world; they grow soy to fuel it and corn to sweeten it. Today, these commodities do not grow; they emerge. Meticulously planted and irrigated fields produce horizons worth of corn because they have been engineered to do so.

"You know, people always ask me—I think they're trained to ask or something," Frank says. "They always ask me if my stuff is GMO." GMO refers to a Genetically Modified Organism, but the acronym has become shorthand for a genetically engineered crop. "There's just no reason, as far as I can tell, to grow a GMO vegetable," he says.

In the past thirty years, many farmers have found a reason to grow genetically modified foods. GMOs are made by inserting genes from one organism—say, a bacterium—into the genes of another—say, a tomato—to confer a specific trait. (Genetic modification is different from hybridization, which happens when breeders cross two plants of the same species.) Genetically modified crops often boast better yields—in the forty years after World War II, farmers cultivated 1 percent more land yet increased harvests by 170 percent, mostly because of the combination of GMO crops and fertilizers. Breeders can manipulate seeds to thrive in a particular climate, to grow in drought or flood, to flourish in depleted soils; they can also breed seeds to fulfill a population's nutritional needs—more beta-carotene in rice, for example, or potatoes that absorb less fat when fried. In the late 1980s, tomatoes became the first genetically modified food widely available when researchers at Calgene, a biotech company in California, figured out how to flip the DNA sequence on an enzyme that, when expressed, turned the inside of a tomato to mush. Before then, tomatoes were picked green and shipped to market, where they'd be ripened with a gust of ethylene gas. Turn the mush-making enzyme off and tomatoes could ripen on the vine and arrive to market with their squeezability still intact, no ethylene needed.

I tell Frank what I understand about GMO crops—that, as far as we know, GMOs are less threatening to our bodies than to the land they are planted on. A million acres of corn is not a sustainable landscape. A million acres planted with the exact same variety of corn is amazingly vulnerable to just one persistent pest, one bad storm, one prolific disease. And monocultures of crops create monocultures of pests, which call for monoliths of chemicals. Although breeders engineer crops that can survive the application of chemicals that kill every other living thing in a field—including some living things that contribute huge value to ecosystems, like monarch butterflies—eventually, pests adapt. They come back.

The risk posed to the health of our agricultural system shouldn't diminish the unknown impact GMO produce might have on our bodies. There have been *no* scientifically rigorous studies evaluating the impact genetically modified foods might have on human health. In the early 1990s, when Calgene was trying to get its new tomato to market, it asked the FDA to establish regulations for approval of GM foods, anticipating customer resistance. In 1993, as Canadian and European governments were also trying to evaluate the safety of GM foods, the Organization for Economic Cooperation and Development set the precedent of substantial equivalence, concluding, "If a new food, or food component, is found to be substantially equivalent to an existing food or food component, it can be treated in the same manner with respect to safety." In other words, if it looks like a tomato, feels like a tomato, and tastes like a tomato, then it is a tomato and requires no further testing.

Unfortunately, that's not how nutrition works. The science is unclear, but how GMO crops might be detrimental to human health is by the law of unintended consequences. In the case of Calgene's unsquishable tomatoes, researchers worried that by flipping the gene that controlled ripening, they might have inadvertently inactivated a gene that suppressed toxins as the fruit matured. Although geneticists can pinpoint genes responsible for certain behaviors, they can't yet tweak one gene and one gene only—genes are expressed in unison, or in sequence, in ways we don't yet understand. And if you're adding a gene from another organism into a plant, should that gene be considered an additive and regulated as such? So far, the FDA's answer has been no, as it considers the product of genetic modification more important than the process—the final tomato versus the gene manipulation. What this means is that we simply don't know how the process of genetic modification impacts the foods we're eating.

But Frank is right—most vegetables in our supermarkets are not genetically modified. No organic vegetables are, as USDA regulations prohibit it. But even if every farmer in the United States started planting genetically modified seeds tomorrow, there would be absolutely no way for us to know. California tried to legislate the mandatory labeling of GMO foods in November of 2012, but the voters of my home state—with the help of millions of dollars from food giant Monsanto—decided they did not need the extra information.

As we talk about GMO crops, Frank's gruff voice cracks for the first time with a hint of frustration. "You ask a person, 'Do you want an open pollinated heirloom crop?' and they'll say, 'Yes, of course!'" He shakes his head and leans on the steering wheel. "But then they want all their beets to look the same! They can't. Vegetables are just like people. Some are bigger and some are smaller and some are wider and some are thinner. That doesn't mean they're better or worse. They're just different."

We're still on the furrowed path between two rows of kale. One, the curly kale, grew from a hybrid seed; the other, the purple kale, is an heirloom. "The reason to grow a hybrid seed is uniformity," Frank says, pointing up the row. I can't believe I didn't notice it before now—all the curly kale plants look the same. They're about the same height and approximately the same width. The row stretches in a dark, uniform green: the picture of pristine. The rows of purple kale are, in comparison, the picture of piggly-wiggly. Splotches of purple burst over a handful of the plants; many more are solidly green with only a faded purple outline around the leaves. The row recedes from view, each ponytail of kale swaying with the breeze.

Frank's frustration with the conversation about GMO crops reveals a bigger flaw in our food system, one that begins and ends with consumers. We go to the grocery store and expect perfect produce, and all the time, please. Our expectation—our demand—for tomatoes that are all red and beets that are all round forces farmers to try to grow tomatoes that are all red and beets that are all round. It creates a tug-of-war between producers and consumers and the war is won in the supermarket, when oblong beets are picked over by picky customers and then thrown out by supermarkets.

Heirloom seeds—which are pollinated by birds, bees, wind, and weather rather than direct human intervention—produce piggly-wiggly crops, so growers hybridize, crossing similar seeds with different desirable traits to produce "best of" plants. Hybrid seeds are categorically different from genetically modified seeds; humans have been hybridizing plants since the beginning of agriculture—indeed, often hybridization confers new vigor and vitality on the next generation. But unlike heirloom crops, which have been saved from seeds grown in the same place for generations, and thus evolved adaptive characteristics to those places—more cold tolerance in the north, for example, or drought resistance in the desert—hybrid seeds don't contain the same place-based memory. You cannot save the seeds of a hybrid crop—some are sterile, while others produce wild-card crops—so there is no ecological learning that happens generation after generation, no genetic diversity propagated year after year. Heirloom crops often require less water, and attract fewer pests, having evolved natural defense mechanisms. Planted in their proper place, heirloom crops grow better, so they usually taste better.

Looking at Frank's produce, the word "piggly-wiggly" stays in my mind, and it occurs to me that maybe *this* is why I love getting my food from the CSA. Not because of how it looks, but because the CSA is *not* the Piggly Wiggly, the first self-service grocery store to offer us the dazzling array of choice. Today, that choice has blossomed into a kind of anxiety—what's in season but where did it come from and is it organic but how much does it cost? When I pick up my CSA share, these questions are answered for me. Every Wednesday, I arrive home with a bag full of fresh produce and a weekly newsletter full of recipes featuring that very same produce. Stocked with the right essentials, spices and grains, cheese and beans, it is a matter of knife, heat, and fifteen minutes before I've made myself dinner.

When I ask Frank if he thinks he has the capacity to expand beyond the thousand members the farm currently supports, he doesn't pause before he says, "Yes. It's not that I want more money. I just want to see more people have the ability to eat vegetables. Local, organic vegetables."

We sit in silence for a moment, watching Julie and Rosa, two of Frank's workers, at the far end of a row of Tuscan kale, bending and picking, bending and picking, piling the thick bundles in the cargo hold of the cart. "Mostly we have women working here because they're really good workers," Frank says finally. "But that's my biggest problem—finding labor. There are just not enough people who want to do this work."

"How much do your employees earn?" I ask.

"It depends what they want to do," he says. "It's hard to find people who want to stick around, to make a career out of this. A lot of people pass through for a few months, they'll make ten dollars an hour. Some folks made twenty-five an hour. I had a woman who worked here for eleven years—she was such a hard worker. Not the type to leave if there happened to be a fire at five o'clock. Anyway, she made seventy-two thousand dollars a year."

"Wow," I say. "That's a lot more than writers make."

"You can make good money," Frank says. But Frank's workers are not typical. In the United States, roughly 75 percent of farmworkers are foreign-born, and despite working long hours in what can only be understated and simplified into "taxing conditions," the average farmworker earns between $10,000 and $14,000 a year. Most of these workers are from Central America and Mexico;

half are in the United States without documentation. (One reason you'll find so many Mexican men and women working on farms in the United States is that in 1994, NAFTA, the North American Free Trade Agreement, started flooding cheap, U.S.-subsidized corn and grain into the Mexican market, depressing prices and putting millions of small growers out of business.)

"This is hard work. It's really hard work," Frank says. "It's hard to find young people who want to do it."

Indeed, Frank's problem is the nation's problem. It is a well-worn story, one that begins with this: In 1910, 40 percent of Americans farmed; today, 2 percent do. In 2012, 4 percent of farms sold 66 percent of our crops. Although the number of small farmers getting into the growing game also increased in that time period, the trend is still toward concentration, toward bigger farms and higher outputs.

Or no outputs, as is the case with the increasing number of farms that stop being farms. Between 1982 and 2010, across the United States, thirteen million acres of prime farmland were lost, mostly due to development. A quarter of that land was located in the four states along the Mexican border: California, Arizona, New Mexico, and Texas.

"No one's going to tear that warehouse down over there," Frank says, gesturing to a squat, white warehouse in the distance, "or bulldoze a building to replant a farm. When it gets shrunk, it stays shrunk."

The reason farmland shrinks is that farmers sell their farms. Farming is hard work, but increasingly, it is not work that pays. A recent study of agriculture in southern Arizona found that while farmers and ranchers sold an average of $300 million worth of food annually, it cost them $320 million to produce those products. In 2012, across the country, the average income on farms was *negative* $1,453. And the rising cost of inputs—fertilizer, seeds, machinery, fuel—has forced more than half the farmers in the United States to find jobs off the farm to help pay *for* the farm.

"My neighbor in Duncan put his farm up for sale. I bought it from him," Frank says. "He didn't want to sell it, but his son wanted to be a lawyer, so he just couldn't keep it going."

This small anecdote reveals the second factor in the decline of American farms: Farming is not a desirable career for many young people. According to the 2012 Census of Agriculture, the prairie is getting grayer—the average age of the American farmer in 2012 was fifty-eight years old, compared to fifty-five in 2002 (and fifty in 1978). The statistic *is* changing, as many of my peers, the cohort who matriculated in a time of global alarm, are realizing that growing their own food might be the most radical career they can choose and have begun gardening, leasing land, or building farms. But there are not enough of us—not enough willing to tackle the barriers to entry, to send our roots into damaged soils.

"People talk now about going after other countries for their oil," Frank says. "Just wait until we have to go after them for their broccoli."

One fewer farm does not mean one less eater. Today, the decline of American farms just means that we get our food from somewhere else.

TODAY, IN THE UNITED STATES, that someplace else is Mexico.

In Nogales, Arizona, a few short miles north of the border, in the offices of Vandervoet & Associates, on a brisk Wednesday morning, the phone rings. Prescott Vandervoet picks up the phone. "Morning," he says quickly. "What do you have?" Ten feet away, another phone rings. Brian Vandervoet, Prescott's father and the founder of Vandervoet & Associates, a produce broker and distributor, picks it up, listens for a moment, and says, "They just left the warehouse."

In the winter, 60 percent of the produce on U.S. supermarket shelves comes from Mexico, and most of that produce gets funneled through Nogales, the nation's third-largest port of entry (Los Angeles and New York City are one and two, respectively). Although McAllen, Texas, is seducing an increasing number of semi trucks—with easier access to the Eastern Seaboard and a state legislature that understands that a border functions as a membrane rather than a wall—the Mariposa port of entry in Nogales is still, for now, the Ellis Island of Mexican produce.

Prescott and Brian work with melons. They buy cantaloupe, honeydew, watermelon, and a new variety called orange flesh from three growers in Caborca, in the Mexican state of Sonora, and, depending on the season, another grower or two in Hermosillo. Every day between October and February, the Vandervoets move—receive and ship—nineteen thousand boxes of melons. Warehouse space is tight, so whatever comes in had better displace something heading out; every day, Prescott and Brian manage the movement of 150,000 melons.

Prescott wears impeccable loafers and a maroon polo shirt tucked into blue jeans. Bright blue eyes blink behind no-rim glasses; midthirties, bald, and fit, he says he's the only gringo in his Saturday-night soccer league. His father has gray hair, wears running shoes, khaki shorts, and a baggy green T-shirt; in between fielding orders from other produce brokers, he talks about their last visit to Hermosillo, passing around a corked bottle of *bacanora*—a bootleg agave distillation traditionally made in Sonora—for a quick sniff and fiery swig. The walls at the Vandervoet & Associates office are covered with Frida Kahlo prints and maps of Sonora, Arizona, the United States. An oil painting of faces peering at a newspaper hangs over chairs stacked with *The Packer* and *Produce News*.

Although Brian says that business began booming in Nogales in the 1920s, when Mexican growers found themselves with a surplus of garbanzo beans and started shipping them to the United States, food has flowed across this region since long before a line was drawn to split it in half. Chilies and salt, beans and corns, acorns and agave—all have been traded across the Sonoran desert for more than four thousand years. White Sonora wheat is only one of the many foods Padre Kino and other Jesuit missionaries brought north from the region in the 1700s, swapping fruit trees and olive oil north to south, exchanging turkeys for fish from the Gulf of California.

"Transborder" trade began when the border was drawn in the 1850s with the Treaty of Guadalupe Hidalgo and the Gadsden Purchase, which turned Tucson over to the United States. At the turn of the century, when railroad tycoon Edward Harriman arrived on the scene with a large refrigerated railcar, perishable food could, for the first time, travel across a large distance within a matter of days. "As Harriman's Pacific Fruit Express became the largest operator of refrigerated railroad transporters in the world, fresh produce from the binational Southwest grew from a negligible portion of the U.S. grocery market share to 40 percent of U.S. produce sales in 1929," writes ethnobotanist Gary Paul Nabhan in *A Brief History of Cross-Border Food Trade*.

Now, in early summer, Nogales is quiet. California and Florida are still filling our produce sections with fresh, colorful fruits and vegetables; it's not until October, when our soils cool off and the Mexican harvest begins, that the proverbial fruit will fall. Every day between October and April, three thousand semi-trailer trucks pass through Nogales, arriving with empty holds and leaving carrying forty thousand pounds of produce.

The Vandervoets operate one of about a hundred produce warehouses in Rio Rico, a warehouse district just north of Nogales. Prescott tells us many of them are family owned and operated. As he drives us around the warehouse district, I feel a bit like I'm on a hike with John Muir; Prescott knows the subtleties of this landscape like a naturalist knows a forest. Signs make statements and buildings have personalities. Except for brand logos—Farmer's Best, Cris-P Produce Co.—the white and silver warehouses, like the mass-market produce they'll hold, all look more or less the same. The signs in front of the warehouses and on the sides of stationary semi trucks imply food, but, at least today, there's no feeling of food. Down the road from the Vandervoet warehouse, SunFed's immaculate depot wears its name emblazoned under a field of green rows receding into a brilliant red sunset. Below the SunFed name is the slogan: PERFECT PRODUCE.

"There's no such thing," says Prescott, when I point out the sign. "There shouldn't be. We have a romanticized food production ideal."

"How so?" I ask.

"Our society is based on the fact that when you fly to Atlanta and stay at a hotel, there's a fruit salad at that hotel," says Prescott. "It just has to be there."

What is perfect produce? According to the SunFed website, it is "produce of extraordinary quality, flavor, and shelf-life, resulting in the elimination of shrink from our customer's workplace." Elimination of shrink doesn't sound particularly edible; it refers to quantity—the amount of product lost to rot or ripeness—yet quantity is often at odds with quality, as shelf life competes with flavor for a consumer's loyalties.

Most of the produce we eat is not perfect. It is just there. At Safeway, the food is there, and it seems like abundance. Produce represents nature on our terms; in our supermarkets, nature is generous.

PRESCOTT DRIVES US to the BMV cold-storage warehouse, neither a distributor nor a broker but rather an "in-and-out" operation, a place to put produce on ice while the details are being sorted out. Today, it's got mangoes—too many for me to count, boxes stacked on crates stacked on pallets, hundreds of thousands of mangoes. We walk through an echoing cement corridor of doors and through panels of thick hanging plastic into a freezing room stacked full of mangoes. The mangoes are rock hard, huddled in this frozen place, worlds away from the sweet sweating tropics. The room smells like cardboard. The stacks are taller than my six feet, and the mangoes are huge, like giant marble eggs.

The cold cardboard boxes are stamped FRESKA, one of the largest mango importers in the world. On the underside of the boxes are instructions: *How to Eat a Mango*. Evidently, this is a skill we Americans lack. Cartoon hands demonstrate how to wield forks and knifes to cut surgical cross sections of the thick flesh. Slice it, dice it, with a spoon, on a fork!

I remember March in Nicaragua as the month of sticky fingers and a goopy orange chin. Mangoes in March were a holiday in the middle of a long dry season that began when the rain stopped in December. Ever fond of nicknames, Nicaragua—the Land of Lakes and Volcanoes—had dubbed Rivas, my city, as the City of Mangoes. I learned how to eat a mango the Nica-way. It was warm off a pickup truck and so ripe it felt wet, wobbly like a water balloon. You peeled back a cross section of skin, exposed a strip of raw orange fiber, and dug in, all or nothing. You sucked the juice and bit the fibers and covered your nose in thick orange goo. The mangoes were small enough that two fit into a cupped palm, and I ate mango for breakfast, lunch, and dinner that month.

Now, faced with five hundred thousand mangoes in a freezing storeroom, I forget what Nicaragua's floppy mango trees looked like. It's only later, after we leave the frigid warehouse and walk into bright light, that I remember the thick scribbles of their dark shiny leaves, the bowing branches that bent toward the earth when the world flooded in October, and the pickup trucks that rocked down dirt roads and announced on loud speakers: *mangomango-mangomangooooooo.*

Every mango eaten in the United States is imported, and four out of five of them come from Mexico. Mangoes account for half of all tropical fruit produced worldwide; U.S. imports of Mexican mangoes have gone up a ridiculous 4500 percent since the 1960s, 142,000 pounds in 1967 to 368 million in 2002. The rising demand for mangoes in the United States might have less to do with a sudden mainstreaming of mango margaritas than the increasing number of Hispanic immigrants in the country who remain connected to their homelands by buying the imported fruits of tropical soils.

It's the same physical mango on both sides of the border, but between the two there are often two weeks and a handful of federal agencies. It's the same mango, but shivering in the cold storage, I see only the disconnect. Something must remain between the nodding mango trees of Mexico and Central America and these cold fists of fruit maturing in the middle of a desert. Maybe it is memory, the memory of a sweet mango on a humid night. Or maybe it is the idea of fruit, more than its taste, the idea of fertility, of abundance. Maybe it is the fruit's connection to a lush place full of nature's bounty that makes this freezing fruit, underripe and trapped in a cardboard display case, worth its cost.

AT THE HEIGHT OF THE VANDERVOETS' SEASON, if all goes according to plan, a melon picked at sunrise on Tuesday in Hermosillo is on sale in a Tucson supermarket on Thursday afternoon.

It begins with an agronomist in northern Mexico, walking through acres of fields, day after day. The endless mat of green, tangled vines covered in beefy leaves is startlingly bright against the arid desert surroundings. Receding rows of thick foliage hide bundles of smooth melons, flourishing in the hot, dry soils. The agronomist walks the fields and inspects the melons, noting the diameter of the ripening fruits and taking their Brix reading—the sugar content, measured with a refractometer. The growers watch the weather, report to Prescott and Brian, and wait to hire the migrating field crews who are capable of harvesting a thousand acres of food in a week. They watch, they wait, and then they hire.

Beginning at sunrise, pickers stoop over the low-lying vines and sling melons into burlap bags until noon, when the bulging sacks are thrown into trailers. From noon to 8 P.M., conveyor belts whir under the corrugated tin roof of the open-air packing shed and fifty hands wash, sort, and size melons into boxes. In 9 P.M. darkness, semi trucks are loaded with melons, 1,500 boxes per truck. By 3 or 4 A.M., a truck driver arrives just shy of the Mariposa border crossing near Nogales, and pulls over to sleep for a few hours before the border opens in the morning. If the driver gets in at the front of the line, he's through in an hour and the melons are stacked in the Vandervoet warehouse in another hour.

But produce does not always travel according to plan. Workers pick melons, box and load them onto trucks, and from there, it's all movement, all reaction. Semi trucks laden with forty thousand pounds of produce rock along on rutted roads through Mexico—most aren't paved—and they break down. Melons coming from Hermosillo might hit an eight-kilometer line at the military checkpoint at Querobabi and lose eight hours inching forward so that cargo holds may be given a careful or perfunctory inspection.

Trucks arrive at the Mariposa border crossing in a whirlwind of paperwork: a contract from a customhouse broker in both Mexico and the United States, declare load values, weight surcharges, and export-import agreements. The paperwork must be perfect. On the northern immigration front, the United States Department of Agriculture or the Federal Drug Administration might just look at the paperwork, but they also might take an X-ray or ask the driver to unload part or all of his cargo. Even if the USDA and the FDA wave the truck through, there are over a dozen other federal agencies at the border that might hold things up to take a look around.

Once the paperwork is stamped and the border is crossed, the melons pull up to the Vandervoet warehouse. A beeping semi truck backs up to an open slot, fitting the square of the cargo hold perfectly into the square of the opening. The warehouse foreman slides open the cargo door and the manager zooms over, standing on a forklift. He doesn't pause as he approaches the cargo hold. He darts in, scoops up a stack of eight pallets, and neatly spins into reverse. A quick twist of the wheel and the forklift is in drive again, darting off to deposit a stack of melons in a line in one of four storerooms, where they wait, in the safety of thirty-five degrees, for five minutes or five days.

"Do you ever eat the melons?" I ask Prescott. For the last few hours we've been walking through warehouses, among the brown cardboard canyons of seven-foot produce stacks, talking about melons, squash, and grapes. I'm having a hard time imagining how this mass of melons from northern Mexico—hundreds of thousands of them—ever becomes just one melon in one person's kitchen on the U.S. side of the border.

It's thirty-five degrees inside these warehouses and my hands are so cold that I can barely write on my notepad, but still: This is the source of the produce I smell and squeeze as I wander with my cart around Safeway. I want to try a melon fresh off the semi truck. I wonder if it's even allowed, cracking into these pallets to pull out a single piece of fruit. At the Sigma Sales warehouse, another produce broker, a small sign posted on a steel wall declares: NO SMOKING, NO FOOD IN WAREHOUSE OR COLD ROOMS.

When I ask Prescott for a taste, he nods, unperturbed. "The big companies usually just hire someone for quality control, but I come out here every day and cut into a melon." He walks over to the nearest stack of boxes and pulls a box down, revealing a row of smooth melons with mint-green skin. "Orange flesh," he says, and walks over to a wide, steel table pushed against the warehouse wall. He grabs a knife, slices the melon in half, draws a half-moon shape in the flesh, and stabs out a cross section of juicy fruit. He looks at it for a moment and then pops it in his mouth.

I'm relieved to see someone finally eating a piece of this food flow—relieved that there is some aspect in this process that requires the human action of touch and taste. But the melon that Prescott is eating is a casualty of a supply-chain stall. A fruit's value is a bell curve that builds as the fruit ripens and chains of starches become sweet sucrose—and then dives downward when that sugar turns the flesh to mush. This orange flesh comes from a box stacked in a row of pallets that's been sitting in the warehouse for over a week, waiting for a buyer. The orange flesh is perfectly ripe now, but by the time it makes it to the shelf in a supermarket or into the supply of a food distribution center, it will be rotten. If the Nogales Community Food Bank has an available truck to pick the boxes up, they'll go there. If not, these stacks of melons, hundreds of boxes, thousands of melons, will go to the dump.

WHAT IS THE DIFFERENCE between a cantaloupe picked in Hermosillo and one grown in Phoenix? By all appearances, they are the same fruit; placed side by side, they might be indistinguishable. But a similarity in appearance hides a larger difference, one of planting, process, and movement. Indeed, the most obvious difference between the two is that one is "organic" while the other is what we call "conventional."

Legally, a food is organic if the farm where it grew is certified under the USDA's National Organic Program and if it was grown according to the principles established in the Organic Foods Production Act of 1990. A piece of produce that is certified organic means that a federal inspector has visited the farm where it grew and verified that the farm doesn't use synthetic pesticides, herbicides, or fertilizers; that they don't irradiate food or seed; that they keep records of every transaction, every input and output. A farmer who sells certified organic produce has, theoretically, read several hundred pages of Organic Standards in the USDA's Federal Register, paid several thousand dollars throughout the year-long certification rigmarole, and waited the mandatory thirty-six months before marketing his produce as organic.

You might imagine, then, that small farmers like Frank have not yet found the time or extra cash to endure this process. Frank is a Certified Natural Grower, which means his growing practices are certified and accredited by other farmers that hold him accountable to organic growing practices. Frank scoffs a bit at the national organic standards, which have been considerably loosened due to lobbying from large producers; he says, just because a grower is organic doesn't mean their growing practices are sustainable. (And just because a food is organic doesn't mean it's unprocessed—the domain of certification stops at the source, so as long as all their ingredients originally came from organically certified producers, even ultraprocessed foods can be labeled organic.) Frank doesn't use any of the "bio-fertilizers" allowed by USDA organic standards—they may leech into the water, he says, contaminating it for those who use it downstream, as, by design, the water he uses to irrigate his fields trickles back into the San Pedro River. Instead, Frank fertilizes his soil with a mix of compost and pellets made from chicken manure. When he bought the farm in 2005, the soil was depleted, but rather than cloak his land in quick-fix biochemicals, Frank worked to nurse his fields back to health. Cover crops, like legumes, fixed nitrogen in the soil; stalks of wheat sent roots deep into his fields, building spaces for microorganisms to thrive.

The problem of Big Organic, the industrial-scale organic growers that sell to Safeway and Whole Foods, is in its modifier. Organic food was never intended to fill a place like Rio Rico. Organic growers originally approached the business of growing food in a fundamentally different way; when demand swelled, they were forced to fit this fundamentally different product into an unchanged food system. While there are a few brokers who import only organic produce—Phil Ostram at Patagonia Orchards imports about a semi truck worth of organic produce from Mexico every day—it's a risky business, importing food that can't be sterilized or fumigated while it waits at the border for an inspection, one that incurs extra costs for every hoop that must be jumped through: separate pallets, sterilized machinery, and scale demands of purchasers. "We do a lot to try to not hide behind the label," Phil says. "We aim to build transparent relationships between the consumer and the grower." But, he says, if he can't sell a load on the organic market, if it's about to rot, he might flip it and sell as conventional produce. Who would know? All we know is what we're told on a tiny white sticker.

We fret about what to select from overabundant produce sections. Busy, broke, and overtaxed by decisions, we want a label to tell us—to convey the difference in how a melon does business, even as we know this difference can't possibly fit onto a small sticker. In a sprawling, industrialized society, we don't know—or can't know—everyone who grows our food, so we hold producers accountable by setting up standards and regulations, hoping they will comply. But one size does not fit all, and in our attempts to design a T-shirt that will fit organic growers, we've ended up with the lowest common denominator, a baggy, shapeless thing that does not reveal the differences between bodies or fields of food.

"The landscape of any farm is the owner's portrait of himself," wrote Aldo Leopold in *The Farmer as a Conservationist*. "It seems to me that the pattern of the rural landscape, like the configuration of our own bodies, has in it (or should have in it) a certain wholeness." If Leopold is right, how we divide our landscapes offers an embarrassment of revelations about who we are and how we think. Monoculture is not just a pattern of land use; it is a pattern of mind and body, a pattern of living. Stripped of weeds and cleared of animals, industrial-scale farms are the airbrushed models of our fashion magazines. Firm stomachs, shaved armpits, lean legs: nothing superfluous. Today, a good farm is a clean farm, streamlined and tautly functional.

"WHICH END GOES INTO THE SOIL?" asks Sarah, holding up the flat, unfinished fence post we'd just bought at Home Depot for ninety-nine cents.

"Probably the pointy end," I say.

"Oh, shoot," she says, looking disappointed. We're sitting on the orange cement floors of my casita, painting a signpost to watch over our thirty square feet of soil. Despite all our ignorance and inattention, the plants in our garden plot have begun to grow. Sarah's sunflowers, once shy seedlings, are assertive, beaming yellow faces that peer through the chicken wire like a dog through a fence: *Come play with me.* Buds of future bell peppers huddle below floppy leaves. We are delighted—albeit surprised—and so we are building a shade structure to protect our plants from the summer sun. And we are decorating.

"Why?" I ask.

"I was thinking this curvy end kind of looks like a head." She flips the four-foot post upside down and places the pointy figure-eight curve of the stake next to her own head. "She'd be our lady of the garden."

From her craft box, Sarah produces two googly eyes that dart and jostle about with uncanny expressiveness. She paints a ponytail tuft of green hair that gathers at the sharp end of the stake. Once we pound the blunt end of the post into the dense soil surrounding our plot, googly eyes rolling wildly, there is nothing left to do but wait for the plants to grow into food.

ALTHOUGH IT'S TRUE that many organic growers are not perfect, it's also true that organics matter. If all of our foods were grown without pesticides, there would simply be fewer chemicals contaminating our water, soil, and, most important, our bodies. If everyone bought all organic produce, companies that manufacture pesticides and fertilizers would simply go out of business.

Pesticides are toxic by design—they are chemicals manufactured to kill the organisms on our fields that we have deemed "undesirable." They do quite a good job of this, but they don't eat and run; they linger and infiltrate, sinking into our foods like red wine into carpet. According to the Environmental Working Group, even after a proper washing, 65 percent of conventionally grown produce continued to be contaminated by pesticides.

While representatives of large agribusinesses—and occasionally the USDA—continue to stress that pesticides are not necessarily detrimental to human health, this issue has, unfortunately, long been settled. Pesticides *are* toxic. You can read up on this if you so desire—Rachel Carson has a bit to say about it in *Silent Spring*—but suffice to say that study after study shows a correlation between pesticide exposure and cancer, hormone disruption, and nervous-system toxicity. Or, in the case of Frank, racking coughs.

The question is not whether pesticides are bad for us—it's what to do with this information. Before I joined the Tucson CSA, I tried to buy produce according to the Environmental Working Group's Shopper's Guide, which lists the "Dirty Dozen" of conventionally grown produce: the fruits and vegetables most likely to be contaminated by pesticides. The point of the Dirty Dozen list is to help consumers get the most bang for their organic buck. Conventionally grown onions or sweet corn are doused in pesticides significantly less than fragile strawberries or peaches, so these items arrive to our supermarkets less laden with these toxic souvenirs. Some of our most loved pieces of produce—apples, bell peppers, celery—contain traces of dozens of different pesticides; if you are on a budget, you could substantially reduce your intake of pesticides by eliminating the worst offenders.

Theoretically, of course. In practice, though, strawberries embody the cognitive dissonance that is modern grocery shopping. I would prefer not to know that strawberries have topped the list of our most contaminated foods nearly every year since the EWG started releasing the list—that samples have found as many as thirteen different pesticides on one piece of fruit. Ignorance is bliss when one in four strawberry samples shows residues of captan, a "probable human carcinogen" (in the words of the EPA, an agency not known to play fast and loose with carcinogens).

Is there anything more succulent-seeming, more fresh-brimming and sweet-singing, than a row of strawberries nestled in a clear, plastic carrier? It is not like resisting a carton of ice cream or tray of cookies. Strawberries are sensible—they are healthy! Yet the folate and fiber in a strawberry do not much matter if the pesticides on its surface give you cancer.

So what do we do? Like everything else, produce exists on a scale of process; what makes a piece of produce more processed than another is how much is required to get it from field to table. In some instances, it takes a lot—a lot of water, energy, chemicals, and human labor. I know that strawberries are some of the most processed fruits we grow. Most are grown in the Central Valley in California, picked by some of the lowest-paid earners doing some of the most backbreaking work in a backbreaking industry, and yet, still, once or twice this year, I have been in Target or Safeway buying toilet paper or dish soap and I have forgotten. I have let myself be led astray in the face of succulent strawberries. But what seems more important than resisting temptation always, is resisting it usually; by avoiding situations that might lead you astray. Frank doesn't grow strawberries and I rarely go to Safeway.

In a globalized, industrial food system, Brian and Prescott serve an important function, and they do it well and honestly. As Prescott says, we live in a culture that flies to Atlanta and expects a fruit salad upon arrival. But what we have to consider is the cost of that expectation—the cost of the perpetual melon salad, available year-round and countrywide. Food is now everywhere, and it is expected to be everywhere, from libraries to schools, bus stations to midafternoon meetings. This network of food is like cell-phone service. It exists as background, comforting and noticeable only in its absence; we're not really sure how it gets there in the first place, into those tiny chips or onto plastic platters, but we assume it will be there. This assumption becomes a passive demand and so the supply dutifully burgeons to accommodate it.

I pay Farmer Frank twenty dollars in exchange for two bags of produce. The bounty of food I receive every week is often more than I know what to do with, so I blend cauliflower and kale into soups and stash them in my freezer for the hypothetical winter's rations. I'm lucky that Frank can grow year-round—if my year unprocessed had unfolded in Minnesota or New York, I'd certainly encounter different challenges than I do in sunny southern Arizona. I'd buy more produce in the summer and freeze or can it for the winter. I would probably be *thrilled* to find a melon imported from Mexico in December—a taste of sweet summer in the dead of winter. To some extent, there's nothing wrong with that. In most of the United States today, our foodsheds are the back of a tapestry, strings extending in thick colors across great distances, and our lives are all the more vibrant for it.

I think produce becomes too processed when these strings get so tangled that we forget where the threads begin. I feel about blackberries from Chile the way I feel about molten chocolate cake: Special treats are nice. But if the majority of a day—or a diet—is built on these treats, they are no longer defined as such.

Different figures are batted about, but on average, ninety-one cents of every dollar American consumers spend on food goes to middlemen—to suppliers, marketers, producers. This means that the people who grow the food we eat— even the corn in Cheddar Chex Mix begins as a plant grown by someone— receive only nine cents of every dollar we spend. If everyone in southern Arizona, all million of us, shifted just five dollars each week to food sourced directly from farms in our region, these farmers would earn, on average, an additional $287 million annually—more than enough to compensate for the collective $20 million their farms are currently losing every year.

I roll my eyes at images of the farmers' market pastoral and yet I can't see an easier way to follow my dictum for the year, to spend money better. When I spend money at Safeway, I'm supporting that ninety-one cents; when I spend at the farmers' market, I'm ensuring that the people who grow my food get more than nine cents on every dollar.

As spring melts into summer, after Sarah and I harvest a handful of bell peppers and three watermelons, our garden plot becomes something we dabble in rather than actively cultivate. It becomes more a source of social sustenance than of nutritional—we are inexperienced gardeners, more focused on catching up than digging in. My conviction that I should grow my own food weakened when I met Frank, when I saw how he just *gets it*. How to coax flavorful vegetation out of desert soils and produce beautiful bundles of raw ingredients.

To me, Frank's operation represents an appropriate economy of scale—on twenty acres, he produces enough food to feed one thousand families for a year. Twenty-three people work to get that food to our tables, a bargain given the tangle of people who occupy the in-between spaces of an industrial produce machine.

But what about the rest of Tucson? The one million people sprawled across this desert city? It'd take another thousand farmers like Frank growing produce to supply this population, a large enough number to seem nearly hypothetical until you consider not the farmer but the farm—this scenario would require twenty thousand acres of farmland in a state where two hundred thousand acres grow nothing but water-hungry cotton. Maybe there shouldn't be a million people eating in Tucson, and maybe there will be fewer of us once our water stops flowing so freely, but that's another conversation. For now, even if melons continue rolling across our border, I wonder if we can begin to wean ourselves from the binational commerce that is pulling fertility from Mexico's soils to feed American eaters in order to focus on that which might sustain us closer to home.

WHEN I VISITED CROOKED SKY FARMS, Frank asked Nicole, the farm's marketing manager, to show me around their storage facilities, and she seemed confused—there was very little to show. In two small walk-in refrigerators, two small air conditioners whirred at a breezy fifty-five degrees, keeping crates of produce fresh overnight. One night, that's it—then off they go, to Flagstaff, Phoenix, or Tucson. "We're not in the business of storing produce," said Nicole. "We just distribute it."

Five days a week, fifty weeks a year, workers head out into the fields at

Crooked Sky to harvest food. The lettuce might be soggy from rain; the cauliflower might be covered in ice, the tomatoes might simmer in triple-digit temperatures, but the food must be harvested.

The produce I eat on Wednesday is picked early on Tuesday mornings—if it's too cold and there's a danger of a frost damaging tender leaves, Julie and Rosa will wait until midmorning, but in the summer, they get started as soon as the sun cracks the crooked Phoenix skyline. It's not hurried work, but they work quickly so they have time to harvest two hundred heads of cauliflower, pull up a thousand potatoes, grab two hundred bright butternut squashes off their vines, and another couple hundred eggplants. Two hundred members pick up their produce at Tucson's CSA on Wednesday afternoons, so on Tuesday, it is up to four workers to assemble two hundred shares.

Once plucked or picked, roughly eight hundred pounds of produce travels in the back of a diesel engine John Deere cart back to the small cluster of trailers. First kale, then squash; one by one, the produce falls into a bathtub built for an NBA player and splashes about the cold water. Freed of debris and dirt, the produce is counted again and arranged in black plastic crates. The crates are carried an easy twenty feet across the clearing and into the refrigerator; they're stacked, four or five high, against the short stone walls of the sweet-smelling storage space. A full night's rest or a quick morning catnap; by Wednesday at lunch, the crates are loaded in the back of a ten-foot trailer. Off the farm and onto the freeway, I-17 South to I-10 East—sixty miles and the same number of minutes later, the truck pulls into the parking lot of the Historic Y, where, in the hungry rush of five o'clock, I'll arrive on my bike to fill my backpack full of food and, if I *must,* leave in a better mood.

Unprocess Yourself: Produce

The first rule of produce is to eat more if it. A conventionally grown bell pepper is better than no bell pepper. It's better to eat something fresh and whole—organic or not—than something processed or packaged. If you're really convinced that you can't afford organic food, you can improve your diet substantially just by buying more fresh produce. Check out the Environmental Working Group at Ewg.org to find the most recent Dirty Dozen list.

If you're worried about eating GMOs, check out your state's labeling laws—consider canvassing for groups working to make GMO labeling mandatory. (Incidentally, because three-quarters of processed foods are made from corn, and nearly all of the corn grown in the United States is genetically modified, avoiding processed foods is the single best way to avoid GMOs.) If a food is certified organic, it's not genetically modified.

Visit LocalHarvest.org to find farmers' markets and Community Supported Agriculture programs in your area. Community Supported Agriculture programs tend to offer the biggest bang for your buck—by paying up front, you shoulder some of the risk inherent in growing, which means you reap the rewards when a crop does well. If you're thinking about joining a CSA, ask questions. Some farms deliver straight to your doorstep, which might be appealing if you live in a sprawling city like Los Angeles. Picking up your produce in person offers you the opportunity to ask questions. At my CSA, we have a trading table, which allows us to swap out not-favorite foods. (I have a low tolerance for turnips.) Ask questions of the grower. What's the farm's preferred payment schedule—do they prefer that you invest for an entire season or by the month or week? Does the CSA run year-round or only during the summer? What kinds of fruits and vegetables typically come in a week's share? (The Tucson CSA has a complete harvest history online.)

At farmers' markets, talk to the people who sell you your food. Farmers are happy to have regular customers, so they'll reward you with insider tips—the eggplants are the best they've been all season; there are so many cucumbers, we're practically giving them away.

I am not a very good gardener, so my price per unit of produce grown is not much better than what I might buy at the farmers' market. That said, while it's true that there's nothing more magical than growing your own sustenance from seed, it's also true that there's nothing cheaper. If you think you might have a green thumb, find a community garden, buy some backyard containers or dig up a garden bed, and give growing a gander.

A good way to use up the vegetables you grow, buy, or get in your CSA is to pack your lunch at home. At the beginning of the week, I make a big pot of beans and another of a grain, like rice, quinoa, or barley. In the morning before I go to work, I'll combine beans and grains in a Tupperware, plus any vegetables I have on hand. Most greens can be added raw; otherwise, if a vegetable fits on my little George Forman, I'll grill it—bell peppers, zucchini, or eggplant each take about five minutes. You can also roast vegetables in a big batch when you're making your beans and rice—this works especially well with winter produce like butternut squash, pumpkins, or root vegetables. Once you have the basics assembled—vegetable, bean, grain—think about what flavors you can add. If you've made black beans, make a southwestern-style Tupperware by adding salsa, olive oil, salt and pepper, and maybe pepper jack cheese. Garbanzo beans are the perfect start to a Middle Eastern-inspired Tupperware, with grilled vegetables marinating in tahini, olive oil, dill, and lemon juice. If all else fails, olive oil, balsamic vinegar, and salt and pepper will work with just about anything.

5

SALT

Manipulated food is processed.

Before I settle into Tucson's sweltering summer, I escape for a long weekend at the end of May to visit my parents in Pasadena. My dad picks me up at Los Angeles International Airport and we drive inland, up into the San Gabriel Mountains that hug the eastern edge of the city. The next morning, after I drop my mom off at work and grind back west through rush-hour sludge, the air shifts. I roll down my windows and swing right, northbound, up the Pacific Coast Highway. Traffic thins and the breeze blows straight through me. I wind my way north to Malibu, past Sunset Boulevard and the Temescal Canyon Road until I reach Paradise Cove. Hoping I've made it far enough from the city's runoff, I pull into an empty spot on the west side of the road.

Sundress and flip-flops stay in the car; I'm close enough to the sand that, wearing only my bikini, I open the trunk of my mom's car and hoist out a heavy backpack, laden with the weight of four two-gallon jugs of water. I tiptoe across the hot sand toward the crashing waves of the Pacific, drop the backpack on the sand, spread out my towel, and squint at the ocean's intensity—its blue so primary, so sparkling, so unquestionably *wet*. My eyes adjust, only a day removed from the faded-pastel desert.

I create a momentary man-made lake beside my towel as I crack open each jug and pour the filtered water into the sand. The jugs were full of expired Arrowhead water pulled from my parents' earthquake supply kit; now I grab two of the empty plastic jugs, and head into the ocean.

IN JUNE OF 1862, John Commins wrote in a small piece in the *Charleston Mercury* with instructions on "How to Manufacture Salt for Home Use." "Take a towel, or any piece of cloth—say, two yards long—sew the two ends together, hang it on a roller, and let one end revolve in a tub or basin of salt water," he wrote. "The sun and air will act on the cloth, and evaporate the water rapidly. When the solution is evaporated to near the bottom, dip from the concentrated brine and pour it in a large flat dish or plate; let it remain in the sun until the salt is formed; taking it in every night, and placing a cover on it."

During the American Civil War, salt shortages up and down the fractured country left citizens hungry and soldiers weakened. The primary problem facing salt-scarce citizens was that of preservation—blandness could be tolerated more readily than rancidity. Before refrigeration became widespread, rubbing a food in salt was the most reliable way to keep it from going bad. ("TO KEEP MEAT FROM SPOILING IN THE SUMMER," Confederate soldiers were instructed in 1865, "Eat it early in the Spring.") Although there were a few saltworks in New York State, for most of the nineteenth century, Americans were dependent on foreign salt. Three hundred and fifty tons of British salt arrived to the port in New Orleans every day; that is, until 1861, when the war began and President Lincoln blockaded the port. Facing severe salt shortages, "Owners of large plantations in coastal areas reverted to the Revolutionary War practice of sending their slaves to fill kettles with seawater for evaporation," writes Mark Kurlansky in *Salt: A World History*. "But it soon became apparent that . . . the small amount of salt produced from these kettles was not going to solve their problems."

I'm at the beach collecting salt water to make salt because I am tired of reading ingredient labels and wondering, What *is* that? I am up to my eyeballs in additives and so I wondered, What would it take to make one? I don't think salt is processed, but like so many of the additives in our foods, the process of salt making is invisible to me. I don't know how to make salt, so it seems like it simply *is,* not sourced from a substance in nature but rather found, ready-made, white, and finely crystallized. I want to make salt to understand a process that was once vital but is now obscure and unquestioned.

Salt is one of the most common of the 10,000 chemicals added to our foods. Of these 10,000, 1,480 have been approved by the FDA; 3,600 more have been deemed GRAS, or generally recognized as safe. A thousand more have never been tested by the FDA and a further 3,800 are "indirect additives" and so are totally unregulated.

In the face of such a staggering display of chemistry, I feel powerless. If I was awed standing in Frank's fields, then the astounding array of available additives defeats me. How can one person understand all that's added to our foods, if even the FDA can't get a handle on it? I've been reading ingredient labels for five months, but still I fret. Is citric acid—naturally abundant in citrus fruits and berries—processed? What about sodium bicarbonate—baking soda—or acetic acid—a compound in vinegar? Most of these food additives have been used for hundreds of years and are safe, even if they don't sound like it. But just because a food has been deemed safe doesn't mean it's unprocessed. I'm not a chemist, which is the point of making salt—if I can figure out how to source one chemical, one additive, then I might better understand what's required to make the so many, many others.

Today, the most energy-efficient way to pull salt from the earth is to spread salt water across a broad evaporation pond and wait a few years for the water to leave solid behind. Underground salt deposits, remnants of ancient ocean beds long covered by shifting earth, offer another way to generate salt crystals. Rock salt is produced by mining these deposits, excavating a shaft thousands of feet deep and blowing open a room, allowing miners and their pickaxes access to chip away at the great white walls of a saline cave. Far cheaper—although much more energy-intensive—is solution mining. Rather than send people down into fragile or inaccessible mine shafts, water can be circulated through underground caverns, pumped to the surface, and steamed in tall evaporation towers. Most of the salt consumed in the United States is extracted through solution mining. Of the three ways to produce salt, only solution mining generates the small, uniform crystals that pour like rain out of our Morton containers, the salt that combines easily and uniformly with our processed foods.

While the only processing pure salt undergoes is its removal from water or rock, the table salt shuffling within a Morton canister contains calcium silicate, an anticaking agent that prevents the salt from clumping—as the slogan goes, "when it rains, it pours." Since 1924, when goiter, caused by iodine deficiency, became a problem, iodide ions have been added to all refined salts—except for sea salt—manufactured in the United States.

It turns out that filling a plastic bottle full of the ocean is no easy task. A plastic jug full of air floats with considerable force, so I wrestle each jug below the surface of the water, straddling it like it's a buoy out at sea to hold it steady for the few moments it takes the seawater to gurgle inside. The task is made no easier by the waves that keep breaking on me. I want to swim out farther, to collect less agitated water, but concerns for safety over purity keep me closer to the shore on this particularly empty stretch of beach. After five or six minutes, I stumble back to my backpack, weaving with the weight of two heavy jugs, and then plunge back into the frigid water with the two empty ones. After I wrestle another four gallons of ocean water into submission, I screw their caps on tight and line my four jugs in a row, facing the ocean like sentinels guarding the sand from the tide.

I stretch out on my towel to dry, propping myself on my elbows and inhaling the blue, salty air, the dampness lingering and scratching in my throat. Far down the beach, a small surfer catches a wave, and I watch as he weaves up and down, pressure and release, along the surging white water. I close my eyes. When I open them a few minutes later, the small surfing figure has become a life-size man walking along the tide line. I watch him walk. He watches me lie on my elbows. Just as he passes in front of me, almost over his shoulder, he calls, "Don't get dehydrated today!"

SALT ACTUALLY HELPS *KEEP* US HYDRATED. Salt keeps our electrolytes in balance, which maintains fluid homeostasis in the body. Salt is made up of sodium and chloride, both key elements in the intricate system that keeps our body chemistry balanced. Without salt, which mostly lives in our blood plasma, our bodies can't transmit nerve impulses or contract muscles. But it is a delicate balance. Too much salt means too much plasma in our blood vessels—too much liquid—which can send our blood pressure soaring, upping the risk of heart disease.

Salt is a critical ingredient in food preparation; it preserves food by killing harmful bacteria and enhances flavor by drawing out water and permitting other harmless yet flavorful bacteria to thrive. Salt also preserves food sealed in packages. "Salt is perfect for processed foods," writes Marion Nestle in *What to Eat*. "It is cheap . . . Even better, it binds water and makes foods weigh more, so you pay more for heavier packages."

I hadn't noticed how much salt I'd started dumping into my foods until I went over to Sarah's for dinner one night in April. The quinoa and vegetables were tasty, certainly, but I craved a bit more kick. As I ventured to her kitchen for the saltshaker, she asked, more surprised then offended, "Really?"

"Shoot, sorry," I'd said. "It's delicious!" And then it hit me, why I'd been unconsciously seeking so much salt over the past month. I had never before been a particularly salt-motivated eater. Sugar—you know this—is my white crystal of choice. So why the sudden increase? "Unprocessed foods are relatively low in salt," writes Nestle. "Only about ten percent of the salt in the American diet comes from salt added at the table; the other ninety percent is already added in processed foods."

Give up processed foods, and you give up 90 percent of your salt intake. Give up processed foods, and suddenly it's up to you to shake out the salt your body really needs.

AFTER I DRIVE HOME from the beach and pick up my mom from the high school where she works as an administrator, I unload the jugs of ocean water onto a table on our patio. The afternoon light slants toward evening, warm and breezy, so I leave the sliding glass doors open. It is nice to be home for the weekend, to enjoy the proximity of Tucson to Los Angeles and the luxury of time with my parents. When I lived in Santa Monica, I drove home almost every week, so I am happy for any occasion to relax into home and my mother's presence. If making chocolate got me out of my kitchen and into the community, then making salt has brought me back home.

Zoey leaves her station on the floor below my mom, who's chopping and occasionally dropping vegetables for dinner, and joins me outside, blond tail wagging. A hose rinses out my grandmother's sixteen-liter stove pot, unearthed from a back closet, and I consult the salt-making instructions I've printed.

"It says here that I need to filter the water through cheesecloth," I call to my mom through the open glass.

"Don't have any," she calls back from above the kitchen stove.

I walk inside. Zoey obediently follows. "Well, shit."

My mom looks up. "Try an old pillowcase."

I'm about to pour my first gallon of water into a stove pot that has been swaddled tightly with a pale blue pillowcase when I stop. "Wait," I call back inside. "This won't filter out the salt, will it?"

My mom looks up from her steaming sauté. "Oh. Huh. I dunno."

I walk inside, water heavy in hand, and we look at each other for a moment. Zoey, too, pauses in her prancing about the yard. And then we both realize it at the same time.

"No, no, no," I say.

"That's ridiculous," she says.

I go back outside and start pouring the water through the pillowcase. "If only desalinating water were that easy!" I cry. "Who needs the Colorado River, we've got the Pacific and pillowcases from Target!"

By the time my dad gets home from Caltech, the saltwater saucepot, removed from its pillowcase and a fine layer of sand, is steaming on the stove. He peers into the gurgling liquid and then turns to us, hovering beside him. "You've both gone *nuts*," he says.

I roll my eyes. My mom turns to me. "Can I add pesto to the vegetables?"

"What kind of pesto?"

"It's from Trader Joe's," she says. "Is that unprocessed?"

After I examine the ingredient label and confirm that it passes the kitchen test—with only olive oil, Parmesan cheese, sun-dried tomatoes, garlic, walnuts, and basil—my mom scoops out a great dollop and stirs it in with the vegetables sautéing on the stove.

We turn the stove off when we go to bed. My mom turns the gas back on when she gets up at six and by the time I emerge at eight, the kitchen windows are covered in steamy fog and the water has retreated two inches down the side of the sixteen-inch pot. ("P.S.," writes John Commins. "To make salt requires a little patience, as it is of slow formation.") My mom and I come and go all day on Saturday; every time we return, we set the pot steaming; when we depart, we turn off the burner. Crusty white lines form on the edge of the pot, geologic strata marking the passing of time and increasing salinity.

When I wake up on Sunday morning, the sloshing liquid has transformed into a thick white sludge. I turn up the heat and stir the crystals around, enjoying the crunchy sound they make sliding against the metal. My mom takes over stirring and then we mosey about the house, Zoey at our heels. Finally, around eleven, the salt sludge ceases to gurgle about; it begins to seize and harden. I hover over the pot, steam billowing in my face. I can see small crystals emerging out of the mush. Like rice sucking up the last of its water, the salt exhales its final bit of steam. As my parents watch from the sidelines, I stick my hand into the pot and pluck out a clump of white crystals. I rub them between my fingers—they're sharp, discrete—and then plop the mess on my tongue. The crystals dissolve in a bright burst of saline saliva.

"Salt!" I exclaim. "It's salt!"

"Let me try this stuff," my mom says, and dips her finger into the pot. She licks it and her eyes go wide. "It sure is!" She dips her finger in again and so do I. "It's so *salty!*" we both say.

My dad shakes his head, incredulous. "What did you *think* would happen?"

My mom and I look at each other and shrug. Who cares? We made salt!

MAKING SALT IS A MUCH-NEEDED VICTORY. The complexity of sugar and wheat had tired me out. Although I had eventually succeeded with bread and chocolate, it is fun to make salt on my first try. This fun reminds me that, although I am still overwhelmed by unprocessed, it doesn't have to be overwhelming *always*.

Throughout the morning, while my mom and I continue to insist that we made salt, my dad continues to shake his head, ever the physicist. "You didn't make salt, you extracted it," he says. "Making salt would require some sodium and chlorine and very explosive chemistry."

Although I roll my eyes at him, so smug in science while my mom and I flit in fun, he's completely right. We use the word "make" as if we are creating salt, but like all of the other minerals that augment our food supply, we aren't making salt; we are merely extracting it. Food additives begin when we excavate minerals from the earth, chip away at natural deposits that have accumulated over centuries, and manipulate and transform these raw materials into something less raw, something more specific. We process minerals and only then do they become "chemicals"—only after such industrial processing do they seem to have been made rather than found.

"We say food ingredients are manufactured as if they did not exist before, but the truth is everything comes from something else," writes Steve Ettlinger in *Twinkie: Deconstructed* after he descended into mines and wormed his way into factories to track down the thirty-nine ingredients that make up a Twinkie. "All artificial ingredients came from, at some point, some part of the earth. The extent to which they are manipulated makes them artificial—obscures their source."

In the face of so much manipulation, of ingredient labels that no longer contain words but rather abstract strings of modifiers, polysorbate 60 and FD&C Yellow No. 3, it's too easy to forget that all foods, natural or artificial, are composed of molecules that come from combinations and permutations of the basic atomic elements. A molecule of salt is made up of an atom of sodium smashed against an atom of chlorine by means of an ionic bond, but what makes salt "natural" as opposed to "artificial" is that crystals of sodium chloride occurred in nature long before human-powered laboratories got involved. Salt crystals are what scientists call "basic chemicals," or the chemicals used to make other chemicals. (Another ubiquitous basic chemical is petroleum; the list also includes sulfuric acid, lime, phosphate, nitrogen, and oxygen, all of which occur naturally.) Only 8 percent of the salt we excavate in the United States each year is used for food and agriculture. About 35 percent goes to "ice control," while another 45 percent of U.S. salt goes to the chemical industry. Electrolysis transforms NaCl into chlorine—bleach—or sodium hydroxide— lye. Chemicals that began as salt—as sodium chloride, chipped from the earth or evaporated in the sun—are used to make paper or plastic, to process gasoline or glaze tiles. Salt is used in aspirin, vinyl, shampoo, adhesives; it is used to cure cement and kill bacteria on leather shoes, or in one of another fourteen thousand industrial applications.

Although I'd shown it could technically be made in a home kitchen, as I pack up my suitcase to head home to Tucson, I realize the real question here is not whether or not salt is processed, but rather—is it food?

When does a chemical—a molecule—become a food? If cooking is chemistry, then is processing just industrial cooking?

Give an apple to a chemist and you'll learn it's made up of hydrogen oxide, cellulose, hemicellulose, malic acid, dextrose, fructose, pectin, sucrose, amylacetate, and citric acid. But ask a chemist to assemble this same list of ingredients from his laboratory and you will not end up with an apple. Even in an age of industrial manufacturing and precision technology, something remains hidden, some process of coherence eludes our awareness in the synthesis of "food" from a list of chemical constituents.

My dad, the quantum physicist, who walks among quarks and photons, rolls his eyes at the silliness of pulling salt from seawater. Of course, he says, what did you *think* would happen? But my mom and I are delighted because we have mined the invisible, have sourced the abstract.

Despite our success, ultimately what making salt teaches me is how spectacularly inefficient it is to do individually. Although I'd embarked on this year for precisely this reason, to linger in these so-called inefficiencies, what my salt-making endeavor teaches me is that there is a reason we once decided to cluster together into civilizations. Some processes are best tackled by people working together rather than individuals working independently. I had thought that I might use the energy of the sun to evaporate the water from my salt, but when I learned that this not only requires up to two years' time (a *little* patience?) but also requires some sort of contraption to prevent debris and dust from coating the salt sludge, I turned to the artificial heat of a gas stove. Solitary salt making is not, and has never been, a particularly energy-efficient endeavor, both in terms of human and natural energy, as lots of time and consistent heat are needed to extract salt from its source, something industrial-scale operations do—have always done—quite well. Unlike wheat and sugar, it turns out that the processing of salt is an argument for the industrial food system, for large-scale saltworks that have the time and infrastructure to evaporate salt from seawater using the sun rather than natural gas.

IT'S ONLY WHEN I'M PACKING UP my carry-on duffel that it occurs to me that my plastic baggie full of white crystals might actually raise more eyebrows than eight gallons of salt water would. I decide not to bury the baggie under T-shirts and tennis shoes but instead lay it flat directly below the zipper; the duffel slides through the security checkpoint and X-ray machine at LAX without so much as a glancing bag check. When I get home to my casita in Tucson, I slide the salt into a corner of my spice cabinet, next to my little jar of homemade vanilla extract and in front of the store-bought baking soda. Baking soda survived the great processed purge because it comes from soda ash, a form of sodium carbonate that's been mined from the earth since the ancient Egyptians began using it as soap. Chemically speaking, soda ash is a lot like limestone; if you've ever seen chalky smudges on your fingers after rubbing a limestone wall, you can imagine how the soft rock becomes baking soda. Although soda ash is still mined throughout the world, today baking soda is produced by causing limestone—calcium, basically—to react with the inescapable and ever ubiquitous sodium chloride—with salt.

When I try to cook with my new salt, I find it far too clumpy to incorporate evenly across my sautés or bakes. It's powerful salt, much more saline than salt bought at the store, and so I use it sparingly.

I feel a little silly for having made salt, but it's also making salt that shows me that it is human to want to manipulate the world. We found scattered stands of wild grains and we arranged them into productive rows; we found honeybees filling up combs with nectar, so we built boxes and brought the bees to us. But an inconvenient truth of this human penchant to play with the world's components is that it usually doesn't know how to stop itself. Today, we do not simply transform corn into corn syrup, we manipulate it one step further, adding enriched white flour, salt, and ferrous iron sulfate (and thirty-six other ingredients) to make a Twinkie. The problem is not necessarily in the processing of any one of these thirty-nine ingredients; the issue arises in concert, in the combination all these disparate processes into one single manipulated product we've decided to call food.

Processes of a scale much older and larger than us form sodium chloride crystals. The earth will continue to produce salt, in its oceans and rock deposits, whether or not we mine it up and refine it out, and perhaps this is the key difference between processed and unprocessed foods: how much human tinkering is required to make them. This difference is elusive and intuitive, and yet it is precisely this difference that defines process. If nothing is manufactured—if it is all simply manipulated—then it is simply the *extent* to which something is manipulated that makes it processed.

Unprocess Yourself: Salt

When I buy salt, I buy sea salt, both because I'm now emotionally attached to the idea of the evaporated ocean, but also because it takes significantly less energy to evaporate salt out of water than solution mine it from caves. Sea salt is slightly more expensive than iodized salt, but only slightly.

I buy a lot of salt because I use a lot of salt when I cook. I use a decadent amount of salt. Salt is delicious and so food is more delicious with it. Salt illuminates ingredients and makes flavors cohere—it turns dishes into meals. When you cook at home, don't worry about salt. When you give up packaged foods—or when you eat them very rarely—you earn yourself the luxury to be liberal with your salt usage. When cooking at home, add as much salt as tastes good; your soups or roasts will taste better, so you'll be more likely to cook at home again. And unlike with a microwave Lean Cuisine or bag of popcorn, if you add too much salt, you'll know.

That is not to say that there aren't important health considerations concerning your salt intake. I'm young and active (and I live in the desert), so I lose a lot of salt to sweat—check in with your doctor before you change your salinity too drastically.

To make salt, you'll need a big saucepot and a lot of patience. (If you have access to space that gets a lot of sun and wind—a roof, say, or a backyard patio—you can leave your saltwater to evaporate in a shallow, covered collecting pan.) I got about two cups of salt from eight gallons of saltwater; it'll all depend on the salinity of the water you collect.

At home, filter salt water through cheesecloth (or a pillowcase). In a sixteen-gallon saucepot, bring the water to a boil, stirring constantly—you don't want to scorch the salt. If you want to go do something else, reduce the heat to a simmer; if you're okay standing there stirring for a few hours, keep it boiling—it'll take less time, but requires more attention. Either way, once the salt sludge reaches roughly the consistency of wet sand, you're done—take the pot off the heat and store salt crystals in a cool, dry place.

6

STUFF

Obsolescence is processed.

At two in the morning after a long Saturday night, I'm in my kitchen, hungry. I've just spent an evening with Sarah and our friend Cory hopping around the dance floor of the Cactus Moon bar. Following some yet-to-be-defined unprocessed logic, I'd chosen tequila over Bud Light, and now I am slightly stumbly and very hungry. I stare into my fridge, searching for something ready-made. No luck. I cast around my kitchen. Food. I want quick food. My kitchen contains no late-night unprocessed snacks because I am usually not awake in the late night, but now, at a rare 2 A.M., this seems like a ghastly oversight. Potato! I spot a potato on the counter. A potato reminds me of a potato chip. This potato is raw. I wrap the raw potato in foil, plunk it in the oven, and realize, as the oven clangs to life and I stand swaying over it, that this will take far too long. I grab the foil-wrapped potato out of the oven, toss it into the microwave with the foil still on, and leave the machine to whir while I shower off the sweat and smoke of the Cactus Moon. When I plod out a few minutes later in my pj's, the potato is still cold and quite hard, as if, oddly, it has not cooked at all. I nuke it a few minutes more. The potato remains cold and hard and so, exasperated and still hungry, I go to bed.

It's only when I remove the cold, foil-wrapped potato from the microwave the next morning, when I place a cup of coffee on the glass disk, watch it spin around for thirty seconds, and then remove the ceramic mug, as cold as it was a half minute before, that realization begins to build. I frown at the cold coffee mug. I frown at the cold foil-wrapped potato. Oh. Right.

When I tell my mom that I put a foil-wrapped potato in the microwave, I omit the wee morning hour in which it took place and endure only a minute of her consternation that I put metal in the microwave ("It could have exploded!") before I ask, "Are microwaves fixable?"

"Maybe. But I'm sure it's cheaper to buy a new one."

"That's ridiculous!"

"Well, they're like fifty dollars. You can afford that."

"I know. But everything is fine about this microwave! It turns on, it lights up."

I'm on speakerphone, so after he finishes laughing, my dad chimes in: "It just doesn't *heat* up!"

Come on, I insist. Surely somebody can fix this. My klutziness could not have killed it *forever*. Although it wouldn't be the first time an appliance had died on my watch—I am tall and so my long limbs flail more than most—it seems that everything is so *fragile* these days.

As IT TURNS OUT, this fragility is no mistake. A British real estate broker named Bernard London was one of the first people to use the term "planned obsolescence," which he outlined in his 1932 pamphlet "Ending the Depression Through Planned Obsolescence." Bernard's plan to end the depression—the Great Depression, that is, a "stupid depression" brought on by "people in a frightened and hysterical mood"—offers a sort of madcap confidence in consumerism:

I would have the Government assign a lease of life to shoes and homes and machines, to all products of manufacture, mining and agriculture, when they are first created, and they would be sold and used within the term of their existence definitely known by the consumer. After the allotted time had expired, these things would be legally "dead" and would be controlled by the duly appointed governmental agency and destroyed if there is widespread unemployment. New products would constantly be pouring forth from the factories and marketplaces, to take the place of the obsolete, and the wheels of industry would be kept going and employment regularized and assured for the masses.

In short, London would have us assign expiration dates to blue jeans and laundry machines as if they were cartons of eggs or gallons of milk. And—it gets better—if you were caught using these items past their lease on life, you would be taxed. Taxed! The proceeds from this tax would facilitate the collection and destruction of all the dead products that had passed their expiration dates. And once collected, what would we do with all these dead products, Mr. London? "Throw them into a junk pile."

Reading an electronic version of London's pamphlet seventy years later, it is nearly impossible not to find this idea ludicrous. But as I huff and puff, I try to imagine how it might have seemed rational in 1932, when nearly one of every four American workers was unemployed. London insisted that we change the way we understand economics to fit into a new paradox of plenty. "Classical economics was predicated on the belief that nature was niggardly and that the human race was constantly confronted by the spectre of shortages," he wrote. In 1932, the world's economy was indeed confronting "the spectre of shortages." But by the turn of the century, as technology allowed us to penetrate deeper into the natural world—into mine shafts and oil wells submerged deep in the ocean—nature appeared inexhaustible and brimming. With so many people scraping by on so little, *not* to take advantage of the boundless raw materials offered by the earth seemed like a waste.

London's plan was not formally adopted, but manufacturers have so thoroughly appropriated the premise that it may well have been made official. In the 1950s, a new soldering process developed by Motorola made its handheld radio one of the first "unrepairable products," limiting its life-span to the durability of its components, writes Giles Slade in *Made to Break: Technology and Obsolescence in America*. Over decades, disposable radios begat disposable microwaves (begat unfixable iPods).

When our products do happen to outlast their planned life-span, the culture of style steps in. By 1950, all across the country, American families were happily storing their milk and eggs in perfectly functioning refrigerators, made of solid steel and durable parts. What was a manufacturer to do? They could make new models every year—an idea that proved so successful we now identify our cars by model year—or release special editions, new styles, and seasonal colors.

But the most frugal consumer could resist the allure of style, could refrain, in theory, from purchasing the powder blue of 1955 and instead stick with the canary yellow of 1954. Create an object that would become "functionally obsolete," on the other hand, and you had your customer by a very short leash. Indeed, by "shortening the replacement cycle," a manufacturer was effectively creating new customers. When an object breaks, if it's an object you need, you're left with little choice but to buy another one.

REPAIR OR REPLACE IT? asks an article on ConsumerReports.com: *CR's guide to having products fixed—or not*. The article advises skipping a repair that will cost you more than half the price of a new product: "It doesn't pay to replace counter-top microwave ovens." Upon further digging, I learn that repair doesn't just not pay; most microwave ovens are simply not fixable. They are the single-use appliance for the single-use meal.

Microwave ovens work because when microwaves (waves that are, well, micro) pass through a food, they vibrate the food's molecules and so heat it up. The difference between the way microwaves heat food and the way a flame does has more to do with the source of the wave—creating an electromagnetic field in a metal box versus striking a match—than the actual propagation of heat. During World War II, while Raytheon employees were busy studying radio waves that could be used to detect enemy aircraft—known now as radar—one of their engineers, Percy Spencer, was standing in front of a magnetron tube, which radiated the microwave energy used for radar, and noticed a candy bar in his pocket had started to melt. Intrigued, he started sticking food—kernels of popcorn, raw eggs—inside the tube to see what would happen. The popcorn popped, the eggs exploded, and Spencer showed the world its first microwave in 1947, officially dubbed "the Radarange." This first Radarange cost about $3,000, occupied a space the size of a refrigerator, and sucked up 1.6 kilowatts of energy. By 1967, Raytheon had shrunk the box to fit on a countertop, changed its name to the more palatable microwave, and sold the first hundred-volt device for just $500.

Although it is true that my microwave's untimely demise was more the result of user error than manufacturer intent, the fact that it cannot be repaired seems obsolescence enough. If it does not pay to repair a microwave—if, indeed, it cannot be done—what does one do with a broken microwave?

I could heed Bernard's suggestion and throw it into a junk pile. Although the phrasing itself sounds ludicrous, conjuring to mind piles of dead couches and strangled toasters, that is, in fact, exactly what we do with our garbage today.

"Basically, you dig a big hole in a ground," says Perry Dunson, the operations manager of Los Reales Landfill, as he drives me through the gates in a white City of Tucson pickup truck. "And you put garbage in it."

In 1976, the EPA mandated that these big holes be lined with plastic before being filled with garbage, to prevent toxins from leaching into nearby land and water, but basically, that is how a landfill works. We excavate earth, line it with plastic, and build a pile of junk. Concentrate that pile with a bulldozer, crush it with a compacter, cover it with dirt, and start again tomorrow.

Perry drives a slow lap around the landfill's silent landscape, across packed earth, past quiet bulldozers. It is a world of beige and brown, big sky and scattered debris. We swing a right on a swath of open dirt dotted by drums, buckets filled with paint or pesticides, batteries or solvents, scattered collections of our household hazardous waste. A dozen refrigerators cluster together like sentinels of the landfill, broad-shouldered guards. A tall pyramid of tumbled tires frowns in a corner, deflated and droopy. As we head toward the dumping site, over a wide swath of smooth dirt, he says, "There's fifty feet of garbage below us."

It takes me a moment to understand. "We're *in* the landfill?" I ask, peering through the window at the ground and seeing, finally, flecks of color peeking through tan.

"Or on it. Whatever you wanna call it," he says.

The language of landfills—filling up holes—leads me to believe that this dumping site will look like a crater's edge, but it is nothing more than a line of litter rising into a dirt-covered crest. Trucks drive across an expanse of packed dirt, dump their garbage-laden loads on the edge of a garbage-filled slope; a dozer pushes the refuse upslope and a heavy compacter runs it over, again and again. At the end of the day, the compacter packs heavy earth over the incline of garbage. It is more like building a hill than filling a hole.

"Cool," I say, dumbly. This is not at all what I expected a landfill to look like. It doesn't *look* like the belly of the beast, roiling and noxious, the toxic source of groundwater contamination and greenhouse gases. If landfills account for 20 percent of all human-related methane emissions, and if humans cause climate change by releasing greenhouse gases into the atmosphere—and if methane is twenty times more potent per pound than its more famous sister-emitter, carbon dioxide—then everything I throw into a landfill contributes to climate change.

But this logic is hard to see here. It doesn't even smell like garbage. When we roll to a stop just before the edge of the dumping line, the first thing I think is—birds. There are so many birds, flapping and fat, waddling through waste and soaring over plastic. Birds, and five small cars dumping five small loads against a single, sloped hill. The dozer quietly combs this garbage toward the edge of the hill, arranging it for the compacter. Perry drives a slow loop around this edge, the edge where scattered and temporary debris become the compacted matter of a permanent landfill. The garbage really does seem to disappear, packed into hillsides like cement into molding.

Every day, four million pounds of garbage disappear into this landscape. This seems like a lot of garbage to me, but the number disappoints Perry. "Four years ago, we were getting way more, six thousand tons a day, maybe. It was nice."

"Nice?"

"Yeah, we were making overtime."

We drive past potato chip bags and crushed milk gallons, submerged pizza boxes and Styrofoam takeout containers. Stray shoes, tangled hoses, crushed cardboard—there are so many colors, but it is hard to focus on any one thing. The garbage melts together, until all I can see are plastic bags, so many wispy white plastic bags. "It's too bad, all that plastic. Never biodegrades," says Perry.

"Does *anything* biodegrade here?" I ask. That our trash would biodegrade once we throw it back into the earth, that all of our banana peels and coloring books might just dissolve into humus as millions of microorganisms work their magic, is an idea that calms a worried environmentalist's soul. It is, unfortunately, not true. The aerobic microorganisms that might eat our garbage require sunlight and oxygen to thrive—both scarce resources under packed earth.

Perry shakes his head. "Not really. When those UA folks came over here a few years back, they found a newspaper from 1969. You could still read the front page."

These UA folks are a group of archaeologists who spent over two decades sorting through Tucson's garbage, assembling the most comprehensive record, then and since, of what garbage in the United Sates is made of. A team of hearty graduate students excavated landfills and foraged through Dumpsters, cataloging every item they found. Published in *Rubbish!: The Archeology of Garbage,* the itemized list offers a portal of revelations that extends for more than four pages. The students found Cocktail Mix (carbonated) and Cocktail Mix (noncarb, liquid); Dry Cleaning (laundry also) and Clothing Care Items (shoe polish, thread). Some items came with notes—Potato Peel (note: *Do* not *count peels; weigh them as a group*). Some seemed impossible—Popsicle—and others nonsensical—Slops. TV Dinners (also pot pies) and Electrical Appliance and Items.

MY MICROWAVE SCOWLS AT ME from its perch on the counter as I drink lukewarm coffee and wonder what to do with this corpse of food processing. As I chew over its untimely death, I wonder if my frustration is simply with our disposable culture, in which the objects we accumulate are no longer significant. When a microwave or a refrigerator was expected to last a lifetime, its purchase contained a certain amount of psychological weight. When eating a tomato required waiting until June—when it required, perhaps, planting seeds in March and watering through April and May—its consumption carried more deliberation. When another tomato is always available, that single one that you brought home from a great big pile of them suddenly seems much more disposable.

Today, our industrial food system considers soil inexhaustible, agriculture as conquerable, and food as disposable. If your diet consists of cheap, processed food that doesn't really fill you up, food suddenly seems less valuable—which is maybe why we as a country now throw away 40 percent of our food.

After visiting the landfill, I'm suddenly hyperaware of all the things—cans, cardboard canisters, yogurt tubs, and, well, microwaves—that are cast out from my kitchen. If I'm trying to unprocess my food, I must also reckon with all the *stuff* that surrounds it.

Finally, after a few days of scowling back at the dark microwave, it dawns on me that I don't *have* to buy a new microwave. I've never not had a microwave, but now that I have a microwave that doesn't work, I realize I don't need one. A microwave is not a processed food, but it seems to be an emblem of process as it glows, spins, clanks, and hypnotizes. A microwave prepares Lean Cuisines without supervision, cooks puddles of pasta or hunks of chicken huddled in floppy plastic containers. It bursts open kernels of bright yellow popcorn in a ninety-second ecstasy of noise.

Before the potato incident, my microwave whirred only when I wanted to reheat leftovers, cook oatmeal, or transform my morning coffee into a piping-hot affair; and these functions could easily be accomplished in one of my two heavy steel stove pots, enameled in a bright seventies-era blue, the powder blue of a bad prom suit. My dad bought them when he was in graduate school, and during my third year of college, when I was moving into my first apartment and my mom was cleaning out her kitchen, I claimed them as my own.

As I look around my kitchen, I realize that my parents have supplied me with most of my kitchenware in the years since I'd moved out. I acquired my dishes, a ceramic set from Crate & Barrel painted with blue and yellow swirls, when my mom got a new set. The silverware was my grandmother's, my mom's mom. Even the microwave was a hand-me-down, a relic from my sister's first apartment. It is only the odd frying pan or cutting board that I've chosen to buy myself. While this generational thrift has saved me money—has saved more stuff from being bought—it occurs to me that as things break or obsolesce, it's up to me to decide how I want to populate my kitchen.

EVEN IF I DON'T WANT A NEW MICROWAVE, I still have to figure out what to do with the old one. When humans lived as hunter-gatherers, we just left our trash where it fell and moved on; as we settled down, we had to figure out how to get rid of the piles accumulating around us. It's as true now as it was then: If you have something you don't want, you can burn it, bury it, or turn it into something new and different.

The first public garbage management program in the country began sweeping New York City's streets clean in 1895, when George E. Waring Jr. was appointed as the city's street-cleaning commissioner; twenty years later, 80 percent of cities in the United States offered municipal waste collection. In the late 1960s and early 1970s, "buyback" centers began taking recyclable products in exchange for a small payout; today, determined to absolve ourselves of our waste, more than nine thousand municipalities across the country operate curbside recycling programs that "recover" nearly 35 percent of all solid waste generated.

Everything that goes into my blue curbside recycling bin goes into a big blue truck, which joins a line of other blue trucks unloading their contents at Tucson's Materials Recovery Facility, or MRF, pleasantly pronounced *murf*, where a mess of mixed material becomes crushed blocks of sorted commodities. In between, there are ninety-seven conveyor belts, dozens of steel magnets, and a plethora of sorters—screen, optical, and human. There are twenty-two of the last kind—twenty-two focused faces, bent backs, trained eyes watching over whirring conveyor belts, pulling out items that can't be recycled. They pull out grocery-store bags and Styrofoam containers, which can be recycled but not cost-effectively. Wet paper can't be recycled, and neither can shoes or sofas, garden hoses or Christmas lights, mattresses or dogs.

"Wait," I ask Augie, the scale operator at the Tucson MRF. "People put *dogs* in their recycling?"

"Yeah, it seems like we go through phases when we get a lot of mattresses and animals."

"How? Or—why?"

"People see a bin on the street, they'll throw anything in it," says Augie. "Just last Friday, one of my guys found a dog on the tipping line. It sure stunk up the place."

These twenty-two sorters process fifty thousand pounds of recyclables every hour. The turnover is incredible—it's unbelievable, actually, how much stuff whirs past a single sorter bent over a single conveyor belt. Watching it all, I realize how little notice I pay to the stuff I throw in my recycling bin— plastic, cardboard, glass—as I assume that someone, somewhere down the line, will figure out what to do with it all. This is down the line, one that ends when a baler crushes the sorted material into dense rectangles. "We sell the blocks, just like that," says Augie.

"To who?"

"Depends. The paper and card goes to a Chinese company called ACN. Most of the aluminum goes to Anheuser-Busch. Some plastic goes to Universal Commodities, in New York. But really, it depends on the market. We ship globally."

Although the word "recovery" in the name implies some sort of processing, most MRFs are simply sorting facilities. I'm disappointed that I don't get to see recyclables being recycled, to see them smashed and melted, squeezed and shaped into new life. I wanted to see the reason we recycle—to subvert obsolescence by offering new life to our death-dated goods.

As I'm walking out the door, I ask, "Do you accept appliances for recycling?"

"If a toaster or an iron comes through, we'll process them," says Augie. "But we don't accept refrigerators or freezers, washers or driers."

"What about, say, microwaves?" I ask—just a hypothetical.

"Nope," he says. "Too big."

WHEN JUNE HITS TUCSON, it is hot, it has always been hot, and it will always be hot. Colors tremble under the stern sun; exhausted, they fade into the hot, hard quiet of dry afternoons. I bike across campus as the sun accumulates thick on my skin, lock my bike in coveted shade, and fold myself into a frigid office building. The temperature hits 110, and then crawls on up, to 111, 112. It's so hot that more clothes seem to be the solution, draped layers of white fabric instead of sundresses that leave thin-skinned shoulders exposed.

My microwave has lived in the trunk of my Civic ever since I toured Tucson's recycling center. Without its hulk to occupy my counters, my food life settles into an easy equilibrium. In the mornings, I fill myself with a fruit and yogurt smoothie and pile my lunch into a Tupperware, some combination of grains, beans, and whatever vegetables linger from a week's CSA share. My dinners cook themselves, so bursting is the bounty brimming from my burlap bags—sweet corn and insane tomatoes, eggplant and squash, cucumbers and watermelon. In hot evenings, after late sunsets, I slice the watermelon in thick triangles, fat like double-decker sandwiches, and sit cross-legged on my couch as I slurp cold sweetness and read book after book, plowing through a summer's reading list in a matter of weeks. On Sunday evenings, I soak big batches of beans and simmer them on the stovetop for a week's lunches; if I make chickpeas, then I eat chickpeas all week. I make yogurt, warming a half gallon of milk in a saucepot on the stove, swaddling it with a towel in a warm oven, and delighting when I wake up to a creamy solid.

I eat unprocessed not by intention but by habit, not by choice but by cadence. Just as northern populations bunker down into winter, Minneapolis and Milwaukee girding themselves against subzero temperatures in January, in Tucson, it is June that sends us indoors, settles us down. All nonessential tasks are pushed to a cooler date.

As the six-month mark of my year unprocessed approaches, I feel at ease, complacent, but also like I have barely begun. I've figured out unprocessed in the day-to-day, how to fill myself for breakfast, lunch, dinner, and dessert, but there are so many processes I have yet to crack. I still don't know how milk is pasteurized or grapes fermented, although I've long since decided to consume both. I like eating unprocessed—how it makes me examine all my inputs— but, as empty streets simmer in the sweltering sun, I feel like I haven't yet figured out the bigger picture.

In mid-June, Tucson's Food Conspiracy Co-op is cornered by construction. The City of Tucson is building a streetcar through the heart of downtown and up eclectic Fourth Avenue, lined with gift shops like Pop Cycle and a bar called the Surly Wench. As construction crews lay tracks and we await public transit, the streets are closed and local stores struggle to keep their doors open.

It costs $180 to join the Food Conspiracy Co-op. One hundred and eighty up front and then an extra fifty cents or a dollar here and there, an accumulation of five or ten dollars per trip. Which is precisely why I'd resisted joining for so long. Distance from home and price premiums; the parking was a pain and there were always gray-haired hippies who clogged up the lines with their little bags full of spirulina crunchies.

But then, on a chance evening in June, I hear Kimber Lanning tell Tucsonans to "spend money better" by spending it locally, keeping it close and accountable; and it feels like a revelation. The phrase offers us a way to do something here and now, on our own time and in our own way—something that will reverberate and accumulate with the things that other people might do, elsewhere.

Money multiplies, Kimber says, and the money I wasn't spending locally—

the money I was still spending at Trader Joe's—was multiplying somewhere else, somewhere I couldn't see or know. According to a study by Local First, if you spend $100 at a local business, $73 of it will stay in your community, meeting payrolls, covering rent, creating accountability; spend that same money at a national corporation and only $43 sticks around. Cooperatives purchase 20 percent of the goods they sell from local sources, compared to less than 6 percent at conventional grocers. At cooperatives, employees make more money—about a dollar more an hour than the average supermarket employee—and they more frequently get health care.

Of more immediate relevance to the quest that had taken over my summer, food cooperatives often offer products wrapped in significantly less packaging than foods sold at conventional supermarkets. Since I visited the landfill and the MRF, I can't stop seeing packages. Yogurt poured into thick plastic cylinders; bread shrink-wrapped and then wrapped yet again; dried pasta packed in a plastic bag inside a cardboard box. Trader Joe's baby beets come shrink-wrapped in stretchy plastic and boxed in cardboard; organic, heirloom tomatoes are sold in hard plastic clamshells. Organic food contained by inorganic matter.

The bulk bin section at the back corner of the Tucson Co-op is a U-shaped array of colors. Almonds and oatmeal, pepper and cumin, rice long-stemmed and short, beans black and white. There's a ten-gallon drum of honey. A grinding gear that rumbles and crunches whole almonds into almond butter. You can buy a reusable plastic container or bring your own and weigh it at the front before you fill it up.

Buying in bulk offers the bargain of bulk pricing without the excess of thick containers. Dried garbanzo beans sold from a bulk bin don't have to be branded, which cuts down on a lot of cardboard and ink. You can decide whether to get them home in a plastic or burlap bag, and then remember to bring that package back to the store with you. It also makes sense to buy more food per package for the same reason spaghetti gets cold quickly—surface area to volume. The more volume, the less package per unit. Case in point: A study of a food cooperative in Michigan found that selling a pound of olive oil in bulk reduced solid waste by more than a third of a pound.

For both the makers and buyers of food, packaging, specifically of the plastic variety, serves many useful purposes. It protects products from damage, both en route and in store; it protects against spoilage, keeps our foods safe and clean, and conveys information. Packaging is the "skin of commerce," writes Daniel Imhoff in *Paper or Plastic: Searching for Solutions to an Overpackaged World*. But packaging also "plays the role of divider and conqueror, transforming us from local regions of bulk-buying citizens into a world of more than six million individually targeted, single portion customers," writes Imhoff. Plastic, at least as we currently employ it, is the emblematic substance of planned obsolescence. It takes millions of years to build the monomers that make up plastics, millions more to break them down, and yet often only minutes to fulfill their useful lives carrying our food or drink.

We have come a long way from the turn-of-the-century grocer measuring portions of dried goods to a waiting housewife. In the aisles of a modern supermarket, instead of interacting with counter clerks, with bakers or butchers, now our primary conversation is with a package. We converse with packages and leave them as legacies in our landfills—according to the EPA, containers and packaging make up a third of municipal solid waste.

I wonder if we have started to think of dollars in the same way we think of trash. We send our money in exchange for something we want—often with the simple swipe of plastic, without the physical reminder of a dollar departed—and we don't have to think about what becomes of it. How it influences the contours of our landscape, the shape of our cities.

On the second Friday in June, in addition to a 20 percent discount for anyone who spends more than $150, new co-op members get a free water bottle. The cluttered store teems with people, evidence that I was not the only Tucsonan who decided the prospect of a free water bottle was the appropriate incentive to pony up $180.

I traverse the small store four or five times, wandering up and down its aisles without rhyme or reason, flitting from produce to dairy back to produce and then on to dried goods. I fill a reusable plastic squeeze bottle full of amber honey that oozes out of a shiny metal drum. I fill plastic baggies, vowing to reuse them, with coconut shavings and tamari-spiced almonds; dried beans and lentils. I stock up on cacao powder for the next round of chocolate making and buy a pound—an inordinate amount—of sea salt.

I'm delighted when I find milk sold in a returnable glass bottle; when I find tofu sold in bulk, sans packaging. I fill my cart with three apples, two egg-plants, and a bundle of dandelion greens. When I get to the register, while the ice crystals on a giant bag of frozen peaches puddle on the conveyor belt, I fill out a form and swipe my credit card to purchase a small share of this locally run cooperative. I'd expected to be stressed to lose this $180. In reality, it feels like a contribution.

"No I wouldn't try fixing it yourself," says Neil, an employee manning the front desk at RISE Equipment Recycling Center in Tucson. He shakes his head, at a loss as to how to council me. "The voltage those things pack, it can be really dangerous."

"No," I say quickly. "No, *I'm* not going to repair it. I just want to know if someone theoretically *could*."

Even if it does not pay to repair or recycle my microwave, I am flabber-gasted that it cannot be done, and so I have ventured down to RISE on a fact-finding mission to see if I can find a new home for either the machine or its component parts. The narrow aisles of the cluttered retail store are full of refurbished machinery: round-backed TVs, large-button telephones, DVD players—thirty dollars apiece—and, on a shelf near the back, three dinged microwaves—twenty dollars each. At RISE, a nonprofit subsidiary of COPE Community Services, volunteers spend time and energy on junk. Discarded junk that becomes, once again, electronics—electronics that are sold, deeply discounted, to low-income people who might not be able to afford the machines sold on the front end of obsolescence.

Neil sighs. "Well, you see," he says, "microwaves are really hard to fix. Most people can't do it. But Tim, our electrician, he can fix stuff because he has magic fingers."

"Oh?"

Neil nods, solemn.

"Can I meet him?

"He's not here. But you can come back when he is."

When I return to RISE, Ruben Vejar, the center's manager, gives me a tour around the facilities, through the retail store and then into the guts, a sprawling warehouse of dormant electronics, dusty and silent-faced. Piles of VHS tapes, crates of cables, rows of speakers, islands of office chairs. Outside, across an expansive sorting lot, volunteers untangle the guts of computers and fill crates with motherboards, graphics cards, chips, and disk drives.

At RISE, that which can be fixed is not limited by the capability of the repairman but by cost. "We don't spend too much time trying to fix stuff when the parts cost more than the thing itself is worth," Ruben says. Three-quarters of the stuff that comes in can't be fixed—or rather, it won't be. It's not cost-effective to buy an eighty-dollar part to fix a forty-dollar microwave that'll be sold for twenty.

When we circle back into the retail store, I follow Ruben back into one of the repair rooms. Several middle-aged men bend over the glow of a computer screen. "This here's Serge, he's our programming genius," Ruben says. "And that's Carol, she's a volunteer." Carol looks up and smiles. A man walks out of an adjacent room carrying a Panasonic Toughbook. "That there's Tim," Ruben says. I extend my hand in greeting. Tim's magic fingers are attached to a mid-sixties man wearing a Relay for Life T-shirt. Shaggy hair juts out from a white baseball cap. "He can fix anything," says Ruben.

So I ask him. "Can you fix a microwave?"

"Oh, sure," he says. "With microwaves, either it's a fuse or a safety switch on it. Standard type of switch. They sell fast here. There are a lot of people, poor people, you know, who need a microwave to make their food."

I nod, surprised by his honesty. "What makes something unfixable?"

"Only if the parts are too expensive. If it's really outdated." He smiles a wily kind of smile. "Or if I'm not around."

By the time I bike home and drive back to RISE, the small storefront is closed. Neil had told me I could leave my microwave outside the donations center, but I am skeptical—though what a disappointment it would be if stolen, a microwave that won't even cook your potatoes. Still, I cannot carry this microwave around any longer, so I heave the black box out from the trunk and place it carefully against the white cinder-block wall of the squat donation center. The microwave looks vulnerable and out of place on the hot expanse of parking-lot asphalt as I drive away.

I wonder if the broken objects of our lives are simply collateral damage of our life's haste. We rush to and fro and in our hurry we knock glasses and slam doors and break microwaves because we are unwilling to wait, to do things deliberately. To commit to our choices. While London's plan was not enacted into law, today we are indeed surrounded by his piles of junk. We are surrounded by disposables and left with the tired legacy of those who believed the earth to be inexhaustible.

ON A SATURDAY EVENING a couple of weeks later, I'm sitting around a cast-iron table at La Cocina, chatting with friends in the glow of twinkle lights, microbrew in hand. Noam, a thoughtful, balanced, foodie friend, asks me how my unprocessed adventure is unfolding. I tell him about the microwave's death, my jubilant purchase of a SodaStream home soda maker—no more plastic bottles for my bubbles—and how I am now scheming to buy a food processor. Katie and Tyler own the most basic Cuisinart model and claim it as their most-used kitchen appliance.

Noam nods and says, quite without judgment, in the light way of curious people, "I wonder if at some point you'll have to consider all the processes you bring into your kitchen to unproccess it."

I pause. I say, "Huh."

He shrugs, smiles, and the conversation carries on. I nod and move on—to my left, Sarah leans in and says, "I found the cutest house. I think we might be moving."

So I forget about the food processor until the next day, until I survey my kitchen and wonder: Did I really *need* a food processor to eat unprocessed? I'd just gotten rid of my microwave, after all. Could I make do with something a little less plastic?

The antithesis of the food processor—or rather, its antecedent—is a mortar and pestle, which is what we used for thousands of years to pound corn into meal, grains into flour, and herbs into pesto. (Indeed, the word "pesto" comes from "pestle.") I send out a call on Facebook: Does anyone I know own a mortar and pestle and can I borrow it? Within the week, I am at Rani's house, holding her heavy stone set and trying to explain to her and her husband, Jay, why grinding my own peanut butter is a perfectly sensible thing to do.

"Maybe I'm just trying to prove a point," I say.

Rani laughs. Jay continues to sit on the couch, slightly less enthused than his wife by this weird intrusion into their Wednesday evening. "I swear, I've had that thing for ten years now, and every year I say I'm going to get rid of it," Rani says. "And then someone asks to borrow it!"

"What do you use it for?"

She shrugs. "I don't know, grinding herbs, I guess? Pesto, spice rubs."

When I get home, a cup of peanuts crowds into the stone basin. After a minute of crushing, the peanuts are reduced to a fine powder; after another few minutes of a pound-and-twist action, heavy on the wrist, the peanuts begin to cohere into a kind of paste. Pound, turn; pound, turn-twist. The paste begins to become a kind of butter—a knobby, disjointed butter that tastes sort of like peanut butter but doesn't coat the insides of my mouth with quite the same smoothness.

I spend a few weeks browsing Tucson's numerous secondhand shops with an eye for a processor, but to no avail. Browsing halfheartedly, it is true; buying a used food processor felt uncannily like buying secondhand underpants. And so I turn to the Internet and find that the only Tucson-based retailers that sell Cuisinart products are Target, Cost Plus World Market, and Sears. And, of course, there is Amazon.com, undercutting them all with a $75 Cuisinart DLC-2A Mini-Prep Plus Food Processor for $33.56.

The thing about planned obsolescence, about designing products that don't last, is that they are cheap. As my checking account swings from paycheck to paycheck, the cheapness of this legacy does not go unappreciated. I want to pay more for things that last—for goods made in my community—but it seems like every time I gear up to buy something of substance, my paycheck has dissolved into rent and electricity, locally grown groceries and a couple amber ales on Saturday night.

I couldn't afford a plastic food processor if I had to pay for all the externalities ingrained in its production. If its price reckoned with nature's limits, with all the fossil fuels embedded in its polycarbonate, it would be out of my reach. Low price, high quality—isn't that what we all want? After the first Cuisinart debuted in 1973 at Chicago's National Housewares Exhibition, the new food processor promised, in the words of a sales pamphlet, that "the highest level of raw materials and engineering have been employed to make your Food Processor the finest quality machine at the most reasonable possible price."

I can't even consider the finest-quality food processor. I earn less than $1,200 a month; that a food processor is being sold for $34 is a relief. It is indeed the promise of economies of scale—that there will be an abundance of goods that don't cost us very much money. It doesn't even feel like a defeat when I click purchase. Rather, it opens a cascade of new windows promising new food adventures. If I've chucked my dollars into the landfill of Amazon, at least there will be unprocessed salad dressing and homemade pesto.

An amazing two days later, the processor arrives, flouting its own irony as I pull it from a flurry of packaging. The brushed-chrome base emerges from the box pristine and poised. An S-shaped, stainless-steel blade slips over the three-cup plastic bowl and locks the unit in place with a quiet *thunk*. A cup of peanuts again crowds together, awaiting their lacerations. One hand holding the top in place, I push grind. The blade whirs to life and hums merry circles. The peanuts crunch and crumble, thrum and thud. Two minutes later, all of the peanut bits have been siphoned into a whirlpool of spinning beige. A minute later, a silver spoon collects a warm bundle of creamy pulverized peanuts.

I had thought, while mash-grind-twisting peanuts into a sort-of paste, that limiting my consumption of peanut butter to the manually prepared might be a handy way to limit my consumption of peanut butter in general. Patience before craving. But I realize, spreading the warm butter over my tongue and into the corners of my mouth, it is precisely because of this craving that I should not use a mortar and pestle to make peanut butter. While the logic of working for your treats makes sense for most of the hours of our lives, it fails at very particular moments—say, in the face of 2 A.M. hunger. There is a day or two every month in which I simply must eat peanut butter by the heaping spoonful, and these are days when I have no interest to stand in my kitchen slamming a pestle.

And, my sister is right—the food processor soon becomes my kitchen's favorite device. When a profusion of dill arrives in my CSA, I blend it up with garlic, olive oil, balsamic vinegar, and mustard, provisioning a jar in my fridge with a week's worth of salad dressing (dressing that does not contain, it's worth mentioning, maltodextrin, hydrolyzed soy protein, or monosodium glutamate). I roast a big batch of green chilies, sweet corn, and tomatoes and spin them into a spicy-sweet salsa. I make pesto from anything green—basil and dandelion greens in the summer; kale and Swiss chard later in the fall.

When I pile chunks from two frozen bananas, a tablespoon of cacao powder, and a heap of almond butter into the food processor, I'm skeptical they will cohere into anything resembling frozen yogurt, as a post on Pinterest has promised me that they will. After the first few pulses, the bananas become grainy beads, the powder fluffs into the lid, and the butter sticks to the sides. But I keep faith, and after a minute on grind, the disparate banana suddenly turns smooth. The almond butter gathers and grabs. The cacao powder spreads and dissolves, turning the whole spinning circle into a creamy chocolate brown. A spoonful reveals that my fellow pinner did not lie—this might be *better* than FroYo.

There is space in our lives and in our kitchens to compromise between instant gratification and responsibility, between convenience and consequence. A food processor feels like an appropriate middle ground, somewhere between a mortar and pestle and a microwave. I give up the microwave because it's easy to, and I keep the food processor because it's useful—because it allows me to be intentional and careful about processing my foods at home, a practice that is, for so many, becoming obsolete.

Unprocess Yourself: Stuff

Putting so much energy into examining the foods I bought forced me to also examine the *things* I bought. Buying unprocessed starts with being an unprocessed consumer, which for me means acting as if the things I bought were the things everyone bought, as if the choices I made were the choices everyone made. If I didn't buy toilet paper made from recycled paper, who would? If I didn't buy chemical-free cleaning products, then, I decided, the companies who make those products might deduce that there simply isn't a market for sustainably produced cleaners.

When I learned about planned obsolescence, I took a deep, dark detour into plastics. Convinced that they were processing my foods by slow, toxic leach, I spent a frantic two weeks trying to eliminate plastics from my life. *Plastic Free* by Beth Terry is a great starting point; so is the documentary *Bag It*. I splurged on a SodaStream to save on plastic bottles full of soda water. (Target accepts and recycles spent carbon dioxide cartridges.) I bought stainless-steel storage containers for storing leftovers and packing lunches and finally invested in several stainless-steel coffee tumblers for my to-go beverages.

It's worth mentioning that my favorite Local First Arizona study—the one that shows that a 10 percent shift in spending to local businesses could create $140 million in new revenue for a city the size of Tucson—applies to *all* goods and services, not just food. If we want to build strong, sustainable communities, then spending money better applies not only to eggs and vegetables but also earrings and handbags. Seek out local businesses for any wares that can be produced locally.

Pesto is reason enough to buy a food processor. It's both insanely easy to make and outrageously more expensive to buy—and a great way to use up any green things you have piling up in your fridge. If you're using winter greens, roughly chop and either sauté or blanch before adding to your food processor. Add garlic, lemon juice, a generous amount of olive oil, and any nuts you happen to have lying around—pine nuts are superexpensive, so I usually use walnuts (almonds tend to be a little too hard). Pulse until the mixture becomes smooth, and store in the refrigerator for up to three days, or in the freezer for up to a year.

7

OUT

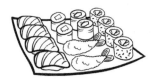

Try your best.

My date, Dustin, orders the tempura before I have a chance to say otherwise. He has blazing blue eyes—broad shoulders, a solid six-four—and so, when asked, I agreed to meet him for happy hour, thinking drinks not dinner. But he swiped the menu before I'd glanced over it, swiftly ordering an eel-avocado roll and vegetable tempura with the kind of assuming male authority that hinted at future incompatibility. Blazing blue eyes aside, of course.

We make small talk—work, weather, news—while an unprocessed debate rages within me. Do I tell him now? Wait for the food to come? Feign such fullness that a mere nibble of a flour-battered vegetable will push me over the edge? I could fake vegetarianism—that'd get me out of the sugar-glazed eel roll, at least, but I don't know how to avoid the tempura without becoming the Girl Who Doesn't Eat.

I hadn't figured out how to go on an unprocessed date before now because I hadn't needed to. I wasn't *not* dating; I was just reading and writing. No one interesting demanded my attention, so I kept reading and writing, happily ensconced in my apartment, comfortably attired in marvelous sweatpants. And then June arrived and with it summer, the stifling skin-exposed summer of the desert, and somewhere in the restlessness of hundred-degree days and breezy nights, it became time to get back into my body—to put my body back in conversation with another's.

The problem of an unprocessed date is the problem of an unprocessed social life. We convene around food and drink. We convene to do other things, too—around work, or the arts; around movement and sport—but for the most part, across the world, food and drink are the nucleus around which our social lives orbit.

All too soon our waitress returns. She approaches with two platters held at right angles like oven mitts on beseeching hands: a platter piled high in deep-fried vegetables and a plate dotted with syrup-slathered eel and avocado rolls. She slides the two plates to the middle of the table. Dustin slides a small plate over to me. He gestures—ladies first. I pause. The waitress pauses. Dustin looks at me. The waitress looks at me. I look at the pile of tempura.

IN THE MOVIE *NOTTING HILL*, Hugh Grant plays a foppish midthirties British bloke who owns a travel bookstore. Hugh's character stutters, all floppy brown hair and rumpled oxford shirts and skinny, slouching charm. About an hour in, Hugh has survived a very painful breakup and believes he will be alone for the rest of his life. So begins the montage of blind dates: the same dinner table, the same companions—best friend and best friend's wife—and a series of increasingly nutty women. The culmination comes when a perky, pigtailed woman named Keziah refuses a platter of woodcock.

"No, thank you," she says. "I'm a fruitarian."

Hugh looks at her and exhales a polite, "Oh." Then, "What is a fruitarian, exactly?"

"We believe fruits and vegetables have feelings," she says. "So we think cooking is cruel. We only eat things that have actually fallen from the tree or bush and are, in fact, dead already."

Hugh's jaunty smile fades from his face and he stammers around for a bit. "Ah. Well. All right." He pauses. "So these carrots?"

His date nods, and looks away with a grimace. "Have been murdered."

I STARE AT THE TEMPURA, Dustin and the waitress stare at me. A TV buzzes quietly in the corner over Dustin's left shoulder—it *is* a nice shoulder, bound by muscle and a blue polo shirt. The waitress stands at the edge of our booth—what is she still doing here? Finally, I can take it no longer. As I pull one of the two small round plates toward me and select a small piece of tempura and a single eel roll, I formulate the unprocessed dating clause, a clause that allows a murdered carrot in the name of socialization. Released, finally, by my action, Dustin quickly loads his own plate with several rolls and a piece of tempura.

"What do you write about?" he asks.

"Right now I'm writing a lot about food."

"Cool," he says. "Like restaurant reviews?"

"Sort of. I'm interested in how our food systems affect the climate."

He nods and thinks this over. "Do you think this whole climate change thing is going to catch on?"

"What do you mean?"

"You know, 'global warming'?" His voice wears italics and, though his hands don't leave the table, his fingers become bobbing quotation marks. "The idea that the world is warming."

"Well." I consider a few phrases, examine a few sentences, and finally settle on: "It is."

"Maybe, but not because of us. The earth's temperatures have fluctuated throughout the Holocene. The increase we're witnessing now is no more drastic than past variations." As Dustin starts explaining why the "idea" of global warming is a hoax foisted upon us by Wall Street traders, I lose focus. I watch as the tempura collapses into a soggy pile of vegetables and crumbled batter; the rice kernels of the final eel roll become brittle and dry, slowly tumbling to the ceramic plate.

"And the best part is, when we left, he said he wanted to go out again!" I tell my sister, when I get home and call to report that I've just gone out with a climate denier.

"How did you meet him?" she asks.

"A coffee shop."

"Climate deniers drink coffee?"

"Evidently."

"You need a better screening process," she says.

"How do you screen for 'acceptance of climate change'?" I ask.

By the time I hang up the phone and gleefully return to my pajamas and the couch, I realize that an unprocessed dating clause is a total cop-out. Allowing myself a nibble of something that I have committed a year of my life to avoiding simply because I want to save face—because I want to make a good first impression on someone who very well may turn out to be a buffoon—is an evasion of what felt so important about this project in the first place.

Unprocessed is like global warming, or some microcosm of it, anyway. How could I talk about something as big as global warming—so crazy as unprocessed—on something so small as a first date? And yet, how can I *not*? For those of us who live in the desert Southwest—indeed, for all of those who live in extreme climates around the world—it is impossible to ignore the fact that annual temperatures and precipitation levels have already swerved far away from the norm.

Part of the point of forgoing processed foods is to take a small stand against the inertia of a popular narrative that has handed us these foods in the first place. I don't feel awkward or prissy when someone offers me a cigarette and I say, "I don't smoke," even when sixty years ago, this refusal would have been considered peculiar. An unprocessed dating clause allowed me to dodge precisely the attitude I wanted to cultivate—that not eating processed foods was just what I did, a new way to imagine normalcy. An unprocessed dating clause undermined the premise of the project: Small decisions *can* accumulate into something big.

Just as "acceptance of global warming" becomes a dating prerequisite I never knew I needed, I decide that eating unprocessed will become a screen to filter out the uninteresting or unimaginative.

MY FIRST UNPROCESSED MEAL IN A RESTAURANT was with Hilary and Sarah at Pita Jungle, an organic sort of restaurant chain in Arizona. Hilary worked at a Phoenix location when she attended Arizona State University and says, "I think they'll be friendly to your endeavor," when she calls to suggest we swap a potluck for an evening out and treat ourselves to matching silverware and proper water glasses.

I hadn't been to a restaurant for the first month of unprocessed eating—busy, broke, and anxious about venturing into unknown territory with unidentified ingredients. When I told Hilary about my apprehension about bringing unprocessed into a restaurant, she said, "Yeah, I know. But we haven't seen you for weeks!"

I moved to Tucson knowing no one, and Sarah and Hilary were my first friends. They were simply women I knew, quick acquaintances for passing conversations, until I invited them over to my apartment to make pizza. Although I was thrilled to leave Los Angeles when I finally was offered an escape, my excitement was quiet. I had just found my way out of an ill-fitting relationship, a too-tight shoe that blisters so slowly you don't notice it until the skin breaks. I moved out of the apartment I shared with drama-absorbed roommates and drove to the desert, sinking into a thick relief as soon as I saw my first saguaro, blinking with wide eyes through my first dark desert night. My traffic-tensed shoulders relaxed as I padded through the hushed apartment I could rent for myself, neat and mine alone.

It was awkward, at first, to invite Sarah and Hilary over, but as soon as they arrived, shuffled off their shoes, and crowded into my tiny kitchen; when we began to measure flour, spill olive oil, scoop cheese, and simmer sauce; after we had sipped wine and listened while the oven clanged: Something clicked. Moving to a new town is always a hard thing, and I remember that night, over hot pizza and burned tongues, something shifted or cohered. I called my mom the following day and announced: "I have friends!"

When we drove out to Pita Jungle, I was nervous for a different reason. I looked at the menu online before I left but ended up with more questions than solutions. I knew to avoid refined grains—pastas and sandwiches were out—as well as sweet sauces and marinades—no teriyaki tofu for me—but what about all of the additives that were unknowable?

I was nervous about going to Pita Jungle because, in the words of Samuel Johnson, "Abstinence is as easy to me as temperance would be difficult." I'd first encountered the line, in Gretchen Rubin's best-selling book *The Happiness Project,* with a flash of self-recognition. People are, Rubin writes, either abstainers or moderators. When trying to change a habit, conventional wisdom says to take it slowly, bit by bit—be moderate. Go to the holiday party, but eat only one appetizer. Don't deprive yourself; eat dessert occasionally. But for Rubin—for Johnson, for me—abstaining is the easier choice. "If I never do something, it requires *no* self-control for me; if I do something sometimes, it requires *enormous* self-control," writes Rubin, and indeed, if my year unprocessed has shown anything, it is that my personality is that of an abstainer. I wanted my year to be *perfectly* unprocessed, no ifs, ands, or buts slinking in unawares.

After our server had presented us with water and three iced teas, I began my bombardment. "Do you know if the sauce on the chipotle chicken has sugar in it? What about your salad dressings—are they made in-house?" When the server nodded, I ventured one more question: "Do you know what they're made with?" To this, I'd gotten a look that said clearly, *Whaddaya mean?* "Like, the honey vinaigrette? Is it made with honey?" She didn't know, but if I *really* wanted her to, she would go in the back and ask.

"What are you guys going to order?" I asked Sarah and Hilary when our waitress has departed.

"Veggie burger," said Sarah.

"Salad, not sure which," said Hilary. "You?"

"I don't know! Everything has sugar in it! The organic chicken breast with steamed veggies seems like the safest bet, but I'm not really eating meat. I wonder what's in the marinade."

"Yeah," Hilary said, contemplating my conundrum. "I mean, you'll never know the exact ingredients of *everything*."

"I suppose," I said. "But that seems crazy."

After our waitress returned to inform us that the honey vinaigrette was sweetened by sugar rather than honey and I'd asked, "Do you know where you get your whole-grain hamburger buns?" her cheerful demeanor began to crack. Finally, I ordered a grilled vegetable salad: sautéed vegetables, tomato, garlic, and ginger on a bed of mixed greens with house-made lemon vinaigrette.

As soon as they handed their menus back to the waitress, Sarah and Hilary turned to catch up: Why was Hilary's ex-boyfriend flying out to Tucson and will he soon be a non-ex? As they chatted, I sipped my unsweetened iced tea, my frazzled brain turning over all of the unprocessed options of my order until finally I realized: I should have skipped the dressing entirely. Should have just asked for oil and vinegar. Of course, I'd just entirely missed Hilary's analysis of Andrew's pending visit, but if I could just catch the waitress's attention, maybe it wouldn't be too late. When Hilary saw me peering over her shoulder, she said, sternly, "Megan. Your order is *fine*. I'm sure it's unprocessed."

"But what about the salad dressing?"

"What about it? What if they marinated your veggies in high-fructose corn syrup before grilling? You're never going to be able to know *everything* in your food. I think you did the best you could."

"You think?" I said, finally returning my focus to her face.

"Yes," she said, as confident as I was faltering. "Besides, you just ordered a fifteen-dollar salad. I think your best bet at this point is just to enjoy it."

INDEED, PART OF THE POINT of unprocessed was to find more joy in food—joy and connection, both to food's source and also with the people around the table. Just enjoy it: a simple command that's so hard to follow. Especially when eating out, when food is richer, portions bigger, and ingredients harder to trace.

At home, I know exactly what goes into my food. I know that the extra-virgin olive oil I cook with is *actually* extra-virgin olive oil and that my aged balsamic vinegar hasn't been aged alongside food coloring or thickeners.

Out in the world—or at a Sustainability in Higher Education conference in Phoenix—it's impossible to know if the brown-spackled tortilla wraps stacked on plastic trays on a long foldout table are *actually* made with whole-wheat tortillas, as their little sign declares; if the vegetables that fill them are organic and the hummus holding it all together is additive-free. A best practice for eating unprocessed is: If you don't know what's in it, don't eat it. This advice, as it turns out, is not super helpful when you're standing in a buffet line in front of your boss; when you've been stuck in the same over-air-conditioned conference room since 8 A.M. and won't be let out until 5 P.M. Best practices suggest you bring a bag of trail mix and an apple in your purse, but reality suggests that this bag of trail mix might not sustain you until you get home at seven. So you take a wrap and return to your table. (And you always offer to share your trail mix.)

When I am not stuck in a conference room in Phoenix; when I'm at home, cooking for others, or when others cook for me, food is so much more delightful than it's ever been. When a friend invites me over for vegetarian chili; when his girlfriend makes jalapeño corn bread and generously lists the ingredients—cornmeal, honey, butter, eggs, cream, and jalapeños—I'm inappropriately delighted. Perhaps because I'm now so accustomed to refraining from food—pizza at a brewery or cake on a coworker's birthday—I am ridiculously thrilled by shared food when I'm able to partake.

And after six months of unprocessed eating, my relationship to food has changed. I eat when I am hungry and stop when I'm full. I'm eating whole foods, so what I eat satisfies me—it lingers and sticks in my stomach. Full, I focus better, exercise stronger, and sleep deeper—my mind mulls over the possibility of dinner rather than the repercussions of lunch. As I feel more confidence in my grasp of *that which is processed,* I start to enjoy the expansiveness I'm allowed in that I can eat *anything* that is unprocessed.

But what about my relationship to my body? As I shed my sweatpants and don shorts and sundresses, I fret over how all my unprocessed enjoyment might be affecting my body's ability to enjoy clothes that still fit. I wonder, in spite of my reclamation of wheat, my delight in chocolate, if I am still settling into this new way of eating, of being with food. I weigh myself daily, watching for a shift in the tally of a body's accumulations. I let myself eat anything that's unprocessed, and yet still I worry that I'm eating too much of it.

But I'm trying. At a midsummer sale meant to turn our minds toward fall—a futile exertion in Tucson—I buy a stretchy black dress, cinched at the waist, and start wearing it so much that Sarah takes to calling it my "date dress."

WHEN I SHOW UP for the first seminar in a course about sustainable ranching in Arizona, I sit next to a dark-haired, dark-eyed, messenger-bag-adorned anthropologist. I run into him at the Tucson Food Co-op filling up on quinoa at the bulk bins, and then again, by chance, at Cartel Coffee, where we sip

espresso and work on our laptops, side by side. He says, "We should hang out."
We meet for a Monday-evening drink—in summer, there are no weekends—
and after I order a beer, Jonathan orders a gin and tonic. "Have I told you about
this?" he asks. "I'm not eating gluten. Or dairy."

I am impressed, thrilled to find his crazy-diet flag waving so soon.

"Why not?" I ask. "Are you intolerant?"

"Trying to figure it out," he says, running long fingers through thick hair. A
shaggy chunk falls back across his face as he picks up his drink and we walk
outside to the patio. "I've had issues for years, but before I moved to Tucson,
I was the manager of this locally sourced organic restaurant in San Francisco
and we got all sorts of people with these crazy high-maintenance diets. I didn't
want to be one of those people."

I start to say, "Funny you mention," but Jonathan keeps talking, talks for a
while about his Ph.D. program in anthropology, before the conversation finally
shifts back to me—to my writing, how I might just be one of "those people."

"Cool," he says. "Is it hard?"

"It's been fun, mostly," I say. "Sometimes hard, but fun. I make my own
chocolate now!"

"Why?" he asks. "I mean, awesome. But why?"

"There's refined white sugar and weird emulsifiers in all the bars they sell
in stores."

"Emulsifiers?"

"Um, like food binding agents. They hold the stuff together, make it so it
doesn't melt in the package."

"You going to teach me how to make chocolate?" he asks, raising his eyebrows and smiling. My stomach leaps. Jonathan is tall; he bikes, meditates,
and gardens. We will be perfect together!

"Of course," I say, smiling back.

Instead, Jonathan invites me to an underground supper club organized by a friend of his, a local chef. We each pay twenty-five dollars—so do a couple dozen other people, friends and friends of friends—and we sit together on a bale of hay in front of a long picnic table in his friend's backyard. We nibble on grilled corn on the cob, suck the meat off grilled artichokes. We eat portabello mushroom pizza and I quietly refrain from the molten chocolate cake that comes out for dessert.

After dinner, we bike back to Jonathan's place; we sit on the porch in his backyard, watching his chickens shuffle their feathers and sway in their chicken coop. He kisses me while they cluck their approval; when I leave, he hands me a paper bag full of freshly laid eggs.

"My aunt called me the other day," he tells me, over a date of coffee and chess. "She owns some land up in Northern California. She's looking for some-one to farm on it and I'm starting to think that someone should be me."

"Whoa. Sweet!"

He nods.

"How do you even do that?" I ask.

"I'd probably have to do a farm apprenticeship first."

Week after week, I had sat next to Jonathan in class and learned about the farmers and ranchers who are working to link wild ecosystems to domes-ticated food systems—about those farmers and ranchers who are taking a stand against monocultures and degraded land. Week after week, I'd scribbled notes about restoring riparian ecology, native pollinators, and crop biodiversity. Now, as Jonathan talks about farm apprenticeships, I glimpse the possibility of something else, some other future that does not involve struggling in a city or chasing a job around the country. Putting down roots. I fall head over heels for this dream, the romance of moving to a world of wet dirt and sprouting seeds. I'm enchanted as much with the idea of farming as I am with Jonathan. With *doing* the thing rather than just talking, writing, reading around it—leaving behind Safeway and cement freeways in exchange for farm stands and rocking rutted roads. I love the idea of being a practitioner rather than an observer peering in from the sidelines.

But this idea proves stronger than its reality. Jonathan's interest falters or it never quite focuses on me. He stops suggesting dates. When I finally ask him what's up, he says, "I'm just not feeling it. The chemistry's not there."

I feel ridiculous when I disagree—like I have fabricated the feeling of his kiss. Finally, I say, "I guess there's no sense forcing it."

He nods and says, "Cool, glad we can be mature about this."

It takes a few days of bruised ego moping and unprocessed brownie baking before I realize I hadn't fallen for Jonathan; I fell for his food, his farm, his hypothetical future, the fuzzy future we would forge together. We cared about the same things, so it was easy to imagine a future—forgetting, of course, that first we had to care about each other. The reality is trickier than the recipe. Any farmer would have seen it, how I'd ignored the wild game of chance that is coaxing sprout from seed.

Monoculture is not just a pattern of land use; it is a pattern of mind and body, a pattern of living. My impatience to enact change is the impatience of quick-fix farming. I dream of grand solutions, love at first sight, the sweet possibility of a life's changed course. Flight from city to farm, from a homogenous life to a weedy wild one. I tunnel vision on work, and when I am not working, I tunnel vision on play. I am gardening and then I am at the grocery store; driving and then working on my laptop. I wrap wire around the stakes of my mind, along the edges of my mental spaces; I mono-crop my own mind, segmenting thoughts like fence-rowed fields, and perhaps this is why I hadn't dated all year—because dating, I'd thought, took me away from the real work of my year, the work of unprocessing.

The promise of the chemical revolution, which brought fertilizers and pesticides to our fields, was the promise of convenience, of instant gratification and consistency across acres. The promise of monoculture has been to kill every wild thing in a field, save one. If there are lots of fields in a place, and each field contains one thriving wild thing, then collectively, across many fields—so goes the logic—there is an ecosystem diverse enough to remain healthy.

Unfortunately, save for the stalks of corn and hardy grains that thrive in this segmented system, wildlife does not work like a stack of LEGOs, each block clicking on top of the next to form a complete whole. A healthy wild ecosystem is like Play-Doh. It is smooth, supple, and cohesive, salty-sweet and pliant—until it isn't. Play-Doh is Play-Doh until it's not, until someone forgets to snap the lid shut or someone else leaves it near the oven; until it becomes brittle like cold cheese or hard like brown sugar. Play-Doh is like wildness because all it takes is one change, the right change, and suddenly you are left with a hard lump of red dough and you don't know why.

"Monocultures of the mind make diversity disappear from perception, and consequently from the world," writes Vandana Shiva in *Monocultures of the Mind: Perspectives on Biodiversity and Biotechnology*. "Conservation of diversity is, above all, the production of alternatives, of keeping alive alternative forms of production."

MY FRIEND DAVE makes fun of me for *deciding* to date. For thinking that dating is something that *could* be decided—could be planned, arranged, organized; that it could be accomplished over the course of a summer.

"It's like you put it on your to-do list," he says as we stand on his breezy porch, leaning on the cast-iron rail, suspended over city lights and dogs barking in the distance.

I laugh. "Yes, well. It needed to be done!" The anxiety I'd felt about restaurants was the same as what I felt about dating. I couldn't control if a restaurant put sugar in their sauce, just as I couldn't control the reciprocation of romantic interest. Restaurants and relationships—both required some relinquishing of autonomy, some relaxing of control, and I realize, standing here with Dave, that perhaps my year could benefit from a dose of flexibility. A mindful flexibility, that is—not the careless kind that made me eat flour-battered tempura because a man who didn't believe in global warming had ordered it. For if we convene around food, and if that food is sometimes processed, then I had to learn how to try my best and simply accept the outcome—perfect or not.

And so Dave is right about my to-do list. Summer *had* seemed to me like the perfect time to date. "It was my summertime extracurricular activity!" I say.

He laughs. "Of course."

Dave and I have been friends since we met the year before. He had a girlfriend all year, one who moved from Minneapolis to build a relationship in a two-bedroom apartment in Tucson. Our interactions have always been comfortable and unassuming, platonically pleasurable. Now, in August, he's invited me over to make dinner because he's heard about how ridiculous my foray into dating has become—I recently went out with a fellow who, after one drink, sent me a picture of his groceries and asked me to analyze them—and because this live-in girlfriend of his is now an ex-girlfriend, an ex-girlfriend who has gone back to where she came from, and Dave is stuck alone in their ex-apartment babysitting their ex-dogs.

Dave is all clutter. He paces, he mutters, he forgets where he parked his car; he leaves on time but arrives late. Dave drinks carbonated water out of miniature plastic water bottles—he goes through two eight-packs of mini plastic water bottles, bound together with those horrible fish-strangling loops, every *week*. It's not that Dave *isn't* interested in recycling or the environment. He's just more interested in soul music and travel writing, politics and public radio.

This is, explicitly stated, a "nondate," the second of such. A couple of weeks earlier, we met at an Italian restaurant in downtown Tucson, at a restaurant prescreened for unprocessed approval. After a year of friendship, Dave knows far too much about my unprocessed project, so after we sat down, after the server greeted us with a charming *buona sera!* Dave said, "Your call, I'm good with whatever." With so much fluffy white flour folded into spaghetti and penne, Italian restaurants are tricky for unprocessed, but our server assured me that Caffé Milano's house-made gnocchi were gluten-free (i.e., flour-free). The potato dumplings arrived nestled in the center of a broad platter like little pillows tangled in silky-cheese covers. Dave and I split the entrée, split the check, and went our separate ways. A lovely nonprocessed nondate.

But tonight, when we convene in his apartment to cook ourselves dinner, it begins to glimmer of something else. "Regardless of the particulars, the minute we include even one other person at the table, everything changes," writes Deborah Madison in *What We Eat When We Eat Alone*. What we eat when we eat alone is an odd and scattered affair—oatmeal with salt, chopped tomatoes with corn, a slab of meat. When we eat alone, we eat what we want, whether that's sardines from a can, a stacked sandwich, or an exquisite roast. When I eat alone, as I usually do, my meals require no justification or explanation. I heap giant salads into stainless-steel mixing bowls, fry eggs on burned toast, and lick honey straight from the jar. The presence of another person changes food. It becomes more elaborate, not about a coherence of ingredients but rather one of tastes, of additions and flourishes *just because*. Just because you have an audience and a glimmer.

I scrape out the spongy innards of a giant eggplant as Dave slices tomatoes and arranges cheese. He had texted me a few hours before, asking if I was okay to tackle our main course given my complicated directives. *I'll do cheese and crackers,* he wrote, and before I could respond, I'd gotten another message— *Wait, are crackers processed? Shoot.* And, five minutes later—*Never mind, we're doing tomato slices.*

Dave's kitchen is broad, but as we share the space—I stir my sauté of eggplant, summer squash, and onions and he reaches across me to grab the pepper grinder—it glimmers. After filling two excavated purple shells with steaming vegetables, I slide the brimming bowls under the broiler. We sip wine and nibble cheese while we perch on bar stools and lean on the kitchen counter.

"Nice work, Kimble," Dave says, when I turn off the oven and slide a color-fully stuffed eggplant onto each of our plates.

"Thanks. Can't say I cook like this every night."

"Well, of course. You think I make myself a little platter of cheese and crackers on a regular basis? That's the point of cooking for someone else. Makes you up your game."

Dessert is a bowl of cherries on his porch. We stand on the warm Saltillo tiles; we lean on the cast-iron rail over the city, talking about the year before us.

The problem with my abstainer personality is that you don't know until you try. The problem with a monocultured mind is that it allows no weedy corners that bear unexpected fruit. If I didn't try to engage in the messiness, of eating out and eating with another, then even if I ate perfectly unprocessed, I wouldn't really have *lived* unprocessed. Abstain though we try, today's world is one of moderation. Of trying and failing, and then trying and half succeed-ing. There are so many processes that we *cannot* remove ourselves from—the natural gas heating my stove, the coal-fueled air-conditioning cooling Dave's apartment—and so I construct an eating-out version of my kitchen philosophy: Don't let the food be the enemy of the company.

The Sahara Hotel sign blinks on Stone Avenue, miles away; the white head-light of a late-night biker slides silently across Alameda and Church. It's breezy and quiet and the city sighs, thankful for a reprieve from the day's sun. The silence breaks with the slow, soft hoot of a cargo train passing through town.

"Hello, train," Dave says softly as the sound thickens and arrives underfoot. The train's guttural hoots slide so easily through this thin, brittle air that it's impossible to escape the reverberations, impossible to situate yourself in rela-tion to the sound. It is silence and then sound everywhere, a hollow deepness, until, finally, the train slides to the south and the sound follows it like a trail of steam.

Dave and I have never spent this much time alone, save our jaunt to the Italian restaurant, and this fact whirls through the warm air, nine stories aboveground, like the cooing train—and then it fades, forgets itself as we sit and sip, joke and chatter. Dave rambles and repeats himself, telling stories I've already heard and recommending reading he's already suggested. We don't talk about unprocessed food, about global warming, farming, or urban chickens.

Midnight clicks past and I have to be at work at nine, so I slide my empty wineglass onto the glass table with a soft screech. I look at Dave and begin to stand up. "Time to go?" he asks.

I nod.

"I'll walk you out." We lean against opposite walls in the elevator, quiet as it clicks down nine floors. Across the lobby and an open door and I'm almost out into the warm night when he stops me and says, one foot still propping open the front door, "I know this isn't very nondate, but—" and then he kisses me, quickly, and looks at me to see what I'll do. And then we are kissing, less quickly, the brittle summer air wandering through the open doors of his apartment building.

Unprocess Yourself: Eating Out

If you're eating at a restaurant you've never been to, look up the menu online before you go. You're looking for foods that don't contain refined sugars, refined grains, or chemical additions. Identify a couple of unprocessed options beforehand and ask questions when you get there. Where do they buy their steak, fish, chicken? What's in the sesame ginger marinade? Do they make their bread or buy it? (Yes, you might feel like you're in a *Portlandia* sketch. But we all have our neuroses—luckily, food is a trendy one to have.)

In Tucson, it's impossible not to eat tacos, so I asked around, did my research, and figured out a handful of restaurants that make corn tortillas in-house and use fresh ingredients. Whatever your regional food happens to be, figure out the purveyors that sell some unprocessed version of it, and you'll have an easy default for eating out.

It's worth saying that I don't eat out very often, so when I do, I'm picky. I simply don't eat at some restaurants. I don't think it's possible to order unprocessed at Chili's. Ditto at the Cheesecake Factory. It's not that these restaurants don't offer some sensible items on their menus; it's that, because they are chains, they have to make sure a Luau Salad eaten in Bozeman tastes the same as one eaten in Boston, and the way that they do that is by adding chemicals and stabilizers to their recipes.

It's a happy convergence of priority and practicality that it's often easier to order unprocessed at a locally owned restaurant. As the local food movement gains momentum, there will be more chefs, in more cities, paying attention to where their ingredients come from. Support those restaurants that are themselves supporting local growers—because, if you don't eat there, who will?

Eating unprocessed in a world full of processed foods means being prepared, planning ahead, and asking lots of questions. That said, the point of eating out is the occasion—connecting with another person, be it friend, colleague, or the quiet part of yourself that gets neglected in the hustle and bustle. Try your best and ask questions, but above all, enjoy the company of whoever you happen to be eating that food with.

8

DRINK

Unprocessed alcohol takes time.

One of my favorite references to the early process of alcohol making comes in the *Kalevala,* a nineteenth-century epic poem that put Finnish culture on the map, so to speak. Just about halfway through the poem, our narrator introduces us to a maiden in a kitchen who must brew ale for a large wedding celebration. Evidently she has been sent to the kitchen without clear instructions, as we meet her in the depths of a conundrum, fretting over a pot of steaming barley water that is *not* transforming itself into ale. A splinter of wood, a handful of pine needles, a pinch of hop pods—no additive seems to work to set the stew a-brewing. Finally, distressed, our maiden sends a marten to gather handfuls of yeast "from the homestead of the forest bear." While she waits on the marten's return, she asks a honeybee to collect the stalks of "honey-hay" waving by the loins of a virgin sleeping "with her copper belt unfastened."

The honeybee and the marten return with their assigned bounty of yeast and honey. The brew bubbles.

The food processes we have made uniform—steel vats connected to steel pipes in sterile factories, small or large—began with such inexactitude, with yeast gathered from the forest and honey snatched from the loins of a sleeping virgin. Today, most of the processes behind cooking are simply known. Yeast leavens bread and ferments sugar into alcohol. It is so, and so we buy beer in cans and wine in bottles and we don't have to wonder, don't have to puzzle over the mystery of it all.

It is one thing to know that yeast organisms break down sugar polymers into chains of alcohol; that once consumed, these alcohol molecules penetrate the membranes of our own cells and interfere with their normal operations. When enough of these molecules accumulate in a person—in the collective entity of cells that constitute a nervous system—that person becomes intoxicated. It is one thing to know this, but it is another entirely to imagine how innocuous grains or grapes might become, after time, patience, and heat, a substance that so beguiles our minds and bodies. As much as there is to be said about how to make alcohol—we are endlessly fascinated by the nuance— perhaps we say so much about the making because we cannot quite articulate what alcohol makes of us.

WE'RE DRIVING SOUTH FROM TUCSON, Dave and I and this new thing tangled between us called "we." We roll through ranging grasslands and ascend into cooler air. The town of Bisbee leans and edges, sinuous streets winding toward mountains and descending into copper canyons. Dave drives while I fail to navigate—Bisbee loses us in its winding streets, past the Mimosa Market, Café Cornucopia, and, to my delight, a candle store called Bliss-Bee. "It *is*!" I exclaim. Finally, two one-way streets and a U-turn later, we find the

Old Bisbee Brewing Company, music and chatter wafting across the brewery's open-air patio.

Months after we began, Dave and I are both still surprised at how well we get along. He stays up late, I get up early; he prefers salt to my sweet, beer to wine, music to science, and so we are surprised, pleasantly, at how easy it is to be together, how much chemistry and how little friction we share in spite of all that we don't.

At the Old Bisbee Brewing Company, my request for a tour is granted in a matter of minutes; brewmaster Tim leads us across a narrow alley and into a small room, angled to fit into the steep mountain. It's cluttered with the chrome of brew tanks, full of the sweet smell of fermenting grains. Stacked in a corner are hundred-pound bags full of barley.

As we stand feet from the gristmill, Tim tells us that brewing begins when he pours the premalted grain into the hopper. Ground into grist, the grain is augured up a steel pipe and deposited into a three-hundred-gallon lofted tank where it's mixed with water and heated up. "That's basically it," Tim says with a relaxed shrug. "Water, grain, heat; a little time and filtration, and you've got beer."

It is, of course, much more complicated. Still in the first tank, the hot grain sludge called wort simmers around "like tea," says Tim. Once the wort has steeped for a bit—"How long, about?" I ask, to which Tim says, "Oh, an hour or two," sounding Canadian even after Dave-from-Minnesota finds out that he's from Maine—it travels one tank over, where it's brought to a boil and mixed with some hops.

"What exactly *are* hops?" Dave asks. "I mean, I think I know what they are in relation to beer, but, actually, what are they?" I realize as soon as he says it that I have no idea what hops are either. Hops are the thing that makes a beer hoppy.

"Hops are a type of flower," Tim says, and then adds, "They're actually closely related to the marijuana flower, so they sort of look like a marijuana bud, if you happen to know what that looks like."

Dave and I both nod noncommittally.

"They're bitter, but they add a sort of citrus, banana-type quality to beer," says Tim. "When monks first started making beer, they'd flavor it with whatever sacks of herbs and flowers were lying around but eventually realized that the hop flavor complemented the grain really nicely." Hops, as it turns out, smell like beer. A whiff of a bucketful of green, pelletized hops, looking sort of like rabbit feed, is the whiff of a pint of beer.

After the wort is steeped, the hops are added and the sludge moves into a new tank; once it cools, "We pitch the yeast in," says Tim. Yeast arrives and the grainy tea begins to ferment—starts to become beer. "You have to watch your pH and temperature here," Tim says, pointing to the three fermentation tanks lined up along the wall. Dave and I swivel our heads and then our feet follow. I'm scribbling in my notepad but Dave's just checking it all out, hands in his pockets and chatting it up with Tim. Dave's curiosity complements mine, normalizes it. He puts his hand on an elbow and a palm on his chin and asks, "So, here's a question I never thought of—" I stop scribbling and Tim stops talking and we both look at him. "Where in this whole process do the types of beer split? What makes the difference between, say, a stout and an ale?"

"Great question. It depends first on the roast of the barley, after you malt it," Tim says. "The higher the roast temperature, the more robust flavors you're going to get. We use black barley for stout—it's roasted at really high temperatures so the sugars break down. For amber ales, we'll try to caramelize the barley, maybe do a sixty-minute roast. For a light beer, like a pale malt, you don't roast nearly as long. You rely more on hops to create the flavor profile."

Dave and I turn to each other and nod in illuminated interest.

I turn back to Tim. "So, wait, do you malt the grain yourself, before you brew?" Malting is basically sprouting, which makes a grain's sugars more accessible to yeast. To malt grain, you soak it in water and then leave it in a warm spot until it sprouts thin tendrils. The process activates an enzyme that breaks the grain's starches into smaller sugars, into glucose and maltose, which become fuel for hungry yeast that metabolize those sugars into alcohol. As soon as this enzyme is activated—but before the sprout eats up all the sugar—you stop the process through heat.

"We get our grain premalted," he says. "There are a lot of malt houses around the country; our malts come from a place in Canada."

"Does that mean the grain grows there?" I ask.

"Yup," Tim says, as casual as I am shocked. If the barley was grown and processed a thousand miles away, how could the drink it became be called local in Arizona? If the hops were grown there, too, then the most local ingredient in the beer might well be the water. I struggle to formulate another question, but Tim has moved on. "So anyway, the beer ferments for about a week, depending on the variety. You want it hot, but not too hot to kill the yeast. But you don't want it so cool that bacteria start growing."

"So then, after a week, is it done?" Dave asks.

"Mostly. Most of the sediment, the bits of leftover grain, sinks to the bottom and serves as a sort of filter. Then we cold-clarify, which just means that we let the temperature down gradually so we don't shock and kill the yeast. And yup, we have pipes that lead directly from these tanks"—Tim pats one with his right hand and points with his left—"under the street and into the taps at the brewery."

We walk across the street and order a flight of beer each. Six different samples straight from the fermentation tanks. As the first few ounces of beer settle in my stomach, I ask Dave, "Are you hungry?"

"Very," he says. "Will you be able to eat anything here?"

I don't want to leave, don't want to crack the moment and leave the breeze behind, so I say, "Let's just see what they have."

At the far edge of the brick patio, a broad grill holds a line of organic brat-wurst. After a quick Google on Dave's phone, I decide the bratwurst itself is reasonably unprocessed—that it might contain sugar, but also might not—but that the bun it comes in is most definitely processed. Although our waitress tells me that bunless is actually the more traditionally German way to eat a bratwurst, when she brings it out, it rolls around the broad white plate danger-ously. Dave's bratwurst looks snug and filling couched in a fluffy white bun, but even after I cover mine in sauerkraut and mustard, it looks naked, and naked is not how you want a shiny brown bratwurst to look. Still—we finish our flight, the breeze flutters my hair, and Dave touches my neck.

"FROM THE START, it seems that beer had an important function as a social drink," writes Tom Standage in *A History of the World in Six Glasses.* "Shar-ing a drink with someone is a universal symbol of hospitality and friendship. It signals that the person offering the drink can be trusted, by demonstrating that it is not poisoned or otherwise unsuitable for consumption. The earliest beer, brewed in a primitive vessel in an era that predated the use of individual cups, would have to have been shared."

Since I started eating unprocessed, sharing liquid—beer, wine, coffee—has become a mainstay of my social life. I can't grab a slice of pizza at Brook-lyn Pizza or stop for a Sonoran hot dog at Rob Dog's. I can tag along—I can mingle and observe—but I can't partake of the subtle, accumulated bonding that begins with the sharing of food. So instead, I share drink.

Drink gets me out of my kitchen and into the world. I meet friends at the Shanty, a shabby sort of Irish pub; we migrate to Plush, a tacky, tchotchke-adorned bar with felt seats and live music, or we convene at La Cocina, my favorite twinkle-light-adorned patio. It's on this very patio, sitting at a cast-iron table and drinking a beer, that Noam asks me about my food processor; months later, milling in the kitchen at a friend's party, sipping on red wine, he suggests a recipe for homemade ketchup. When Sarah becomes single, again we convene at the Cactus Moon for tequila and dancing. When Hilary's new boyfriend comes to visit from St. Louis, he's introduced across bar stools at the District Tavern. The action of unprocessed unfolds in the grocery store and in my kitchen, but I'm still trying to live it here, out in the world. I eat, drink, and shop unprocessed; I read unprocessed and think unprocessed; and so sometimes, occasionally, at a bar, I can sit with a glass of wine and escape the process of being unprocessed.

And indeed, I'd allowed myself the escape. Had sipped on microbrews. Indulged in the occasional gin and tonic. Stuck by my red wine standby. Alcohol, after all, *seemed* unprocessed. Mysterious though the process remained, it was an ancient one, from mead halls in the Middle Ages to the wine splattered throughout ancient Rome. But of course, the way we prepare food has changed since the rise of the Roman Empire—why wouldn't alcohol have changed along with it?

As It Turns Out, the question I'd struggled to articulate at the Old Bisbee Brewing Company—how can your beer be local if it's made from grains grown and processed somewhere else?—is actually very easy to answer.

"A lot of people ask us, 'Why don't you use local grains?'" says Tristan White, a founder of Tucson's Dragoon Brewery. "Well, nobody in Arizona malts barley. And even if they were, no one is growing enough for us."

It's pouring rain on a Tuesday afternoon in August, the long-anticipated monsoon season finally in full swing. Hair sticks to the back of my neck. Sweat slides down my back. The taproom at Dragoon opens at 4 P.M.; with fifteen minutes to spare, a handful of employees cluster around the bar. The thick air is punctuated by laughter and thunder, by sweet-smelling brew and sour-smelling yeast.

"Oh," I say, disappointed that I drove twenty minutes through skittish rain to find that the answer to my question could have been addressed in an e-mail—that the answer is so easy, so obvious. I'm suddenly and irrationally annoyed by these brewers, faces hidden behind beards and brews ensconced in impenetrable steel tanks. Where were all the women—what happened to my maiden in the kitchen?

And then Tristan corrects himself. "Well, we do use some White Sonora wheat in one of our brews," he says, referring to the grain I watched Jeff Zimmerman mill all those months ago. But because there are no maltsters in Arizona, the grain goes into the brew, called Ojo Blanco, unmalted, without adding any fermentable sugars to the mix. "It adds flavor and creates a good mouth feel," Tristan says. "But it's hard to do on a large scale."

And, for a microbrewery, Dragoon is brewing a lot of beer—fifty-five thousand gallons a year. To make just five hundred gallons of their signature brew, the Dragoon IPA—enough to last a local bar just a few weeks—they need 1,100 pounds of grain. Which is a lot of grain.

Some Arizona farmers do indeed grow barley, but most, if not all, are growing the six-row variety used for cattle feed instead of the more easily malted two-row barley that most brewers prefer. "A lot of commercial brewers will use six-row barley because it's cheaper," says Tristan. "And it mixes more easily with adjuncts."

At the mention of an adjunct, my interest piques. An adjunct, I learn, is anything brewed into beer that's not barley or wheat, used simply to lower costs. Anheuser-Busch uses rice; Miller uses corn. There is nothing inherently processed in this substitution—in the Southwest, Tahamara Indians have been making corn beer, called *tesguino,* for centuries. But the ingredient label of Miller Lite does not *say* corn. Indeed, there are no laws that require brewers to disclose their ingredients. (Oddly, the Department of the Treasury, not the Food and Drug Administration, regulates alcoholic beverages.)

Caramel coloring, high-fructose corn syrup, and "natural flavors" are three ingredients you might find on a beer's ingredient label, if it had to wear one. But then again, maybe not. Many additives are used to filter out impurities in a brew and so they stay behind in the tank when the beer is bottled. Many more, like sugar, are digested by yeast long before we digest the beer.

"Wait, so if you're only using a little bit of White Sonora wheat and not Arizona barley, where does the rest of your grain come from?" I ask.

"Our barley for our IPA comes from a maltster in Canada called Rahr," Tristan says. The rest comes from regions you might imagine would grow grain—England, Belgium, Germany. Regions with climates conducive to growing grain and hops have had thousands of years to build an infrastructure to support small breweries—an infrastructure southern Arizona doesn't yet have. Tristan tells me that although a local winery recently became the first in Arizona to grow and harvest hops, Dragoon can't use them because no one in Arizona yet owns the machine required to pelletize the hops.

Of course, there is a reason most hop and barley growers are located in the cooler, wetter north—"Arizona isn't the best place to grow either of those things," says Tristan. "Local is great, but it's only great if it's actually good."

And because brewers—even the small ones—use so much grain, large companies, like Cargill, have long dominated the malting industry. Even if someone in Arizona started growing a thousand acres of two-row barley, "We really can't use it until it's malted," Tristan says. "And very few breweries malt their own grains."

IF FEW BREWERIES MALT GRAIN TO MAKE BEER, then even fewer distilleries— only five in the United States—malt grain to make liquor.

"I think the coolest thing we're doing is malting our own grains," says Stephen Paul as he walks me into the brew room at Hamilton Distillers. "We've got the whiskey distillation down pretty well. But malting sure is an adventure."

Stephen Paul is—there's no other word for it—nice. He's wearing thick cowboy jeans and a long-sleeved button-down that looks freshly pressed, but he's happy to linger in the steam of a simmering pot of grain as he asks me what, exactly, makes food processed. He's weeks away from moving into a bigger warehouse across town; he's missing labels for a dozen cases of already-bottled whiskey; he's working with a company in Portland to design the country's first tank-based malting system. But he's unrushed. He's curious.

"That sounds daunting," he says, after I outline the year's parameters.

"I had no idea what I was getting myself into," I say. "I'm kind of glad I didn't."

"You're telling me," he says, gesturing at the scrap yard around him—the former home of Arroyo Design, a carpentry company specializing in fine furniture made from mesquite, the signature wood of the Southwest. Today, that wood is the source of the smoke that turns sprouted grains into Whiskey del Bac—the whiskey of the pueblo.

Stephen learned how to malt grains out of necessity. One night, he and his wife, Elaine—he calls her "Idea Woman"—were sipping Scotch before a fire fueled by mesquite scraps discarded from the workroom when Elaine wondered: Why couldn't they make their own Scotch? Scotch made from barley smoked not over peat, but rather mesquite?

"If we had called up a malting house and said, 'We want you to make us mesquite-smoked malt,' we would have totally given up our concept," Stephen says, sidestepping a puddle on the edge of the workroom floor. Before Stephen started, there were only four other distilleries in the country malting their own grains—and none smoking barley with mesquite.

Stephen slides open a heavy metal door and I follow him into a small cool room. Five forty-gallon fermenters stand, clustered, in the corner—they look like miniature grain silos, upright column falling into a tapered cone. "To make whiskey, first you make beer," he says. "A basic nine percent brew. And then we distill it in the sill."

At the other end of the cold room, we peer over two shelves full of shiny, wet-looking barley. Stephen runs his fingers through the mass; the tiny, beige pearls scatter and tumble around his palm. Wispy white tendrils peek out from the tip of each grain, seeking light and fuel to begin a new plant.

There's usually a five-gallon bucket below the barley, Stephen says, which is where the process of malting begins. Order a bag of barley from a farmer—Stephen gets his from southeastern Colorado, although he's talking to a farmer in Marana, just north of Tucson—and then set it to soak. After a day, you clean the barley and spread it, eight inches deep, across a cement floor or on a series of stacked drying shelves. You turn it to make sure the grain is aerated; you keep an eye on the temperature and humidity. Four or five days later, when the enzyme is activated and the sugars are available but not yet consumed by the new sprout, you stop germination.

"And you do that by smoking the barley," Stephen says as we walk outside. Three or four feet from the wall of the warehouse stands a tall black box with a removable front and a stack of shelves slotted within. "It's basically a glorified meat smoker."

A broad corrugated tin tube siphons smoke from a small woodburning stove stacked with mesquite scraps into the smoker and across the soaked barley. Heat kills the sprout, halting enzyme production—and soaking the grain full of flavor.

"After that, we mill the barley in a basic two-roller," says Stephen. "And then we make our beer."

"Beer that becomes whiskey," I say, leading him into the next process as he walks us back into the first room, the brew room, where beer begins as barley and ends as whiskey.

A whiskey still looks like magic. Burned copper, round midsection, Hershey's Kiss top, with a swirl that ends in a tube and a tube that ends in a slow, clear drip of moonshine. Distillation works because alcohol evaporates at a lower temperature than water. "Lucky for us," says Stephen. "Because what's left after the first spirit run is water." The next spirit run—I love the image of the spirit running up and out of the genie lamp just to drip, drip, drip into a glass jar below—they separate the good alcohols from the bad ones, "the ones that make moonshiners go blind," he says. After they discard the bad and collect the good, they blend the liquid with distilled water until it hits 60 percent. After it's aged in an oak barrel for six months, after it's diluted, again, to 45 percent alcohol by volume, the country's only mesquite-smoked whiskey is bottled, labeled, sold, and, finally, sipped.

We leave the swelter of the brew room and return to the air-conditioning of Stephen's office. Stephen asks, "So what do you think? Is whiskey unprocessed?"

I smile, touched that he's remembered to ask the all-important question. "I think so," I say. "I mean, you buy a sack of grain from a farmer and then turn it into spirit, all right here—you can sort of see it all." As soon as I say it, I realize how important the visual was for me—that I could see, or at least imagine, how grain becomes beer becomes clear distillate becomes smoky brown in a barrel. It's no more a miracle than a small, yellow flower turning into a tomato, but this transformation captivates me: the drip-drip-drip of whiskey out of a shimmering still.

The first time I'd tried Whiskey del Bac, I was out to dinner with Dave. He discovered the smoked whiskey long before I had, so he'd ordered us a single glass, neat. Swirled, it smelled like campfire—of thick, sweet smoke and syrupy grain. When I finally took a small sip, it didn't kick, simply warmed. The smoke built, lingered, mellowed. "Yeah," Dave said, responding to my wide eyes. "I just love that smoke."

When I tell Stephen Paul about my first sip of smoke, he smiles and says, "You know, I get a call once a week from Ultra-Pure, trying to sell us NGS."

"What's NGS?"

"Neutral Grain Spirits. Or sometimes they're called Grain Neutral Spirits."

"Um . . ." I say, still at a loss.

"Basically it's a neutral alcohol made by big distilleries and shipped in bulk for use in gin, vodka, whiskey," he says. "They're made mostly from corn. Corn has a lot of starch, so it's easier to break down into fermentable sugars." Commercial distillers can do repeat distillations on any kind of grain and filter out flavor and odor to make completely neutral booze. Sell that "grain-neutral spirit"—the name acquires more meaning when you figure out what it is—at a bargain price and "distillers" can then reflavor, rebrand, and flip it as something not so neutral.

"Wait," I said. "Can you age NGS in a barrel for a year and call it whiskey?" Stephen nods.

"Or add sugar to the distillate and call it rum?"

Again a nod.

"That's insane!"

"So Elaine and I went to this distillery in Portland," he says. They were selling nine "award-winning" spirits, including a new Oregon marionberry whiskey. "On the description, they were careful to say that it's 'handmade with local marionberries and aged whiskey,' but they don't say where the whiskey was made. Maybe I'm inferring incorrectly, but it seems like they would be claiming the whiskey as their own if it was."

I'm stunned. If microbreweries were importing barley, at least they were *brewing* locally. I peer at the bottle of aged whiskey sitting on his desk. There's no list of ingredients—just a description: handmade in small batches in a copper-pot still, using house-malted, mesquite-smoked barley.

"We went to another distillery, up in Portland," Stephen continues. "They've been open for six years. And they're selling a fifteen-year aged whiskey. Now, how do you think that's possible?" His grin answers his own question.

I LIKE HAMILTON DISTILLERS WHISKEY, but I'm not really a whiskey drinker. I really liked Dragoon's Sly Amber, but I also don't often order beer. The process I was nervous to investigate was wine—which always, inevitably, calmed me.

I am something of a type A, and a glass of wine helps me melt from the sharpness of a day's A into something more like a rounded, evening B. Wine helps my brain puddle instead of rush; it pulls flavor from food and spills relaxation into weekends. I love the feel of a wineglass cupped in my hand—adult—how the roundness of a narrow lip touches my own—cold—how liquid rolls around my mouth—lingering. Before the fear of a blank page, wine emboldens me. ("Quickly, bring me a beaker of wine," said Aristophanes, "so that I may wet my mind and say something clever.") Wine initiated the pizza party I hosted for Hilary and Sarah, the first venture into a friendship. Wine facilitated the awkward "nondate" that became a date that became a relationship. ("I am tempted to place the craving for fermented liquors, which is unknown to animals, with anxiety regarding the future, which is likewise unknown to animals," wrote Jean-Anthelme Brillat-Savarin in *The Physiology of Taste*.)

The difference between beer brewing and wine making is simply the source of the sugars that fuel yeast's sweet munching. Unlike barley, which requires soaking and heating to release its sucrose and maltose, grapes comes full of the sugary juices that yeast thrives on. To make wine, you extract those liquids from grapes, remove the bitter seeds and stems, add some yeast, wait a bit, and voilà. There is wine. Of course, like beer, it's a bit more complicated. Temperature and time are finicky companions to sugar and yeast. The hotter and longer the grape pulp—called must, a word about as appetizing as "wort"— remains in contact with the grape skins while fermenting, the darker the wine will be. White wines hang with their skins at a cool sixty degrees for about four to six weeks, while red wines ferment at a hotter eighty degrees for two or three weeks before the skins are removed and the must continues to ferment. After a month or a year in a barrel or a tank, must becomes wine. (Wine must become!)

I thought, at the starry-eyed inception of my year, that I would just *make* wine and so it would be unprocessed. People make wine, I thought—surely people who are not professional wine makers can make wine. But then I visited Brew Your Own Brew, a home-brewing store near the University of Arizona, and learned that a home wine-making kit would set me back $124.99. When I asked what I'd get for this amount of money, a hipster sales clerk rattled off a long list of stressful-sounding equipment: drilled rubber stopper, econolock, wine hydrometer, five feet of siphon tubing. And, of course, grape juice concentrate, as well as small paper packets full of powdered chemical stabilizers and clarifiers, which seemed to miss the unprocessed point of brewing at home.

So instead I made mead. I found an article online titled "Cheap and Easy Homemade Wine," bought a plastic bucket, an eight-dollar air lock, a package of brewers' yeast, a liter of raw honey, and invited my friend Rani over with the promise that there would be already-brewed wine. We'd filled the five-gallon bucket halfway full of warm water, stirred in thick gobs of room-temperature honey, and stirred until the honey dissolved and the water swam in foamy, caramel-colored circles. A few weeks before, we'd both attended a fermentation workshop hosted by Sandor Katz, the author of *The Art of Fermentation;* we had learned that when making mead, look for bubbles. (The word "fermentation" comes from the Latin *ferveo,* which means to boil.) We stirred for a few minutes, clicked the lid shut, slid the air lock in place, and called the endeavor a success. The bucket sat on a chair in my kitchen, like a silent dining companion, for weeks. After a month, I cracked the lid and ladled out a cup of pale golden liquid. It tasted vaguely alcoholic, sort of sweet. It was good—it bubbled and brightened—but it was more like maybe-mead, like fizzy juice, than anything that resembled wine.

WINE BEGINS WITH GRAPES GROWING IN SOIL; when the fruits of that soil are gathered and intensified by fermentation and time, you encounter a wine's *terroir,* or the taste of a place. While many vintners wax poetic about the taste of *terroir,* the sword of *terroir* cuts both ways. For every wine maker now calling attention to the particular textures and tastes of their growing region, there are many more who, through modern fermentation technology, are trying to cover their *terroir,* to minimize the taste of a degraded landscape or shoddily harvested grapes.

Before my year began, the only time I looked at the back of a wine bottle was to find its price tag. If wine wore an ingredient label, surely it must have read: *duh,* wine. But when I finally look on the back of a bottle of Trader Joe's 2011 Costal Syrah—a refined $4.99 bottle that comes with a "lush mouth feel"—I find this: ALC 13.8% BY VOL. And, after that, CONTAINS SULFITES.

Sulfites are any sulfur-based compound, produced naturally both in our bodies—about a gram a day—and in grapes. Because all wines are made from grapes, all wines contain trace amounts of grape-sourced sulfites. The reason the disclaimer appears on the label is that many wine makers add synthetic sulfur dioxide or potassium metabisulphite to their grapes before they ferment them, a "treatment that may sound antiseptically modern, [but] it is centuries old," writes Harold McGee in *On Food and Cooking.* Sulfites inhibit the growth of bacteria and unwanted yeast strains, and also prevent the oxidation of flavor and pigment molecules in the final product, producing tastier and more consistent wines.

What wine makers don't have to include on an ingredient label are the more than seventy other additives that can facilitate a grape's journey into spirit. These additives might include enzymes, to extract more juice per grape, or clarifiers, such as gelatin, egg whites, or casein, which help pull grape sediment out of the wine after fermentation. If a wine's yeast digests too much alcohol into sugar, wine makers might add tartaric or malic acid to pull back the tartness; they can also add ammonium salts to slow down sugar-munching yeast. If the yeast continues to go gangbusters, metabolizing all the grape's sugar into alcohol, the wine must be retroactively sweetened. Simple syrup of sugar and water often does the trick, though honey and fruit juice are sometimes used.

When I learn this, half a year and many dozens of bottles of wine into my year unprocessed, I feel like: Damn it, wine—you, too? Unlike with sugar or wheat, when I learned about bone char and bleach, rancid grains and Humpty-Dumpty parts, with wine, this revelation of process does not elicit the same moment of *gotcha,* the same impulse to fix and restore.

Admittedly conceived from a place of great bias, one argument in the case for wine (for a case of wine!) is that most of the aforementioned additives are included in such minute quantities as to be barely detectable in the final product, which is why none have to appear on ingredient labels. Yeast will metabolize most added sugars and stabilizers, and many of the clarifiers are pulled out along with the sediment. Even sulfites continue to be "ingested" by the wine after bottling, and there's little evidence to show these additives have any cumulative effect on our health. (Contrary to popular opinion, sulfites do not cause hangovers; more likely, it's the histamines in alcohol firing those headaches.)

Of course, there are many wine makers who add nothing to their fermentation tanks except for yeast and time. The problem, though, is cost. Mass-produced California wines are the supermarket tomatoes of alcohol: bright, sweet, and so, so very cheap. But unlike heirloom tomatoes at farmers' markets, good wine costs so much more than its cheap counterpart—not twice as much, but four or five or six times more. Cheap wine is so cheap that it asserts itself as right—it recalibrates our expectation. And if you are broke, and there is wine that is cheap—and it is not just drinkable, but enjoyable—then why spend more?

ON THE FIRST DAY of the grape harvest at Flying Leap Vineyard, Marc Moeller is cleaning. On a slab of cement behind the winery, he sprays a squat, shallow stainless-steel collecting pan with a high-pressured hose. He cleans the destemmer; he scrubs hoses and washes filters. "Clean, clean, clean," says Marc. "That's all I do." That, and move stuff around. For a small winery, space comes at a premium, and if the crusher is in the way of the bottler, they have to move it. "Rolf spends a good part of his day moving stuff around," Marc says. Rolf-Peter Sasse, a taciturn German who describes himself as the winery's "secret weapon," is cleaning the crooks and crannies of a ten-foot-long grape crusher. He looks up and offers a curt nod—yes, I move a lot of stuff.

A cell phone buzzes in Marc's pocket. He pulls it out with his left hand. "Tom's on his way," he tells Rolf. If Tom is on his way, that means that the grapes are on their way—three tons of them, hand-harvested at Flying Leap's fields in Willcox, ninety miles northeast of Sonoita.

When I first moved to Tucson, I assumed grapes growing in the desert's summer swelter would just melt off the vine. As it turns out, on the plateau southeast of Tucson, hot days and cool nights combine to create a climate entirely amenable to wine grapes. (Gordon Dutt, a soil scientist at the University of Arizona, was purportedly the first to realize this in the 1970s, when he went to France with a sample of Sonoita's soil and realized the two disparate regions were actually quite similar belowground.)

In anticipation of the grapes' arrival, Marc and Rolf start preparing for the crush. It takes both of them, at full strength, to heave the collecting pan and crusher from the hot cement slab outside onto the cool concrete of the covered warehouse. The destemmer rolls in parallel to the crusher, a thick plastic hose connecting the two.

As Marc and Rolf catch their breath and pause before heading back into the sun, I ask if they've thought about farming their grapes organically. "Growing organic grapes is really hard," Marc says. "Your yields go way, way down.

The bugs go for the grapes, for the vines. And you'd just get killed by weeds." He pauses. "If we switched to organic, we'd be out of business within two years."

He tells me that Flying Leap, along with most of the wineries in the region, practices something called integrative pest management, which is basically a form of spot treatment—you do not carpet-bomb a field with pesticides when you could instead take more time to apply judiciously and seek alternate solutions. Growing grapes and making wine is a slow, deliberate process; small wineries like Flying Leap are it in for the long run—which means they have to live, for the long run, with decisions they make about their soils.

I'm surprised at how quickly the concern is dismissed. There are viable organic wineries—Trader Joe's sells an organic red blend for $4.99—and, like the rest of the organic market, demand is growing. Of course, I don't know grapes—what it takes to grow and harvest a healthy field full of vines. Unlike barley or wheat, which can be stored, grapes are finicky fruits, tiny water balloons of sugar just waiting to be burst.

As we talk, Marc gets grape updates—they're thirty minutes away. Then fifteen. Five. And then, finally, "They're here!" Marc says. He turns to me. "It's just so *exciting*."

By the time I get outside, Rolf's already behind the driver's seat of a forklift, pulling a crate of grapes from a trailer hitched to a pickup truck. The grapes are green, with a bruised, hazy sort of yellow rimming the juncture between stem and skin. Rolf shuttles the last crate of grapes over to the lofted opening of the destemmer, where Marc waits, perched and leaning on a twelve-foot ladder, plastic shovel in hand.

"Ready?" Marc calls down to Rolf, who's situated himself among the hoses.

"Yes," he says, calm.

The destemmer switches to on, and with it, the warehouse transforms from the tasting room's backdrop into a rumbling, rousing factory where things are *made.* Marc scoops grapes from crate to machine, crate to machine. They tumble into the turning gears; stems shoot out one opening, careening to the ground, hard, while a mass of partially crushed grapes slithers through the translucent tube into the crusher. The grapes have already become less fruit, more juice. As they splatter into the crusher, juice drips out the perforated surface into the collecting pan below, each droplet shimmering across the surface as the pan fills with beige liquid—cloudy, cold, and sweet.

When Marc climbs down the ladder to take a break between crates, I ask, "What's your best value wine?"—emphasis on the word "value."

As he rattles off varieties, my pen scribbles nonsense in my notebook, so focused am I on the question I have to ask next.

"The better question might be: How is anyone making wine that's so cheap?" he answers, when I finally muster the courage to ask: Why does their wine cost so much? "Well, we're doing everything by hand. We do small batches. We pay attention to our grapes—we take care of our land."

Cheap wine is commodity wine, he says. "That wine is produced on a massive, industrial scale, with an industrial harvest. Those big producers have thirty-five-thousand-acre fields that are all harvested by machines. Everything goes in there. Leaves, rodents, green grapes, rotten grapes. And they ferment thousands of gallons at a time. They don't age—as soon as it ferments, they bottle it."

"And the fermentation just, like, takes care of all that extra stuff?" I ask, appalled.

"To a point," he says. "Yeasts are pretty powerful organisms. But because the wine isn't pure, they add all sorts of ingredients to make it taste the way they want. Like, flavors. They can say, this wine needs more vanilla. Or something else. They can add sugar and make it sweeter."

Damn it, wine, I think.

"Yup," Marc says, reading my expression. "When you buy a seven ninety-nine bottle of Chardonnay from Trader Joe's, or anywhere else, it may taste good, but those tastes are not coming from natural processes."

Rolf checks me out at the tasting room counter and suggests his favorite blend, a 2009 Sangiovese. As he runs my credit card, I watch as Marc checks the hose siphoning the juice in the collecting pan into a fermentation tank. Again, I am thrilled at the visual—at the chance to see grape became juice become, with time, wine.

I am decidedly less thrilled when I sign a credit-card slip authorizing the purchase of a $27.25 bottle of wine.

Part of my resistance to learning this process is that it feels like there is no way to give up cheap wine without sacrificing a staple of my social life. Twenty-seven dollars is actually a bargain for a bottle of fine wine, and Flying Leap certainly makes fine wine. But I don't drink fine wine. *We* don't drink fine wine—absolutely no one I know, no one I might share this wine with, can afford to spend twenty-seven dollars on a bottle of wine. We spend six or seven dollars on a glass at a bar; we spend eight or nine for a bottle at home. And maybe the wine we're drinking is made from shoddily harvested grapes; maybe it's thickened with a few fermented leaves and a dash of corn syrup. But apart from the story we're told on the label—the myth of the mysterious process—there is no way to know.

WHAT MAKES CHEAP, COMMODITY ALCOHOL so seemingly processed is not necessarily the actual process of how it's made—it is all fermentation, writ large—but how little we know about what's in our beer, wine, and whiskey. All the corn in Miller Lite has to come from somewhere; probably, it comes from a farm in Nebraska or Illinois. But we don't know. And so maybe the addiction to *terroir* by small brewers, wine makers, and distillers is as much about place as it is a reaction to the nameless, neutral booze most of us are drinking.

But *terroir* comes at a price. A liter of mesquite-smoked whiskey from Hamilton Distillers costs forty-eight dollars. A bottle of Sonoita wine hovers around thirty. A pint of Dragoon costs twice as much as the same glass filled with Miller Lite.

This sense of place also comes with time—*terroir* takes patience. It comes from thick roots and deep investments.

"We have a lot of history here," says Todd Bostock. "But we don't have hundreds of years." At Dos Cabezas Wineworks, even after ten years in the business, Todd and his wife, Kelly, are still trying to figure out what varietals of grapes to grow, when to plant them, how to train the vines, and when to harvest the grapes. "We're trying to make stuff that belongs to the place that we are," says Todd. "We don't want to be a cover band. We want to be the best in Arizona. The best *of* Arizona."

On a Saturday afternoon in August, Todd and Kelly are mixing varietals. Behind the tasting room, across a dusty patio, inside a shaded warehouse, Todd siphons wine from small barrels into large aging tanks. Kelly hauls the empty barrels outside and heaves them in place over a barrel cleaner.

The wine they're blending today is their signature Dos Cabezas Red—my favorite local wine, I tell Todd, because it's the most affordable. A bottle retails for $18.50, which is still out of my price range, but a glass in a local restaurant is reliably the cheapest wine on the menu at seven or eight dollars. "We could charge more, but we won't," says Todd. "The whole point of making wine is so that people can drink it. We want this wine to be precious, but not *that* precious. It's an encapsulated moment in time. But then it's gone."

One reason Arizona wine is still more expensive than wine from California is simply that the industry is new. "We're working to build a local wine infrastructure," Todd says. If you're in Napa and a barrel breaks, you drive down the street and get it fixed. In Arizona, you pay to ship that fifty-pound barrel across the country and suffer the loss while it's gone.

While Todd siphons wine and Kelly hauls barrels, friends visiting from

Phoenix throw a football across the dusty courtyard with the youngest Bostock. Five-year-old Griffin squints into the sun, focused on the spinning plastic football. "Our kids are growing up here and on the vineyard, and I love that," says Todd, pausing in his work. "Our kids will grow up thinking that this is a viable career choice. As that happens generationally, there will be huge growth in this kind of production. All this stuff takes time."

Back at Flying Leap Vineyards, Marc Moeller had said basically the same thing. You want affordable Arizona wine? Wait fifty years. "I like to compare Arizona wine now to how Napa was in the sixties," he said. "One fourth of one percent of wine consumed in Arizona is local wine. There is a market for Arizona wine in Arizona. We just don't produce enough of it."

Yet. In fifty years, when production increases, not only will Arizona wine be more affordable, drinking it will also confer its own sort of social experience, particular to this place. In the meantime, while I wait for a rise in income or a drop in price, I continue to buy cheap wine from California, Australia, and Portugal. It tastes good, but more important, it gathers friends at dinner. It relaxes me when I am knotted up, comforts me when I am out of place. I stand at bars and clutch its glass, happy to have something to hold on to.

Wine making takes time. So does brewing, distilling, and mead making—so, really, does building local food systems and unprocessing individual ones. Making alcohol takes trial and error—yeast and honey, foraged and found. Mistakes and experiments and then waiting—waiting for fermentation, for a good harvest to become good wine. It takes patience and slow-growing vines. "That's how durable, important stuff happens," says Todd. "Over generations. All of this is building on stuff other people did. We want the winery to be dense. To be durable."

Unprocess Yourself: Drink

It's true that wine, beer, and liquor made locally are often more expensive than the homogenous brews manufactured somewhere else. But as more local producers get into the game—and as communities rebuild the infrastructure needed for production and distribution—prices will go down.

The explosion of microbreweries and wine makers across the country means that it's very likely that there's someone in your state brewing beer and fermenting wine. The Brewers Association has a comprehensive list of local breweries on its website at BrewersAssocation.org. Check out the Winery Passport app in iTunes to find local wineries and wine tastings. But ask around in your community, at favorite restaurants and markets, if they have local liquor recommendations. At the very least, it'll let them know that you're interested.

Look online for home-brewing classes, courses, workshops, and home-brew stores. There's a pretty significant up-front cost for equipment, so consider gathering a few friends to split the cost (and share the brew).

I don't drink much hard alcohol, so when I do, I try to drink the good stuff. Local distilleries are spouting up across the United States—ask questions and check the label to make sure what you're drinking is really small-batch liquor.

When I'm out in the world, at restaurants or bars, I always order local wine if it's on the menu; but if I'm at Trader Joe's or the Food Conspiracy Co-op, I'll leave with a few bottles of $7.99 Syrah (organically produced, if possible). After all, I am still young and broke and good wine takes time—a $30 bottle of locally produced wine gives me something to work toward.

If it sounds like fun, experiment with making your own alcohol. Making mead requires the smallest start-up cost. Start with a three-to-one ratio of water to honey, but feel free to tweak after a few tries. Make sure your honey is raw, as pasteurization kills the yeast needed to begin fermentation. You can make mead in basically anything with a cover—a bucket works well, although a large canning jar with a loosened lid works, too. Combine warm water with honey, stirring vigorously. Once the honey is dissolved, cover loosely and leave somewhere clean and warm—a kitchen counter is a good spot. Check on your mead every few days, stirring each time. As soon as it begins to froth and foam, it'll taste more like kombucha than wine; let it go for a few more days—or weeks—and it'll become drier and more alcoholic. You can make flavored mead by steeping herbs, spices, or dried flowers in the mixture, either before or during fermentation. But really, if you want to make mead—or any fermented beverage—you should just go ahead and buy Sandor Katz's *The Art of Fermentation*.

9

REFRIGERATION

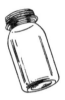

Good work is unprocessed.

We are a quiet bunch, hovering around the expanse of stainless-steel counter at the Mercado San Augustin kitchen. Loraine, a midsixties woman whose curly blond hair is pulled loosely back with a blue-and-yellow-striped head-band, tells us that she's been canning for thirty years. As she talks, she un-screws lids from mason jars. Her hands shake as she works—Parkinson's, I wonder, or fatigue from thirty years of canning? The class begins early, five before nine: Evidently those who sign up for a canning class at 9 A.M. on a warm Sunday are also a punctual bunch. We are a group of nine women and two men, one clearly a husband supporting a wife. The other man arrives late, dripping sweat, and hovers near the back, worrying his wedding band around his left finger, and I wonder about his wife, the wife of a man who cans.

We are nervous. Loraine begins the class in this nervousness. She says, "People don't can anymore because they're worried they're going to kill someone." We all smile and sigh, the elephant of botulism thus acknowledged. "You won't kill someone!" Loraine insists. "If you follow the tenets of canning. Cleanliness, temperature, and organization. That's it!" she says, washing her hands. The premise of canned foods is that hot food deposited into a hot jar submerged in boiling water will seal itself from oxygen's decaying grasp; so we begin by boiling water.

Today we are going to can onion relish, prickly-pear syrup, and tomatoes. While prickly-pear syrup and onion relish are lovely garnishes to a food supply, I'm here because of the tomatoes. Because it is tomato season now, in the thrumming heat of Tucson's August; because, for most of the country, summer is bounty's season. Unlike this sunny, irrigated desert, in which a rotating variety of plants bursts forth year-round, summer in the majority of the United States, for most of our country's history, has been the season to plan ahead—the time to preserve.

I am here because my grandmother canned her own produce. She lived on a farm in West Texas, and if she didn't grab freshness when it exploded in the late summer, harness this explosion of nutrients, and siphon it into a can, that was it. There were no grocery stores to dash to, no produce departments to supply her counters. What little freezer space she had was given over to summer's other harvest, the slaughtered cow. So she canned.

"There are few things in modern life that are as reliable as the modern canning jar," Loraine says. The lowly mason jar, that now-stylish symbol of "alternative" culture that graces the tables of hipster wine bars and coffee shops. I realize now that perhaps this is why the mason jar has made a comeback: because it feels so timelessly reliable.

Loraine informs us that our canned food will last a full year in our cabinets, but I don't jot this down on my "How to Can" work sheet. Although the premise of preserving food in jars is to create a steady stream of vegetables throughout a year when produce might not flow so steadily, I am not here intending to stock my cabinets with mason jars full of a winter's rations. I am skeptical of the premise that I could feasibly preserve a year's worth of wares without dropping out of school or quitting my job. Or perhaps I don't note it because it feels hypothetical; I don't live in New York, I live in southern Arizona, where my CSA provides fresh produce year-round.

Rather, I am here to prove that I *could*. Preserving food without cold storage makes me more nervously stubborn than anything else I've attempted—I *like* my refrigerator—and so I'm here because I'm curious to find the line between process and progress.

As Loraine begins unwrapping the skin off each tomato—first scoring its ends, dunking it into a bath of boiling water and then into ice water before she peels away the flesh—we cluster around her, notepads at the ready. One woman says, "I can't imagine doing this in the old days with no air-conditioning in a hot kitchen." We all laugh.

"With dirt floors and ten kids," says another, and we chuckle again.

Ten kids and dirt floors: Isn't this every modern woman's nightmare? I don't even have to imagine it, I can feel it on my skin—the back of a palm swiped across a sweaty forehead, the frizzy-haired resignation pulled back into its own headband, the falling away from your own self's sovereignty and into the needs of your family. I remember the cramped kitchen of my dad's home in West Texas, and imagine my grandmother corralling her clan of stubborn boys into the kitchen at the end of summer to help her can the winter's wares. My grandfather owned a farm, and though he leased most of his land to cotton growers, some of it was still dedicated to food production and livestock. A cow would be butchered at the end of the summer, and the meat freezer would fill with sirloin and brisket. Tomatoes would flourish, along with corn, zucchini, and okra, and the kitchen would fill with the sound of mason jars rattling around a tub of boiling water and four boys jostling for space as they slipped hot produce into hotter jars.

When her boys were young, her husband still alive, and my grandmother was tasked with preserving the foods that would populate her family's meals throughout a year, a mason jar was not a symbol of unprocessed, of counterculture. It was a small piece of technology that had better not fail.

I miss my grandmother, miss her drawling voice wavering over a telephone line. I wish I could hear her say "my word," pronounced *whirred*, the syrup of Texas speech finally catching her after so many years. What is odd about taking a class to learn how to can tomatoes is that this used to be simply known, passed from kitchen to kitchen like stories through a family. My dad remembers the agony of being twelve and being forced to can food with his family instead of running across rivers; I remember grocery shopping with my mom and the anticipation of spongy microwave pancakes clasped between small fingers. When we visited my grandmother in Texas, as thunderstorms built across summer skies, we didn't cluster in the kitchen. Rather, Katie and I sprawled on a knotted carpet in the living room, my grandmother perched in her electric throne above us, and we watched *I Love Lucy* reruns. I was young and my grandmother was old and it simply never occurred to me to ask her how she had once preserved food for her family.

IN 1795, WHEN OPTIONS FOR PRESERVING FOOD consisted of chucking it in the ground with something cold or smothering it in salt and hanging it from a hook, the French military offered the hefty sum of twelve thousand francs to anyone who could figure out a better way to preserve food for the nation's overextended troops. Nicolas Appert was a Parisian confectioner who had been fiddling with preservation for years; he fiddled for another fourteen years—claiming prize money was evidently a bit less urgent back then—and in 1810, he announced the innovation that transformed modern diets. Put food in a jar, cork it, and boil it.

Fifty years before Appert won his prize money, human diets had already begun rolling toward a colder modernity. In 1748, a Scot named William Cullen let ethyl ether boil in a partial vacuum and created the first artificial refrigeration system, though it took another century before the technology was available to the masses. In 1914, the DOMELRE (Domestic Electric Refrigerator) first becomes available, complete with an ice cube tray, and in 1944, the U.S. Office of Education released a film titled *Principles of Refrigeration* to remind the American public that "the process of producing cold is the process of removing heat"—that coldness is defined by the absence of heat energy. When molecules move to and fro—like the cartoon bacteria wiggling within a cartoon chicken leg—they produce kinetic energy, or heat. The difference between a solid, liquid, and a gas is the difference in this movement, in the relative vibrations of a substance's molecules. When a liquid changes to a gas, it absorbs heat energy from its surroundings; when those surroundings happen to be a cartoon leg of chicken, "heat is withdrawn from it." While we say that food becomes cold in a refrigerator, the truth is rather that it becomes less hot—its molecules slow down, and so, therefore, does the growth of bacteria that might spoil a cartoon chicken leg.

The chemicals we've used to chill our fridges and freezers have run the gamut from abrasive (ammonia) to downright toxic (sulfur dioxide), so it was quite big news when, in the 1920s, a team at General Motors synthesized a new carbon compound—a chlorofluorocarbon, or CFC—that seemed neither abrasive nor toxic. In 1937, Freon was deemed "the ideal refrigerant" and "a milestone in modern refrigeration history." This "safe refrigerant, which is harmless to human beings and to products, and which will not burn or explode" offered a real advance in food storage: Freon was stable and it was cheap. In the 1920s, relatively few homes had refrigerators—as few as five thousand in 1921. Within two decades, a General Electric pamphlet declared, "America's 20,000,000 mechanical refrigerators represent a vital part of our national economy."

Freezers captivated a generation of homemakers, promising to liberate them from the seasons that reigned over their kitchens. "Imagine eating fresh peaches and cream while winter winds blow snow against your windows—imagine perfect ears of fresh golden corn to coax your family out of the March doldrums," exclaimed a General Electric home-freezer instruction pamphlet. "The miracle of frozen foods makes these and many other delightful dishes possible all year round!" (The pamphlet also cautioned the overexuberant food freezer, *"Freezing will not improve low-grade foods!"*)

By the time I was growing up, the promise of Freon—the promise of CFCs—had come to fruition as a giant hole in our ozone layer. Unlike Bernard London, unlike my parents, I came of age in a time of nature's limits. By the time I was born, the drudgery avoided by the technology of convenience had simply been billed to my generation, the generation that had to learn how to live in an increasingly cluttered world, to reckon with convenience's waste. By the time I knew to ask where things came from—the cotton in my blue jeans, the plastic in my hair dryer, the gasoline in my mom's Volvo—it was understood that nature did not produce with such reckless abandon, that the raw materials of the world were not boundless. That they might, in fact, soon become scarce.

WHEN ORGANIC TOMATOES GO ON SALE for seventy-nine cents a pound at the 17th Street Market, I buy six pounds, nearly enough to fill a plastic shopping bag to the brim for only $4.74, and set aside a Wednesday evening. To prepare for my evening of canning, I find a used sixteen-liter stove pot—tall enough to submerge four one-pint mason jars in boiling water—and spend $4.99 on a new pair of tongs required to excavate my jars from below the boiling water once they have been sterilized.

"I don't get how canning tomatoes proves anything," my sister says. "You don't live on a farm, you live near a Safeway."

She has a point—especially since I've just spent more on my canning supplies than I did on the tomatoes. Of course, if the tomato seedlings that Sarah and I planted all those months ago, now swathed in burlap shade cloth, protected from the beating sun, had actually born fruit, I'd have a more urgent incentive to preserve my bounty. While we'd harvested a total of six fat watermelons and a profusion of bell peppers, the cucumber seedlings seem to have been strangled below the watermelons' suffocating vines, and the tomatoes—well, the tomatoes *had* grown, into spindly stalks of coarse green matter that we had searched up and down for the sign of a flower, to no avail.

Why can my own food, besides just to show that I could? In 1943, the U.S. Bureau of Human Nutrition and Home Economics issued a guide for Wartime Canning of Fruits and Vegetables, encouraging the country's fledgling canners to do their patriotic duty. "Every jar of garden-fresh fruits and vegetables you put up at your home this year will do double duty. It will help your family to keep well-fed next winter. And it will help the Nation by easing the load on transportation and commercial food supplies." Today, it's hard to read the pamphlet without the screen of irony, as today we are supposed to help "the Nation" by *increasing* our consumption of commercial food supplies. Maybe this is why canning is back in style. It's no longer a patriotic act but rather one of subversion, as we withhold our support from a commercial food supply that has failed to keep us "well-fed."

I skin and slice my own beefsteak tomatoes as Loraine demonstrated. I wash my hands excessively, sweating in the clean steam of a stove pot full of mason jars that quietly clang and dance around the boiling water. Standing over my counter, listening to music, scoring, dunking, unraveling the skin of tomato after tomato, I relax into the motions of this task. Canning is hard enough that it requires my mind to stay attentive, but not hard enough that I must train my attention on it and it alone.

My grandmother never wanted Texas. She grew up in Chicago, and her stomach sank when her new husband, John, a hunky World War II veteran, brought her to Floydada for the first time. Floydada, a name that's hard to pronounce unless you're slow on your vowels—*Floy* like cloy, *day* with a twang, *duh* with a lift—with only three thousand people and so much sky. That dismay must have ballooned like a thunderstorm rolling over cotton fields when he died two decades later, leaving her to wrestle with the family farm. Left her to reckon with the neighbors, to correspond with the creditors, and to collect the accounts payable. Dickens, no!—no woman in West Texas could, would, *should* possibly run a farm *all* by her *lonesome*. So my grandmother rewrote her letterhead and changed her signature from "Joyce Kimble" to the genderless "J. Kimble" and she plowed ahead, undeterred.

I'm going to Lubbock, Texas, in a few weeks to present a paper at a literature conference. My parents don't want me to drive—it's so far, the landscape so lonely. But like my grandmother, I am stubborn, and that is why I want to drive—so I can escape the conference early and visit Floydada, a short sixty miles northeast of Lubbock. When we were kids, we flew into Lubbock almost every year, leaned into a grandmother's waiting arms, and pressed against windows for the hour drive back to Floydada. A long road through long cotton. My grandmother blinked at the road through bright blue eyes and slouched over the blue-beige steering wheel with increasingly concave shoulders. I think about those shoulders as mine mimic their shape, slouching over a too-short counter, peeling tomatoes.

I peel and dice six pounds of tomatoes. A slice down the middle of each tomato, three quick scores across its body, and then a scoop into a saucepan simmering over heat. I slip the cooked tomatoes into jars along with a tablespoon of lemon juice and a sprig of rosemary.

The top of a mason jar has two parts. The lid, a plastic rimmed metal disk that suctions to hot glass, creates the seal that protects the food inside from the outside air, while a metal ring secures the lid in place while the jar boils underwater for forty minutes. After forty minutes, Loraine said, after you pull the jars out from underneath their water baths, the lid will click. You can hear it, she said, so wait for it: It sounds like a whispered *thunk,* a quiet gasp. The jars are heavy when I pull them out of the boiling water, but I hold on tight, worried I'll shatter the hot glass on my exposed thighs. They both make it safely to my kitchen counter. (After sterilizing four pint-size mason jars, I'm shocked when six pounds of tomatoes fill only two to the brim.) I watch. It's only a minute before the jar to the right—it's so quick I nearly miss it—thunks. It thunks, and I peer over it, gleeful, to see that the lid has collapsed, concave, the seal set. Lefty isn't ready to thunk, but Loraine says this sometimes takes a few hours, so I leave him to his business and head to bed.

The next morning, the lid of the left jar is concave—it is thunked. Picking it up, I am impressed by its heft. I shake it about and then hold it up to my face and see, finally, tiny air bubbles scattered throughout. I see air bubbles in what is supposed to be a vacuum-sealed jar, and I realize—shitshit*shit*—that I forgot to smash the tomatoes down into the jar, forgot to exhume these tiny fingers of oxygen that sit there, latently ominous, capable of growing nefarious bacteria to poke into one of my carefully sterilized tomato chunks.

I pick up the other tomato jar and it, too, is infested with oxygen. I glare at them. I pause. And then I glance at my refrigerator, ye beacon of progress and process, of preserved safety and cold storage. The jars are probably fine. The tomatoes are probably sterile and will likely remain so until I eat them. But the nervousness that began our canning class creeps back across my counters. It would really be a bummer to give myself botulism. I stand there with my two jars, torn between cabinet and refrigerator. I waver on the line between progress and process—between those processes that offered real progress for the safety of our food supply and those that only isolated us from real food's pleasure. I am not my grandmother—I live, as my sister said, closer to Safeway than soil. As much as I try to opt out of this modern system, as I try to eat seasonally, to enjoy the root vegetables that will populate my CSA share all winter, when push comes to shove, this safety net exists. There are still fresh tomatoes for sale at Tucson's food co-op; when they go out of season, I can buy their canned compatriots a few aisles over. I will not go hungry if these tomatoes go bad, and I realize that this experiment, this unprocessing of food, with all its successes and failures and late-night microwave breaking, depends upon that safety net. I slide my two heavy glass jars full of ripe, red tomatoes onto a bright, cold shelf. The fridge gives an automated grumble of assent as it whooshes shut.

THE QUESTION OF WHETHER OR NOT we should can our tomatoes in August rather than rely on cold storage to transport them in January—the question of whether or not we should reclaim any of food's other processes—is as much an environmental question as it is one of work and what makes for a pleasurable Wednesday evening.

Whether or not you think cooking is a pleasurable way to spend a Wednesday evening determines how you respond to the fact that the average time we spend preparing our food has plummeted over the past century—about three hours a day in the 1920s, down to about ninety minutes in 1965, to a precious thirty-three minutes today. One interpretation of this decline is that it has liberated us to do other things—rather, it has liberated *women* to do other things. While in 1926, women were spending on average twenty-three hours a week preparing food and cleaning the home, in the late 1950s, that total had dropped to seventeen hours. By then, women had help—the housewife could rely on the assistance of food manufacturers to do more food preparation for her. (A woman is, by the way, always referred to as a housewife in the food literature of this era.) In the 1950s, the American Can Company published a series of pamphlets exalting this new culture of convenience: "There's a new kind of cooking developing in American kitchens today . . . we call it 'Quick Trick Cookery' because food canners and manufacturers have done all the drudgery for you . . . This modern processing leaves you free to spend your time using your creative talents and imagination in the classroom or in the kitchen."

Even as I scoff at this yellowed pamphlet's pride at liberating the housewife from kitchen drudgery to pursue these expansive options, my coffeepot grumbles and I scuttle out the door to work.

The point of unprocessed is not to return to some idealized moment in our food history, to a time when my only option for pleasurable work was in the kitchen. As much as I savor the image of my lanky dad and his three brothers slouching while they slipped diced vegetables into mason jars, I don't envy my grandmother's task: feeding a household of hungry men on the grace of her good planning and an acre's harvest. Our nostalgia for the foods we used to eat often fails to take into account the work required to make those foods—and who's going to do it. Progress has been made in the kitchen since the time when "woman" and "housewife" were synonymous terms, and I am grateful for it. It is indeed the legacy of packaged foods—first it was already-churned butter, then already-baked bread—that gave us time, and therefore choice, to step out of the home and into the world. Now that we have Cheese Whiz and crackers, we flit away to work and play, freed from the work of feeding our bodies (and the bodies of those who might depend on us). But what was it that I was rushing out in the world to do, exactly— what was I so eager to achieve?

"I do not believe that 'employment outside the house' is as valuable or important or satisfying as employment at home, for either men or women," wrote Wendell Berry in his famous 1987 essay "Why I Am Not Going to Buy a Computer." The man got some serious flak when he declared that his work didn't require a computer—thus reducing his addiction to the energy corporations, freeing him from contributing to "the rape of nature"—because his wife transcribed his handwritten manuscripts on a Royal standard typewriter, editing and correcting as she typed. Originally published in the *New England Review,* the essay appeared next in *Harper's* magazine with reader comments alongside the piece. "Wendell Berry provides writers enslaved by the computer with a handy alternative," wrote one reader. "Wife—a low-tech energy-saving device. Drop a pile of handwritten notes on Wife and you get back a finished manuscript, edited while it was typed. Wife meets all of Berry's uncompromising standards for technological innovation: She's cheap, repairable near home, and good for the family structure."

Berry responded: "If I had written in my essay that my wife worked as a typist and editor for a publishing house, doing the same work that she does for me, no feminists, I daresay, would have written to *Harper's* to attack me for exploiting her . . . It would have been assumed as a matter of course that if she had a job away from home she was a 'liberated woman,' possessed of a dignity that no home could confer upon her."

As we know it today, work takes place in a realm outside the home. Work is something directed to an outside end; chores are something we must do in here. But what makes for good work? If a wife edits her husband's manuscript because it contributes to the economic well-being of a shared household—and because she enjoys it—is this better work than what she might do for someone else, somewhere else, to earn a paycheck to contribute to that same household? The better question might actually be: Is it more pleasurable? "More and more, we take for granted that work must be destitute of pleasure. More and more, we assume that if we want to be pleased we must wait until evening, or the weekend, or vacation, or retirement," wrote Berry in a later essay, "Economy and Pleasure." "We are defeated at work because our work gives us no pleasure. We are defeated at home because we have no pleasant work there."

Since the first half of the twentieth century, women have exchanged work in the kitchen for work in the world—and thus so did I, without ever knowing it was a decision to be made.

MY FAMILY ATE DINNER TOGETHER almost every night when I was growing up. And almost every night, my mom cooked that dinner. It was enough of a struggle to tear my dad away from the lab, to break his laserlike focus on some new frontier in quantum physics. I don't know if they ever discussed the division of labor—maybe it just emerged naturally. Katie and I were tasked with our own breakfast—mini pancakes, please—while my dad made our lunches and took us to school. My mom did the shopping and so she made dinner.

After I can my tomatoes, on a Sunday afternoon early in September, I call home and ask my mom what it was like—shopping, cooking, and cleaning while also working. She says, as if she's still slightly irritated with me, "Oh, you were *such* a picky eater. You went through a phase where you'd only eat noodles covered with blue cheese dressing and bacon bits."

I remember, as soon as she says it, the taste of bacon bits covered in blue cheese—delicious. "Did you worry about getting healthy foods on the table?" I ask.

"Well, I think what I considered healthy back then is really different from what I consider to be healthy now," she says. "The problem was that you guys wanted pasta most of the time, so we made a lot of pasta. Do you remember what the girls ate, Jeff?"

My dad's sitting next to my mom on the couch and we switch to speakerphone so he can chime in. "It was a constant struggle between giving you something you'd eat and something healthy." As if to substantiate my mom's earlier irritation, he adds, "You were *so* picky. That was part of the reason to send you to the store with your mom. It was clear those Lunchable things you'd buy were not a very good choice, but you'd eat them. I made all the lunches—so okay, throw *that* in a bag and I'm off the hook."

I press my mom on the time issue. She was on her feet all day, commanding a classroom full of seventh graders. Wasn't it hard to work all day and then come home and cook dinner? She's noncommittal—I can almost hear her shrug. "I don't know. You know, we'd do all the shopping on Sunday, so the food would be there."

I'm surprised at her nonchalance. The fact that my mom cooked dinner every night seems now, in adulthood, like a defining feature of my childhood, and she is literally shrugging it off.

"Your mom was always reading cookbooks and nutrition stuff, to help get good ideas," my dad says. "We weren't hippies, but we've always been on the healthy end of the spectrum."

"What'd *you* eat growing up, Mom?" I ask.

"I grew up on Velveeta. Meat and potatoes. On Sunday, my mom would cook a big roast. Monday, she'd chop it up and make a casserole and Tuesday she'd do something different with it."

"Did you or Grandma ever can foods?"

"No, no, I lived in the city," she says.

"So?" I ask.

"I guess we never needed to," she says. "We went to the grocery. I think frozen vegetables were just becoming popular in the sixties. There was an evolution of cooking. Everyone started steaming their vegetables, instead of boiling them."

My dad chimes in. "Growing up, every vegetable I ate was soggy. You didn't need teeth to eat them. I remember the first time I had steamed broccoli. It was still crisp. I didn't know broccoli could taste like that."

"Food has changed immensely in my lifetime," my mom says. "Back when I started cooking, if you wanted salad, you took a head of lettuce, washed it, tore it, and chopped it up. I remember when we began to get different kinds of bagged vegetables that were cut up. Bagged lettuce—that was crazy! When was that? Maybe the nineties."

"Was that a good thing for you, as a cook?" I ask.

"Yes," she says. "Of course. But it was more expensive and those were the days I had to pay attention to every penny."

"But it also meant that coming home, your mom could cook stuff up faster," my dad says. "It was more expensive, but it was convenient."

Today, I can come home and assemble dinner in ten minutes from a bag of precut broccoli, premarinated tofu, quick-cook rice, and a bottle of sesame sauce. While all these foods pass the kitchen test, the processing that happens behind the scenes is as new a contribution to cooking as flash freezing was to the 1960s. Mildly processed foods are indeed more expensive—per pound, a head of broccoli will always be cheaper if you buy it whole—but the precut ones are undeniably appealing in their convenience. More money at the store for less time at home.

The problem with this convenience is in its excess. Instead of combining discrete, identifiable foods into something like a meal, we outsource this combination to someone else. We buy Stouffer's frozen lasagna and end up eating modified food starch. We go to Chili's and end up with a plate full of high-fructose corn syrup instead of the enchiladas we thought we'd ordered.

What I remember about our family dinners is not what we ate, but rather the events around eating. My mom scolding us when we got in her way as she rushed around the kitchen. Bickering with my sister about whose turn it was to set the table. I learned to cook hovering over my mom and I learned respect (more so in retrospect) when she'd get up to do the dishes, too.

Feeding a family requires compromise, and in the modern supermarket, compromises abound. My mom has paid attention to food her whole life—she became a vegetarian in college because she didn't like how animals were treated; she shopped at Whole Foods back when it was a garage-size natural food store in Austin. So of course, when it came time, she'd try to cook healthy meals for her family—it was work, but work that contributed to a household's well-being.

ON A LOLLING, SWEATY SUNDAY IN PLAYA GIGANTE, I found a book left behind by a hotel client: *More Than Money: Questions Every MBA Needs to Answer,* written by former Harvard Business School professor Mark Albion. Starved for media, I read anything in English that crossed my path in Playa Gigante—decade-old *Surfer* magazines, recent issues of *Men's Health,* trashy novels, or aged guidebooks. *More Than Money* promised to tell me how to find "real wealth" in the business world, encouraged me to "think *differently* about career possibilities." Albion poses a question to all those budding businessmen out there, in school to learn about *how* to make money but not necessarily *why.* He asks, "What will your contribution be?" and tells an anecdote to prove his point.

> An American businessman was at the pier of a small coastal Mexican village when a small boat with a lone fisherman docked. Inside the boat were several large yellowfin tuna. He complimented the fisherman on the quality of the fish and asked how long it took to catch them. "Only a little while," the fisherman replied.

The businessman then asked why he didn't stay out longer to catch more fish, certain there must be a demand.

> The fisherman smiled. "I catch enough to support my family and I live a full and busy life. I rise with the sun, fish a little, play with my daughters, have lunch with my family, and then teach children

how to fish before I stroll into the village each evening where I sip wine and play guitar with my wife and friends."

Listen, said the budding businessman. I have an MBA. I could help you. He told the fisherman how he could expand his small fishing business into a *big* fishing business. How he could buy a fleet of boats, turn a profit, invest in expansion. He could move to the capital, fund an Initial Public Offering, and eventually—become a millionaire.

> "Really? A millionaire? Then what?"
> "What do you mean?" asked the MBA, a bit surprised.
> "I mean, what would I do if I were a millionaire?"
> "Whatever you like, of course. I'd imagine you'd retire, move to a small coastal fishing village where you would rise with the sun, fish a little, play with your granddaughters, have lunch with your family, and then teach children how to fish before strolling into the village each evening where you'd sip wine and play guitar with your wife and friends."

I remember reading this passage on the Brio deck, cradled in the hammock of a wicker chair, watching the sun flirt with the ocean horizon. I knew, even then, that the fishermen in the village below were not sipping wine and playing guitar; that they were stringing nets and preparing for an early morning, hoping for a good catch. But as the round belly of the sun eased into the water, I wondered. At what point does our work advance or enrich us, materially and spiritually, and at what point does it remove us from the activities—intellectual, communal, emotional—that accumulate into a life lived well?

There's no easy fix. No way to say to women—or men—that they must work *and* cook. But I can't help but wonder if, when we outsource the process of making food to someone else, we also lose something essential in the process of living. In the name of economy, of time or capital, we have outsourced to others those key activities that define the day-to-day. Don't want to make a lunch? Buy a Lunchable. Don't want to help your kids with algebra? Hire a tutor. But what is life if not the day-to-day? Sunsets in Nicaragua and family vacations in the Canadian Rockies are spectacular, but if that's what we're waiting around for, what is the point of a Wednesday evening? The tasks we have decided to label mundane—as tasks!—are that which accumulate into relationships and memories. Cooking dinner or helping your kids with homework.

If what we do every day is more important than what we do once in a while, then outsourcing our day-to-day demands to serve the goals of the once-in-awhile—those big-ticket purchases we save our time and money for—seems like a net loss. A little chipping away at the fullness of life, in all its messiness.

Although canning tomatoes felt like an antiquated endeavor in an age of supermarkets and flash freezing, I wondered if the point of eating unprocessed was to start to reclaim some of these outsourced activities for myself. To strip away all those assumed yet invisible outsourcing decisions we all make every day with our dollars, pushing the processes of life out of our personal domain and into the abstract. I buy a loaf of presliced bread, make soup from a can of preskinned tomatoes, and it is too easy to forget that these foods have sources, that *someone* processed them, and that not too long ago, that person was a housewife.

A FEW WEEKS AFTER I CAN MY TOMATOES, a new semester begins and I step back into busy days. I look down into work, and when I look up again, my weeks have flown into fall and it is time for me to drive from Tucson to Texas. I drive because flights are expensive, but really I drive because I want to *do* distance. I want to know, to feel and see, how it is that Tucson becomes Willcox becomes Deming becomes Las Cruces becomes Artesia becomes Brownfield becomes Lubbock.

During the days of our summer visits, I rode my grandmother's bike around Floydada. Her bike didn't have brakes, but it didn't need them: Gravity pulled you to a stop on the flat gravel streets, if you had the patience to let it. In the mountains above Los Angeles, I was barely allowed to venture two topsy-turvy blocks to a friend's house, but in Floydada, the flat roads let me roam, alone. I biked down to the Conoco station on Tennessee Street; I glided to the Dairy Queen and maybe all the way down to Lowe's Supermarket on Farm Road 284 to buy vanilla ice cream and chocolate syrup.

Fifteen years later, the Lowe's supermarket seems fuller somehow. The kaleidoscope of the interior—bright, packed aisles, a symphony of selection—is incongruous with the dust-faded, cotton-strewn streets of the town. Lowe's sells both canned and fresh tomatoes, as well as Floydada Whirlwind T-shirts, emblazoned with the high school's tornado insignia, alongside copies of the *2012 Old Farmer's Almanac, Southern Edition.* I haven't been to Floydada since my dad's youngest brother died two years ago, when we buried him next to his mother and father in the Floydada cemetery. I am nervous and lonely, paled by a dark drive across eleven hours of desert and flat plains, and so I dally in the supermarket aisles, comforted by the crowded bounty of all this food. This Lowe's wasn't open when my dad was in high school, didn't sell fresh spinach and broccoli when he left Floydada to go to college. When my grandfather died in 1976, leaving behind four sons and a young widow, if you wanted food in Floydada, you grew it yourself or went someplace else to get it.

As I wander around Lowe's, I think about buying a bar of chocolate to put on my grandmother's grave, but find only bars of Hershey's Milk Chocolate for sale. Remembering her righteous outrage whenever we offered her anything less than the darkest of chocolate, I leave the bar on the shelf.

I buy a bag of minicarrots, munching as I walk to the parking lot to my white Civic, incongruous in this small town of big trucks. My peppy car with its Arizona plates: I do not belong here, and so the man outside the gas station waves at me as I roll past on the way to the cemetery.

John, Joyce, and Joel are in the back row of the Floydada Cemetery. Their short gravestones face away from the manicured graveyard and onto an open field, into the open sky. Wisps of cotton accumulate against the upright stones like snowdrifts. I unfold myself from my car and settle onto the gravel before their marble placeholders. The marble is hard and cold against my dry fingers as I trace their names. I sit, cross-legged, in front of Joyce and John and Joel and let the wind whip my hair into great tumbleweed tangles. I sit still, silent, for a moment, and then, craving contact, to feel the solidness of the earth—to feel strength in matter rather than the erasure of wind—I crawl toward my grandmother's headstone, shimmy my weight around, and then lie on the earth, facing skyward, my head resting on the slanted gray stone.

The broad, blue sky is too much to ingest at once, so I diminish it with glances at my stretched-out body, black jeans, and a gray sweater; a flat stomach and bendy legs. A young body—my body is young and it is an odd thing to know this, to know that its youth will not last, that my smooth skin and running energy will fade into my grandmother's brittle hands and fragile gait. A body's increasing limits, its tangible demise, must feel very odd when your mind does not fail along with it. However trapped my grandmother felt living in West Texas, she must have struggled so much more with being trapped in the body that confined her to a wheelchair for the last years of her life, a sharp mind shut in a broken body.

I lie on my grandmother's headstone for a while, long enough for my cheeks to burn soft pink under the autumn sun and hard wind.

WHEN I GET BACK TO LUBBOCK, before I canvass the streets of this deep-fried, Tex-Mex city looking for an unprocessed dinner—the best option turns out to be a Chipotle salad, sans dressing—I stop by the National Ranching Heritage Center, a twenty-seven-acre park hanging on the edge of the Texas Tech campus. Founded in 1976, the Heritage Center is populated by fifty historic ranching buildings salvaged from around Texas—Milk and Meat House, circa 1880; Slaughter Round Pen and Nance Snubbing Post, circa 1900; Old Block Ranch Drift Fence, late 1880s.

I peer, wander, lean into the buildings, and then step into the Pitchfork Cookhouse, built in 1900, salvaged from Dickens County, Texas. A stark informational plaque reads: "The cookhouse began as a one-room structure. The dining area was added later. There are no frills. This was a working ranch kitchen."

Two heavy picnic tables, set end to end, span the length of the room. Eighteen plates and eighteen cups sit loosely on the wood planks. I duck through a low doorway and walk into the kitchen, sized to the same scale. Cast in silver steel and whitewashed wood, the kitchen revolves around a large island in the middle, a steel expanse cowering below a hanging array of cast-iron kitchen implements: spatulas, knives, tongs, flyswatters. Above the double-door iron oven—the doors fall open with a loud clang when I peer inside—beside the eight-burner stove, is a quaint line of tin containers, arranged from small to large: salt, pepper, tea, grease, coffee, sugar, flour. At the end, a fifty-pound tin can—large enough to hold a few basketballs—wears a label of KRAFT PURE VEGETABLE SHORTENING. The whitewashed, wood-panel walls of the kitchen try to be cheery. Bright light spills in from the glass windows, spreading sun across the countertops; but even now, on a fall afternoon, the decor seems to cringe at the sound of the wind grinding against the old structure, to flinch into the sagging linoleum floor, dirty, cracked, and cold to the touch.

This is it—this is what my fellow canner was talking about when she joked about "the old days." This is the modern woman's nightmare. A roomful of chattering family and friends could drown out the dismal wind, but standing alone in this century-old cookhouse, I feel no desire to return to these early days in our nation's settlement. This same wind was blowing across the plains when the first settlers arrived, when they gazed across the land and began to build the infrastructure that would protect and nourish them.

Finally, I notice it: a white appliance nudged into a white corner. A rounded rectangular General Electric freezer-fridge combination, with a steel handle attached to a heavy door that exhales like a secret when I pull it open.

As I stand, alone, in this kitchen, I feel the scattering of my family across the country. It is not just my nuclear family—my parents in Los Angeles, my sister and brother-in-law in Seattle—but also the extension of uncles and cousins spanning the country. Not one of my dad's brothers returned to live in Floydada after high school, landing in Oregon, Tennessee, New Mexico—and, of course, California.

The geography of my recent drive makes it hard to ignore how right in the middle I am between the far-flung and its source. Eight hours from Los Angeles, west on the Interstate 10—eleven from Lubbock, east on the Interstate 10. I am straddling something, some sort of decision of distance, and although I don't know what this decision is, it occurs to me, as I walk back to my car through a landscape of re-created history, that a scattered life is, by necessity, a processed one. Young, modern, and urban are the qualities that define my relationship to food more than any distance I traverse along the processed-unprocessed spectrum, and it is precisely these three qualities that make un-processing my foodways so difficult.

In January, I started a project that I believed would be quiet and personal. I tried to bake bread alone in my apartment and I failed. I started with a sad sack of wheat and realized its rancidity only when I ventured out and met Kyle the farmer and Jeff the miller. Chocolate and vegetables showed me that it was only when I combined forces with other goals, other projects and personalities, that I could start to unprocess my food.

Community is both the blessing and curse of urbanity. With so many people in one place, we can create our own communities wherever we happen to land, but as we move away from our families, we have to decide to build these support networks. If our natural families are so scattered, what else is there to do but outsource some of the processes that relatives and neighbors have provided for so long? It takes a village, of course; now we are simply paying for that village.

We slip away from our families so easily; we get into college, hire moving trucks, and inertia intercedes. Two decades ago, when my mom sent Katie and me to our rooms for childhood transgressions, we shimmied our bellies into the adjacent hallway, our hindquarters firmly in-room as ordered, and bowed our heads together in whispered giggles. Small decisions accumulate—jobs and significant others—and now we live two thousand miles away from each other. I am twenty-six and happily childless, but occasionally I think about it, what I might do when I have kids. I want my hypothetical children to grow up around their grandparents, around their aunt and uncle. It's not really even a want—it is, like heat moving to cold, an act of chemistry. Katie is twenty-eight, two years married, and on the brink. We talk about it, and she jokes that I should move into their furnished attic—she has named it, in my honor, the Writer's Attic. What we don't ask each other is how it might even be feasible to create and raise a new life when we are both so severed by distance from the lives that shaped our own.

I wanted to can my own vegetables to remove myself, however slightly, from the refrigerated boxcars and semi trucks that shuttle another region's seasons to our supermarkets. But if a point of unprocessed is to recalibrate the work I have outsourced in order to live my urban life—without forgoing that urban life, without relinquishing the intellectual work offered to modern females, the work that distinguishes me from my west Texas ancestors—then I will work with refrigeration.

Unprocess Yourself: Refrigeration

The easiest way to unprocess your kitchen is to cook your own food. What exactly constitutes cooking will vary significantly from person to person. The difference between my cooking and your cooking has to do with where we start—with a whole shoulder of pork or presliced bacon; with tomatoes off a vine or skinned in a can; with presliced bread or a bag of flour.

I view the trade-off of process for convenience thusly: The farther an ingredient is from its source when you buy it, the greater the burden is on you to figure out where it came from and how it got to you.

I love to cook and I love to shop for food, so it is easy for me to reclaim many of food's processes. If you don't like to cook, then the trade-off of time or hassle saved is that you have to be able to trust the companies that are selling you your food—which means you have to do some investigating. It is fine to buy food made by someone else—just make sure that someone is someone who deserves your money (and your money's multiplier effects).

There is no right answer to how far an ingredient should be from its source before you cook with it—or before you consume it—but be deliberate in the processes you decide to outsource. I am perfectly fine with buying store-bought bread and store-made tortillas from companies I trust, but there is something I don't like about buying presliced vegetables, premade sauces, or preshredded cheese. One thing I don't like is the trade-off: In exchange for saving a bit of time, I'm agreeing to consume the chemicals that keep these foods fresh once they've been cut or mixed.

Every August, when the Tucson CSA sells twenty-pound flats of tomatoes for twenty dollars, I buy a flat and set a water bath to boiling. I like the process of canning tomatoes as much for the ritual as for the tomatoes. So I can.

To can tomatoes, you'll need: pint or quart canning jars, rings, and new lids; a pot tall enough to fit the jars, plus about four inches; a canning jar funnel, to fill jars; a jar grabber, to pull hot jars out of the water bath; a couple of mixing bowls and a slotted spoon. And, of course, tomatoes, as well as lemon juice. Start by sterilizing the lids and jars by submerging them in boiling water for thirty minutes (a dishwasher works, too). Cook and skin tomatoes—score each end, dunk in boiling water for thirty seconds, or until the skins begin to crinkle, and immediately submerge in a bowlful of ice water. Dice tomatoes. Add a centimeter or so of lemon juice to each jar, and fill to the threads with diced tomatoes and any leftover tomato juice. With the back of a spoon, push the tomatoes down into the jar until they are submerged in liquid. Secure the lids—don't screw the ring on too tightly—and put the jars back into a pot full of boiling water. (It helps if you add a dishcloth to the bottom of the pot so that the glass jars don't clatter around too much.) Leave submerged in the boiling water for forty-five to sixty minutes, depending on the size of the jars. Remove jars from the water with the jar grabber—carefully, as they'll be heavy. Once the jars are cool, double-check to make sure the lid is "thunked," or sucked down, signaling the food is sealed.

10

DAIRY

Milk is a process of scale.

"The goat cheese is in the refrigerator," I tell Dave. "I think there's also Parmesan and blue in there." We're making dinner in my casita's small kitchen; I'm chopping vegetables while Dave assembles a cheese platter. In the months since we first cooked together, our roles have been defined. I do dinner, Dave does hors d'oeuvres. I chop vegetables; Dave assembles cheese.

Dave was an hour late to our third date because of cheese. I offered to make veggie tacos at my casita and he arrived well past nine because, well, as a rule, Dave is late; on this particular evening, he had also detoured to two Trader Joe's trying to find taleggio cheese—his favorite—before giving up and arriving instead with Camembert, blue, and herbed goat cheese. I spun chilies and tomatoes into salsa in the food processor, sautéed fillings for our tacos, and toasted tortillas, all while he'd arranged small trios of cheese on tomato slices. I couldn't imagine what he'd possibly been doing for all that time until he'd offered me a tomato and I slid it into my mouth like an oyster. Three nibbles of three cheeses; honey drizzled on top, red pepper flakes sprinkled over sticky sweetness. The kick of blue cheese, the musty tinge of Camembert, and the smooth-it-over ease of goat cheese—subtle and satiating, unquestionably worthy of twenty minutes' labor. If I am knowledge, Dave is nuance, and with this cheese plate, I learn how to linger in detail.

In October, I finally fall for cheese. In spite of my mother's profuse love of quesadillas, mac n' cheese, microwave nachos—or maybe because of it—I'd never been much of a cheese enthusiast. It was the first food I cut when I started Weight Watchers: Chocolate over Cheese, I declared. Dessert Before Dairy. I still ate cheese, but it was low-point, fat-free, chemically assembled stuff. It was a reference to cheese, a gesture toward curd, but nowhere near the stuff itself. My stomach is finicky and my sweet tooth rages after dark, so I figured it was easier to skip it altogether. Why bother with a cheese plate when there's molten chocolate cake on the menu?

After I began my year unprocessed, the assumption shifted. When sugar- and flour-filled molten chocolate cake is off the table, why *not* try the cheese plate? Cheese that stretches into stringy ropes; cheese that molds into stinky flavor; cheese that coheres into creamy curds. Cheese that comes from milk.

"ROXIE IS FUNNY, SWEET, SASSY, CUTE, AND KIND," says Debbie. "She's what we all strive to be." Roxie is a Holstein cow. Roxie is not just a Holstein cow; she is a stand-in for *every* Holstein cow at Shamrock Farms, all ten thousand of them. Roxie speaks for the masses; or rather, the masses are Roxie.

"She's our mascot, and we treat her well," says Denise, leaning on one of the three life-size cement Holsteins that keep us corralled in the visitor center's lobby. Hilary and I have each just paid nine dollars for the opportunity to tour this dairy farm spread across a thousand acres just south of Phoenix, and I'm surprised to realize, as we shuffle toward the tour tram and Debbie instructs us to "keep our hooves and horns inside the vehicle"—as I notice that we're the only adults unaccompanied by small children—that this will not be a tour geared toward us.

"Roxie's only job is to produce milk," says Debbie. "We take care of everything else for her." Roxie is fed from the "cow cafeteria." She eats feed assembled from house-size piles of flaked corn, soybeans, dried alfalfa, canola, and cottonseed. She cools off in the "Desert Oasis," lounges in the shade of corrugated tin and misting machines, and when her hooves get crusted and dirty, she gets a "cow pedicure." Debbie says, "We don't want her stressed. We want her in top condition to produce high-quality milk."

Debbie tells us that Driver Don won't start the black-and-white-spotted tram unless we call: "Let's get *mooooo*ving." I love me a good pun, but I just can't join in on the halfhearted call mustered by the rest of the tour goers. It's too soon to resort to jokes that go *moo*.

The tram trundles out of the parking lot and rolls along a wide dirt road. A chain-link fence fades into smooth gray as we pick up speed. Beyond the metal fence, pale packed dirt becomes a darker tumble of lose soil and we see our first Roxie. Forty-fifty-sixty Roxies, ambling on clumpy brownness. Air whips through the tram, carrying imperceptible flecks of soil and cow shit. Diluted by so much desert air, the smell isn't a bad one, necessarily; it smells like animal, like sweat and sun, and after a while, it settles on my skin unnoticed.

The tram stops in front of the Desert Oasis, and Debbie selects a blond-haired boy to disembark with her. There's a wooden swing balanced opposite a hundred-pound feed bag like the scales of justice, and as the little boy struggles aboard, Debbie announces, "You'd have to eat five hundred hamburgers and drink five hundred and sixty glasses of water every day to keep up with Roxie!"

"That's a perverse comparison," Hilary mutters as the boy settles on the swing and the sack barely budges. I laugh, too loud; we both stare at our laps when Debbie shoots us a look. I haven't seen Hilary in weeks—we're both slammed with work; she has a new boyfriend who lives in St. Louis, and I, of course, have a Dave who lives in Tucson. So we are having a girls' day at a dairy farm, where every day is for the ladies.

Every day, Roxie consumes a hundred pounds of feed and thirty-five gallons of water. In turn, every day, Roxie releases thirty pounds of waste. Somewhere in there, Roxie also produces eight gallons of milk. When the tram stops at the cow playground and the kids tumble out, I ask Debbie where the farm gets their water.

"We have a well," she says. "It's pumping up from six hundred and fifteen feet, and we have a reserve that goes down to eight hundred and fifteen below."

"So it's all groundwater?" I ask, unrolling the last word too slowly, aware of the political baggage it carries. Groundwater in Arizona is like fossil fuel in the Middle East: precious, finite, and nonrenewable. Indeed, Arizona has pumped more water out of the ground in the past eighty years than it will in the next thousand. The Central Arizona Project, southern Arizona's 336-mile lifeline to the Colorado River, has been built—there's no extra water coming down the pipe.

Debbie doesn't seem to notice the weird tone in my voice. "Yup!" she says.

Not counting the water needed to clean the farm and cool the cows, ten thousand cows drinking 35 gallons a piece means that every day, this dairy sucks up 350,000 gallons of water from the thinning aquifers of Arizona. Every single day, 350 *thousand* gallons of water, a million pounds of feed, and three hundred thousand pounds of waste. What emerges from this convergence of resources is 80,000 gallons of milk: enough to satiate four thousand Americans for a year—barely a gulp in our national consumption, barely a drop in the 6 billion gallons we guzzle up every year.

IN THE DAIRY CASE of the Tucson Food Conspiracy Co-op, you can breeze on almonds, dream of rice, or milk a coconut. You can buy goat's milk, raw or pasteurized. You can buy Organic Valley Soymilk or Earth Balance Soymilk, and still you may choose between original, vanilla-flavored, or low-fat original.

In the dairy case of the Tucson Co-op—where I now shop almost exclusively—you can also buy cow's milk. There are two full double-door refrigerators dedicated to the lactating cow. Conventional or organic; homogenized or nonhomogenized; local or far-flung; pasteurized, ultrapasteurized, or raw. One percent, 2 percent, fat-free, or whole.

Again and again, I lean on the frosty insides of these heavy doors. Time after time, my knee draws a tall triangle on the door, holding it open like a perched flamingo, spilling thick refrigeration into the narrow aisle. I bend and peer; I cradle plastic gallons and cup cardboard cartons.

In January, when I was up to my eyeballs in refined sugar, chemically tainted wheat, and pesticide-laden produce, when I examined the ingredient labels of cartoon-cow cartons, I thought, Milk is unprocessed. Milk certainly *seemed* unprocessed—it was, by all appearances, a whole food, straight from its source. It had been my first food, after all. I didn't have time to wrestle with everything at once, and so I deferred to the labels that now define dairy: organic, hormone-free, humanely raised. If my milk was modified by the correct words—words that I had to trust were true—then, I decided, milk was unprocessed. Then so was a block of artisan cheese; so was a tub of organic yogurt. (Not so for bright orange food-colored cheddar cheese or the silicon dioxide or dicalcium phosphate added to most shredded cheeses to prevent caking.)

But even in January, I had a hazy idea of how many resources it took to support a milking cow, a vague recollection of articles about hormones and antibiotics cropping up in industrial milk. So when I decided a year unprocessed was not going to be a vegan one, it was for reasons I couldn't quite explain. Sugar, sure—that I could do without. Unnecessary additives, no problem. But with milk, something primal and stubborn kicked back at me when I considered opting out. After having decided against so many foods already, when I thought about all the foods that came from milk—cheese, yogurt, butter—I wondered: What, then, would be left to eat?

Were someone to sort through all the grocery receipts that I have kept tucked in a cup in my kitchen since January; if they were to create a word cloud using the words on these receipts according to frequency of appearance, they would see this: small letters spelling "carrots," "unfiltered apple juice," "baking cocoa"; larger letters arranging "onions," "blueberries (org/frz)," "garlic"; and finally, booming from the center, five giant words: "YOGURT." "BANANAS." "WINE." "MILK." "COFFEE." Because produce arrives at my kitchen through my weekly CSA subscription, along with eggs and cheese, and because I stock up on dried goods—beans and rice, oats and almonds—whenever the co-op has a sale, I stop at the store only when I run out of the staples. Which are, evidently—my receipts reveal the truth—fermented grapes, fermented milk, and bananas. My mornings revolve around four of those five giant words, around books and quiet, coffee and cream. Disrupting this routine—bending over books and breakfast, socks and pajamas—disrupts how yesterday turns into today. Breakfast makes me stubborn and milk seems inevitable, like it always has been and always will be.

Cow's milk won out over the many alternatives, both animal—goat, sheep, buffalo—and vegetable—soy, almond, coconut—because it was cheaper, more accessible, and because it seemed simpler. Goat's milk cost $4.99 for half a liter, nearly twice the cost of organic cow's milk; sheep's milk was sold in only the most far-flung natural food stores. Almond and soymilk seemed sensible until I started reading labels. Organic Valley Unsweetened Soy Milk, for example, contains: filtered water, organic whole soybeans, calcium carbonate, organic vanilla flavor, salt, vitamin A palmitate, carregeenan, sunflower lecithin, riboflavin (B_2), vitamin D_2, vitamin B_{12}. (Carregeenan, a texturizer and thickener derived from seaweed, is a controversial additive—it's been shown to cause gastrointestinal inflammation in lab animals, and several scientists have petitioned the FDA to prohibit its use in food because of possible carcinogenic effects.)

I had made my own plant-based milk at home before; almond milk enjoyed a particularly exuberant bout of popularity during my food-processor-enriched summer. Almond milk is, in theory, a simple thing to make. Soak almonds, blend almonds, strain liquid from solid, and you've got almond milk. In practice, it required more dishes than I'd have liked, with a result slightly too watery to turn my coffee creamy. Still, I liked the almond milk I made—it was a nice snack, especially when flecked with cinnamon—but I found myself making it only when I had the time and energy. In the meantime—during nontime and no-energy—I continued to drink cow's milk.

As I had tried to step away from plastic packaging, I'd happily paid the $1.40 bottle deposit to take home a thick glass, cream-top jar of organic, pasture-grazed milk from the California-based Straus Family Creamery. Cream-top bottles are how milk used to be sold, when small fingers might scoop out solid cream from the top of a bottle. A hat of cream congeals when milk isn't homogenized, when fat molecules aren't vigorously agitated to slip in among the milk's proteins. Homogenization came about not as a way to increase milk's safety, but rather to increase consistency from batch to batch. So I scooped the layer of cream off the top of my bottle and thought I had figured it out.

NINE OR TEN THOUSAND YEARS AGO, dairying goats, sheep, and cattle in the grasslands of the Middle East offered an incredibly efficient way to convert the inaccessible nutrients of wild meadows into food humans could digest. While humans get along with just one stomach, ruminants have evolved multichamber stomachs capable of breaking down the fiber of wild grasses into energy. Figuring out how to access this energy from animals without killing them represented a big gain for human nutrition. Unlike meat, milk could easily be fermented into butter, cheese, or yogurt and stored for the winter. For this reason, fluid milk was rarely consumed before the turn of the twentieth century; not only did it spoil quickly, it was also indigestible by most people after infancy, when their bodies stopped producing lactase, the enzyme needed to break down lactose into its simple sugars. Cheese and yogurt contain bacteria that produce lactose-digesting enzymes, which is why those who are lactose-intolerant and can't digest milk—a demographic that includes three out of every four people in the world—can usually eat fermented dairy products.

"Sweet, fresh cow's milk began its real life as an American food in the mid-nineteenth century, primarily as a breast milk substitute for infants and a beverage for weaned children," writes Melanie DuPris in *Nature's Perfect Food: How Milk Became America's Drink*. "It began not on primeval farms, but in the burgeoning city; not with the rise of sanitation, but before sanitary production was possible."

In 1860, when the number of people living in Manhattan hit eight hundred thousand, surpassing the population of most states, the existing food provision system of local farmers delivering to local merchants proved unable to support the city's growing population. Breweries had long dotted the city skyline, supplying the city with spirits, but in the 1860s, in response to urban demand for new food sources, these breweries began building milk stables in adjacent buildings. Brewers would pour spent grain, or "swill," directly into stable troughs, where city-bound cows would slurp it up. This brilliant waste reduction scheme was limited only by the failure of the final product: "a thin, bluish fluid, ridden with bacteria," writes DuPris. So reformers cast the city's milk to the countryside, where cows could eat grass and not beer swill. Although the quality of milk improved, this solution distanced production from consumption, creating the new problem of distribution—how to move a fresh, perishable food along the long road from country to city without spoiling it.

TODAY, IN NEARLY HALF THE STATES IN THE UNITED STATES, raw milk is an illegal food. Raw milk is not illegal like zoot suits are in Los Angeles; it is not an irrelevant law long forgotten. Raw milk is explicitly illegal. In March of 2012, a Wisconsin farmer was sued and threatened with jail time after a Department of Agriculture official staked out his farm and found evidence he was selling raw milk. "We don't sell milk," said the farmer in his defense. "I want to get that clear." Rather, he said, he was *giving* milk away in exchange for a farm subscription. The defense worked and he escaped jail time, but according to a Madison news service, protesters outside the courtroom said that they'd be willing to go to jail in defense of their freedom to drink raw milk. In Arizona, the sale of raw milk is legal as long as the provider has a license and the label wears a disclaimer. (In Kentucky and Rhode Island, raw milk is illegal unless you have a doctor's prescription.)

"There is a *reason* we began pasteurizing milk!" my sister exclaims when I tell her I'm thinking about buying raw milk. "It was making people *sick*." Her husband's brother's friend lived on a dairy farm—he milked his own cows!—and if *he* said he'd never drink raw milk, this unknown person twice removed, well then, case closed.

"Yes, yes," I say. "There are risks. But the risks are not nearly as high as a lot of other foods in our food system."

"Cow udders carry a lot of bacteria, Megan. How clean do you think a cow really is? And think of all the farm equipment!"

Again, she's right. If raw milk contains a few more nutrients than its pasteurized self, it has also historically been far more dangerous. Modern historian P. J. Atkins deemed the milk supply as it existed in the nineteenth century, before pasteurization was commonplace, as "white poison." Throughout the last half of the nineteenth century, every New York summer brought with it the deaths of thousands of babies who had been infected with cholera infantum, a diarrheal disease that doctors eventually linked to contaminated milk. And yet, parents still fed milk to their children; a fair amount of them started drinking it themselves.

As cities grew and demand for milk surged, Americans clamored for reform. The Conference on Milk Problems convened in New York City in 1910 to choose between two alternative visions for milk safety: the certified milk system and pasteurization. Under the first, the Medical Milk Commission would establish quality and hygiene standards, inspect farms for care and conditions of processing, and offer an official certification to qualifying dairies. The certified milk system would be capital- and labor-intensive, thus favoring large operations, but it would avoid the undesirable side effects of "cooking" milk, thus destroying, many doctors argued, many of milk's important nutrients and beneficial bacteria.

Pasteurization, on the other hand, was a technological solution, a quick fix to the much bigger issue of large-scale dairies shipping volatile fluid milk into cities hundreds of miles away. Rather than treating the ailment up front—ensuring milk was produced under hygienic conditions—pasteurization simply treated the symptoms. It's a technique as old as cooking itself: Heat food hot enough to kill germs but not so hot to kill all flavor and nutrients. In 1862, Louis Pasteur simply refined the process. To pasteurize a liquid, you heat it up to 161 degrees Fahrenheit—just below boiling—hold it there for fifteen seconds, and then cool it immediately to stop the growth of new bacteria. If you want a particularly shelf-stable liquid, you can cook your fluid for a second or two at 285 degrees Fahrenheit and call it ultrapasteurized.

By 1917, laws requiring the pasteurization of milk were on the books in over 90 percent of the country's major cities.

Although raw milk has somewhat higher amounts of some nutrients than pasteurized milk because some of its vitamins haven't been destroyed by heat, the reason to drink raw milk is the same as the reason to eat fermented foods—microbes. According to many raw milk proponents, including fermentation expert Sandor Katz, it is the very bacteria already swimming through milk that protect us from any harmful bacteria that might arrive from a cow's udder, a farmer's hand, or a dirty vessel. Some bacteria are bad, yes, but most aren't; bacterial cells outnumber human cells in our bodies ten to one, and drinking foods like raw milk help replenish healthy communities of microbes. And it's not just the Sandor Katzes of the world who are telling us to put down the Purell. An article published in *Scientific American* in May of 2012 stressed that "this mixed community of microbial cells and the genes they contain, collectively known as the microbiome, does not threaten us but offers vital help with basic physiological processes—from digestion to growth to self-defense."

It takes me three separate visits and several passes by the dairy case at the Tucson Co-op before I even pull the gallon of raw milk out of the display case. I peek around an aisle to find an employee stocking bars of natural deodorant. "Hi," I say. He turns to me. "Um, can you tell me more about the raw milk?"

"What about it?"

"Where does it come from?"

"The label says Queen Creek, Arizona," he says.

"Yes, I see that."

"Okay . . ."

"Well, I mean. I guess I'm just wondering if you've had people come back to say they've gotten sick."

"I don't think so," he says. "It's really popular. We get maybe thirty gallons every week and always sell out."

"Oh!" I exclaim. "That's a lot."

He shrugs, but I am relieved—thirty gallons, downright mainstream! Call it crowd-sourcing anxiety, jumping on the bandwagon; whatever it is, I am happy to be a follower here.

When I get home, I pour an inch of cold, raw milk into a mug and take a sip. Raw milk is always sold in its full-fat form—the butterfat suspended in the milk helps protect the liquid from pathogens—which makes it stick on my tongue and the top of my mouth, roll around the inside of my cheeks and down my throat, sticky and sweet. The taste is subtle yet strong; animal and clean. It lingers in my mouth after I leave the kitchen; it sticks in my stomach and fills me up. I drink the milk all week, pouring it into my coffee and smoothies. I don't feel better—a gallon being an insufficient amount to budge a body's inertia—but the milk certainly *tastes* better.

After about a week, the milk stops tasting sweet and begins to turn sour. Which is precisely how cheese making began—when milk curdled. So I pour some in a bowl, cover it with a dishcloth, and forget about it for a few days. When I return, I am delighted to see soft curds of the first cheese likely produced by humans, charmingly called clabber. I lather the clabber on toast, mix it with eggs, and relish my raw success.

Raw milk sourced from a small, local producer feels like a solution to the problem of dairy, but I cannot get over the price tag. It is irrational, a response conditioned by a culture that believes in cheap food, but $12.99 feels like too much to pay for a gallon of milk. Like so many other foods that are now priced as commodities, the true costs of milk production are not contained in the $4.99 it costs for a gallon of Horizon Organic; in the $3.99 it costs for a gallon of Shamrock Farms. (Not to mention the cost of externalities like groundwater depletion or greenhouse gas emissions.) Extensive government subsidies support the cheapness of milk, while the high price of raw milk reflects the cost of doing business outside the system. Twelve ninety-nine for a gallon of milk is not necessarily an inaccurate representation of value. But the receipts piling up in my kitchen tell a different story, one that balks at the addition of another $13 to its weekly tally.

"AT SHAMROCK FARMS, if Roxie gets sick, she's removed from the milking rotation for several weeks, until all the antibiotics are flushed from her system," says Debbie. "We also *never* use any of those scary hormones, the rBGH or bGH—plain ol' BS," she says, with a wink and a nod to the adults in the audience. I want to wink right back at her: You're not a*moo*sing, Debbie.

All Shamrock Farms milk cartons proudly declare NO rBGH! Cows that are injected with recombinant bovine growth hormone have been shown to convert feed to milk 20 percent more efficiently than those without it, which is why almost a fifth of the nine million dairy cows spread across the country receive shots of the stuff every few weeks. Although the milk from cows treated with rbST is not inherently risky—cows naturally produce bST on their own, so rbST is almost impossible to detect—there are many other ways that rBGH-addled cows produce risky milk. Cows are not really supposed to produce eight gallons of milk a day—three or four gallons is considered normal output. The more milk a cow produces, the more likely she is to get an udder infection. When a nonorganic heifer gets sick, she's treated with antibiotics, and although farms are supposed to remove her from the milking system until she's recovered, antibiotics still can slide into her milk, which then slide into us, potentially killing off the friendly bacteria that help our intestinal tracts shuttle happily along.

The tram careens past a metal fence, behind which a smattering of heifers begins trotting after us. "Those are the organic heifers," says Debbie. "There are about nine hundred of them."

"What makes them organic?" I ask.

"Their feed is organic and they have to go out and graze for part of the year," she says. "Oh, and of course they aren't given any antibiotics. The nice thing about Shamrock is that if a cow gets sick, instead of sending her away, we can just switch her over to conventional."

I nod and look back over at the organic "pasture." It is equally brown, equally fenced—equally industrial—as the "Desert Oasis," where the conventional cows live. Enclosed within the metal fence, Organic Roxie seems to have a bit more room to wander about, more room to shake her hooves, but the difference feels like one of degree rather than category.

While there are many small-scale organic cooperatives throughout the country, just two companies—Horizon Organic, with 43 percent market share, and Organic Valley—serve roughly 75 percent of the nation's organic milk market. Organic Valley functions as a cooperative dairy, sourcing most of its milk from scattered small-scale farmers, but Horizon Organic is a different story—two "mega-dairy" farms in Idaho and Maryland, each with over six thousand cows, provide the company with 75 percent of its milk. To keep cows healthy and antibiotic-free in such close quarters, many dairies do what Shamrock does, milking their organic cows until they need antibiotics and are flipped to conventional production.

But like organic produce, organic dairy matters—certainly for environmental health but hugely for human health. When you drink organic dairy, you don't get any of the antibiotics, hormones, or pesticide residues that slip, inadvertently, into conventionally produced milk. There's something rather visceral about the transfer—dairy is, after all, a landscape filtered through a mammal's body. Contaminate that landscape, or the animals that live on it, and you contaminate its milk.

"CAN YOU TELL ME PLEASE if milk is good for me?" my mom asks in October when I tell her I'm wrestling once again with dairy.

"I don't know," I say. "I don't think it's been decided."

"Yes, but it would be good to know. I have that *one* book that advocates for the vegan diet, you know, based on the China Study and all that. But then, you know, Gary Taubes is all *about* the cream and cheese, and I like the sound of that."

Is milk healthy? The FDA certainly thinks so: "Dairy products make important contributions to the American diet. They provide high-quality protein and are good sources of vitamins A, D, and B$_{12}$, and also riboflavin, phosphorus, magnesium, potassium, zinc, and calcium." Nutritionists have been fighting over milk's pro-con list for over a century, and resolution seems nowhere near, given that "the dairy industry is large and united and is especially diligent in exerting influence over anything that might affect production, marketing, and sales," writes nutritionist Marion Nestle in *What to Eat*. Studies suggest that the fat in dairy products might increase our risk for various cancers while others assert that milk prevents cancer; some studies propose that milk consumption increases our risk for heart disease, while others insist that it lowers it. The American Institute for Cancer Research, on the other hand, seems to have just given up: "From a purely scientific standpoint, it would be irresponsible to assert that drinking milk increases a person's risk for prostate cancer in particular . . . but it would be equally irresponsible to insist that the existence of such a link was impossible."

The premise of the 2010 documentary *Forks Over Knives* is that animal-based diets lead to chronic diseases like diabetes, cancer, and heart disease, convincing my cheese-loving mother to begin a Vegan Tuesdays regime. The most compelling evidence offered to support this claim comes from a report known as the China Study, a twenty-year investigation into diet and health that began in 1983. Conducted by the Chinese Academy of Preventive Medicine, Cornell University, and the University of Oxford, the China Study examined blood samples and cancer mortality rates from seven thousand people spread across China. What did they find? "People who ate the most animal-based foods got the most chronic disease," said Dr. T. Colin Campbell, one of the study's lead nutritionists. "People who ate the most plant-based foods were the healthiest and tended to avoid chronic disease." In other words, vegan populations were found to live longer and healthier lives.

But of course, no study is complete without its dissenters, and many nutritionists and food journalists have since dismantled the assumptions inherent in Campbell's conclusions; namely, that cholesterol found in blood samples reliably indicated food intake. The Weston A. Price Foundation responded with a scathing review, writing, "An examination of the original China Study data shows virtually no statistically significant correlation between any type of cancer and animal protein intake."

Sarah drinks two gallons of milk a week. Another vegetarian—except, sometimes, for bacon—Sarah will not, could not, cannot imagine her life without milk.

"Why?" I ask her.

"I don't know, I've always just loved milk."

"Do you just drink it plain?"

"Yup. Don't you?"

"Ick, no. I usually just put it in my coffee. Mostly I eat a lot of milk products. Yogurt, cheese. All the stuff that comes afterward."

When I asked Sarah to come on my Shamrock Farms adventure, she said, "Hmm, no. I don't think I could handle seeing that." Sarah loves all animals—sheep, pigs, emu. She fosters kittens for the Humane Society, nursing six or seven scrawny, scrambling kittens to a healthy weight before turning them over to new owners. Sarah is one of the most politically engaged people I know, an articulate animal-rights activist, and yet she shakes her head when I bring up milk. *"Megan,"* she pleads, when I tell her of milk's accumulating pile of processed facts. "Please don't ruin it."

Rather than ask is milk healthy, we might well ask: Does it satisfy us? Does it make our bodies feel good and full?

As it turns out, health and satiety might be better companions than we thought. New research shows that eating full-fat dairy products actually helps *keep* us slim. No one's sure why—maybe it's because the fats keep us full and eating less, or because compounds in animal fats stimulate our metabolism in yet unknown ways. Other studies show that the fats in milk help our bodies digest its nutrients—that "they act as carriers for important fat-soluble vitamins A, D, E, and K," writes Sally Fallon in *Nourishing Traditions*. That without fats, we simply don't digest these nutrients. "Dietary fats are needed for the conversion of carotene to vitamin A, for mineral absorption and for a host of other processes."

It's the best news I've gotten all month. In October, as I'm falling for cheese, I also fall away from the bathroom scale. At first, I stop weighing myself because the scale seems broken. I've been weighing myself on the same scale since I was in college, since I first started my mornings with the declaration of a body's additions or subtractions, but in September of my year unprocessed, it starts giving a message called ERR. I ignore it for a while, but after two weeks exploring cheese, I want to know. So I buy a new battery and hit reset and there is ERR no more. The number hasn't changed—still 165 pounds, just where I started the year. My pants still fit and yet I'm always full, rarely resisting. I relish this luxury. After years of eating to stay skinny, I am learning to eat simply for satisfaction.

And indeed, since I ate a full loaf of whole-grain bread, since I made snappy bars of chocolate and a frothy bucket of mead, I'd learned that the foods of this year filled me differently. After expending so much mental energy differentiating processed from unprocessed, I have no more resolve to spend on serving size, so I eat by the measure of satiety rather than size. I still slipped up, sometimes still ate more unprocessed food than my stomach really wanted—discovering, as I was this month, my threshold for cheese—but I was learning. And it seemed, so was my body. Without conscious intervention, it was maintaining itself, its weight and its strength. So finally, in October, I stop stepping on plastic and asking for a number.

"**WELCOME TO KINDERGARTEN!**" Debbie exclaims as the tour rolls past a long line of calves. Each calf is contained in a two-by-three-foot pen; there's row after row of them, hundreds of eighty-pound babies swaddled in metal fencing. The calves will live in their cages for four to five weeks, long enough for them to develop the immunities needed to rub hooves with the two hundred full-size cows that live in each section of the "Cattle Oasis" corral.

Like any mammal, in order to begin and continue lactating, heifers must give birth. (A cow is a heifer before she's given birth; afterward, she's just a cow.) "They have to be in a constant state of birthing and calving in order to produce milk," says Debbie. "Roxie lives here until she's six or seven years old and she'll have three baby calves in that time."

"What do you do then?" I ask.

"We'll sell Roxie to a broker," she says. What does the broker do with Roxie? Debbie shrugs. "Any number of things."

Debbie does not want to talk about what happens to Roxie after she leaves the farm, but we learn what happens to her milk when it departs. Milk leaves Roxie in a plastic tube; it leaves Shamrock in the back of a refrigerated semi truck, and it leaves the Phoenix processing plant in a sterilized plastic bottle. We are told, again and again, that Shamrock milk "is never touched by human hands." It doesn't touch our hands and so "it is one of the safest foods you can consume."

"We're headed to the milking barn now, folks," Debbie says. Two hundred cows fit into the milking room at one time, and every one of the ten thousand Shamrock cows gets milked twice a day, every day. When we arrive at the windows that look over the milking room, one batch of cows is queuing up at the door to exit. The next group files up the aisles like obedient cars merging onto a freeway; they've been here before. Before the day is up, every single Holstein will cycle through the milking room two times, pausing for five or six minutes to release four or five gallons of milk into the clasp of a plastic suction cup. Men in overalls and rubber boots meander up and down the aisles, making sure all the machinery is in the right place. The milk trickles, slow and viscous, down translucent yellow tubes that hang like tails behind the cows. Each yellow line sways gently with the pulse of the suction cup. The milk oozes. The cows stand, silent—silent to us, behind the glass, bumping softly against each other. Two hundred in, two hundred out, again and again, all day long, ten thousand cows.

AT THE END OF THE TOUR, we're each gifted a bottle of Shamrock Farms milk. Hilary sensibly refuses her gift, but I don't realize this is an option, so I end up facing Hilary, holding a cold plastic bottle, wrapped crunchily with the image of a smiling cartoon Roxie, hooves raised ecstatically in the air.

"You want it?" I ask, holding it out to her.

"I don't like their milk," she says. "I think it tastes plastic-y."

"I guess I should try it," I say. "Reckon with Roxie." I don't want to drink this milk, but I do have to face the processes that bring me my cartons of milk, the real costs of living in an industrialized society. I crunch open the plastic cap and take a swig. It's strong and weak at the same time; strong in the taste of animal, the taste of warm skin, but weak in the way it rolls around my mouth and into my stomach. I force myself to take another sip and realize that Hilary is right. It tastes like plastic.

"Blegh," I say, twisting the cap back on. I can't imagine how I might throw away this resource, so costly to extract, but I cannot finish this small bottle. I look for a recycling bin. There's only a garbage can.

As we're leaving Shamrock, we drive once again past the long corral of Roxies, and I realize, finally, what matters most in my confusion about milk is not if it's organic or antibiotic-laden; homogenized or cream top; carried in a plastic container or a glass bottle; raw or pasteurized; rather, what matters more about milk is not how its processed, but the fact that it comes from a cow.

In *How Bad Are Bananas: The Carbon Footprint of Everything,* Mike Berners-Lee estimates that the total footprint of a pint of milk—expressed as the carbon dioxide equivalent of all associated greenhouse gasses—is 1.6 pounds of CO_2. Drinking a pint of milk produces more carbon than driving a mile in my Honda Civic; more than tossing out two pounds of garbage or boiling two pounds of potatoes. "Milk is high-carbon stuff for exactly the same reasons that beef is," he writes. Cows are not particularly efficient animals; they waste much of the energy they gain from eating by walking around and keeping themselves warm. Cows fart. They also ruminate—chew up the cud from their first stomach—and so they burp a lot. Both activities release a lot of methane, which nearly doubles a cow's total impact on the environment. According to Berners-Lee, 85 percent of milk's footprint is produced on the farm. (A plastic bottle is barely a toe in the footprint, contributing only 4 percent of the pint's total impact.)

The great irony of milk production is that heifers have to keep birthing calves to make milk. By its very premise—because of nature's gift to mammals, the ability to produce milk for their young—large-scale milk production requires constant growth. Constant birth.

When Hilary and I finally arrive back in Tucson, it is nearly dark. The warm day fades into a fall evening. I am exhausted and so confused. I *like* milk; I don't want to give it up. I should have figured this out already—the incredible process required to transfer feed to cow to milk. How could I have gotten this far *without* questioning this? There is the superficial answer: Shamrock Farm tours were sold out all spring and closed all summer and there are few other dairies in southern Arizona I could have visited—the Southwest is not a region known for its green pastures. The answer I don't want to consider is that I put on blinders and swerved around this issue as a survival mechanism, as a way to even begin this tricky year.

I drop Hilary at her apartment and finally, sitting on the corner of Twenty-Second and Park, in the glow of light from a 7-Eleven, I release a big, sad sigh. So far, my transition away from processed hasn't felt like a sacrifice. I've missed ice cream and Diet Coke, certainly, but I had chosen this year; I had forced these parameters upon myself. Trying to exile sugar from my life was annoying, but it was also a challenge—a puzzle to be solved, like sudoku or chess. But unlike the problem of avoiding foods that contain pesticides—answer: eat organic—the problem of milk doesn't feel like it has a clear solution. Giving up milk feels like an untenable choice, like a sacrifice I'm not prepared to make, but continuing to buy milk feels impossible, an acquiescence to inertia.

THE NEXT TIME I GO TO THE CO-OP, I don't buy milk. I walk past the dairy case, into the bulk-foods aisle and fill up one of my reusable sacks with rolled oats. Chocolate Covered Katie, one of my favorite food bloggers, has just posted about how easy and cheap it is to make oat milk at home—she does it all the time! (She is a favorite blogger because she writes things like this: "First, position yourself so that you're under the oat. Next, pull *really* hard.") So, like Chocolate Covered Katie, I will simply incorporate the making of milk into my Sunday ritual. I have already acquired so many unprocessed habits—soaking beans and fermenting yogurt, grating cheese and grinding wheat. Why should this be any different? This is about routine, I tell myself. It's about a new routine, a shift on Sunday and a morning that no longer needs the milk of an animal.

Of course, plant-based milks, made from oats or almonds, have their own footprints. In drought-stressed California, where 80 percent of the world's almonds are grown—where almond groves alone suck up 10 percent of the state's water—it takes more than a gallon of water to grow a single almond. If you use a cup of almonds to make a gallon of almond milk—say, forty nuts— you're looking at more than forty gallons of embedded water. Then again, if almonds aren't free of a footprint, neither are tomatoes, lettuce, or oats (which require less water than almonds, but more than wheat). Almonds need water, but not nearly as much as cows do (and, when making milk, almond "waste" becomes almond meal).

I start my oats soaking on Sunday morning and quickly cook them while I make lunch. After the oats cool, I scoop the heavy slop into my blender and add water. I whir the blender, round and round, for two minutes. I place a fine mesh sieve over a glass pitcher and pour some of the goopy fluid into the sieve's concave opening. I work the liquid out of the oat gruel with a rubber spatula, grinding the gruel around until the liquid drains. I repeat this procedure five more times, straining liquid from gruel. I add a bit more water, some cinnamon, nutmeg, and vanilla, spin the mix around, and pour the sludge into a pint-size mason jar, filling it about three-quarters of the way to the top. I secure a lid on the jar, slide the jar into the fridge, and then, twenty minutes after I started, I turn back to my kitchen.

Drops of what look like dirty glue speckle the tile counter and amass into a thick puddle near the blender; a smear crosses the tile floor from sink to counter. The dirty blender joins an armada of glue-covered dishes: a saucepot, a glass pitcher, a metal sieve, two spoons, a mason jar, and a rubber spatula. The leftover oat solids sprawl across a large plate.

What a spectacular pain in the ass.

The oat milk, when I sample it from the fridge a few hours later, tastes quite good, but not at all like milk. The consistency is more like porridge than anything I'd want to mix with coffee, but the next morning, a splash of oat milk mixes with hot coffee like batter into water. Whisked about, the coffee does turn a whiter shade of brown, but flecks of oat solid float to the top like they're trying to be foam.

On Monday afternoon, I dash into Bentley's Coffee & Tea. I've been teaching second graders how to garden all day—building raised beds, shoveling wet soil—and I've got ten minutes to emerge out of an exhaustion that feels like a cement sleeping bag before I have to meet with my boss. I need coffee. Black coffee is slippery, too much like dirty water or gritty tea. I want creamy coffee, as the fat in milk slides it slowly down my throat and cushions its arrival into my stomach. If making my own milk is a possible solution to unprocessed milk, it is not a solution on a Monday afternoon when I am tired and I want a cup of coffee at Bentley's. If I want cream in my coffee at Bentley's, my options are 2 percent or whole milk. Not almond or soy, raw or pasteurized. Simply cow, nonfat or full. My habits hold fast and so, despite my recent realization, after my mug returns to me full of steaming black liquid, I pour a small stream of whole milk into it.

Although the making of soymilk is no less a pain in the ass than oat milk—I soak, cook, blend, and strain the soybeans just like oats—the final product carries the consistency of milk much more believably. I liked the almond milk I had made a few months back; genuinely liked it, not just because I had to. But after I make soymilk, as I hand wash yet another armada of dishes, I realize that my like or dislike is beside the point. Deadlines creep, reading piles, e-mails wait. There are too many things to do on a Sunday afternoon other than pull on the teats of an almond or oat. There is no way I can keep this up, the unprocessing of milk, and stay afloat in the ocean of work that surrounds me.

FOR WEEKS AFTER MY SHAMROCK FARMS TOUR, I can talk of little else besides milk, about the great conundrum of dairy. When I run into a similarly food-focused friend and he asks "What's new?" I respond with an indignant, "Do you know how much *water* Shamrock uses?"

"I know," he says, "It's crazy. Hey, I'm going down to Chiva Risa this weekend. It's a goat ranch, just north of the border. I'll forward you the flyer; they're having an open house."

When I mention the goat-farm open house to Dave—we're cooking dinner in my kitchen and I preface the proposition with an eye roll, a "yes, I know I'm crazy"—he says, "Yeah!"

"Really?" I ask.

"Fresh goat cheese, maybe a picnic, some wine? Yeah, that sounds fun."

"Oh. Okay. It's on Saturday."

"Saturday. Goat day!" he says, grabbing himself a beer from my fridge. He begins humming a ditty: It's-a-goatday, goatday, goatday.

The landscape rolls away from desert and into grassland as we slide south out of Tucson. Saguaros become creosote and NPR becomes Mexican *ranchera* as we arrive closer to the border. Chiva Risa's forty acres are spread a half mile north of the Mexican border—the fence is visible from the edge of their property.

After we arrive, J.C., who walks a toe-heel line between borderlands rancher and University of Arizona professor, takes us around the pens to introduce us to the girls. J.C. and his wife, Lissa, bought two goats three years ago, when they had an hour to kill and wandered into a 4-H show in Tucson. Lissa had always wanted a goat, and two weeks after they bought two goats, they had seven. They didn't intend to build a goat ranch, but two weeks after *that,* they owned twelve goats. Two years later, it's a hundred. Cassie Jean was one of the first goats on the ranch and she's still kicking buckets out from under the kids that are trying to pull her teats at their two-year-anniversary open house.

"Cassie is still Lissa's favorite, but she knows all their names, every single one," J.C. says, shifting his weight from boot to boot. He leans against a steel fence, his back to the kid pen, where twenty or so baby goats stare at us, clustered, their confused puppy expressions confounded by the tiny horns curling from between their ears. A hundred goats begets a hundred names; J.C. can't keep track of them all, but, he says, "My favorite is Sammypants. You know, goats are some of the most efficient converters of grain and water into milk."

I did know this, sort of, and I want him to quantify this conversion for a hundred goats. I prepare the question but it stutters around my mind and bumps up against a giggle. Sammypants?

There's a pause in the conversation and Dave asks, nonchalant, "What's her name again?"

J.C. responds, too quickly: "Sam."

I round my mouth and inhale quickly in preparation of a polite interjection. J.C. offers another quick self-correction. "Sammy," he says, and pushes his weight off the fence and prepares to shuttle the conversation onward.

"Wait, was it Sammypants?" Dave asks. "That's great."

"Right, Sammypants, sure," J.C. says. He's embarrassed to have called his goat Sammypants, but how could he not? How could you not nickname, not pick favorites? The gals almost ask it of us—they trot toward us, nuzzle against the fence and our outstretched hands, pickme-pickme. They are endearing animals, social and animated, nudging noses and permanent half smiles stretched across their snouts. The goats have a sense of humor, J.C. and Lissa say. They know what they're supposed to do and they know what they want to do, Lissa says, and they'll make mischief in the space between. "They have this way of neighing, makes it sound like they're laughing."

If there are ten thousand Roxies at Shamrock Farms, at Chiva Risa, there is only one Sammypants.

"Goats," J.C. tells us, "are the most well-adapted animals on the planet. They can live on the least amount of resources." Goats have the highest milk yield by weight of any diary animal, converting the land's scraps to dairy more than ten times as efficiently as cows. But as it turns out, on a farm where every goat has a name, this milk is sold on a limited basis—most of the girls' production goes to goat cheese.

"Do you want to move to producing milk for sale?" I ask.

"Not at all," J.C. says. "The licensing is a pain, first of all—it's outrageous, the paperwork—and I just don't see how it makes the dollars come together." He pats one of the bucks on the head; there are only five of them here, raring to frolic among the ladies. "Goat's cheese sells for twenty dollars a pound," he says. "Goat's milk, you know how much that sells for? It seems expensive at the store maybe, but it's eight bucks a gallon. You can get a whole gallon of cheese from a gallon of milk."

Sammypants' milk is churned into cheese in the hand-built barn with a blue roof. A $14,000 pasteurizer—cheap compared to high-tech models—"gently pasteurizes" the milk for thirty minutes. Lissa adds milk cultures—rennet, or animal stomach lining—to the pot and lets it culture, warmly, for twenty-four hours. A day later, what Lissa scoops out of the great metal pasteurizer is cheese: sweet, creamy curds of goat cheese.

"If producing milk is so cost prohibitive, why can I buy goat's milk at the co-op?" I ask J.C. "Who's producing it?"

"Size," he says. "There are industrial goat dairies. You gotta have enough goats, a large-scale farm with mechanized milking, to earn enough money to support such a small margin."

When I mention that I was just at Shamrock Farms, J.C. says, "Commercial dairies do the same to their goats. It's just the same."

Goats don't fart out nearly as much methane as cows, and they subsist on far less feed and water, but J.C.'s point remains: It is less about the animal itself than their collective accumulation on a giant farm.

"Where do you get your water?" I ask Lissa, once we've stopped giggling with the goats and made it inside for a milking demonstration.

"From the ground."

"Does the Central Arizona Project canal reach down here?"

She laughs. "No. We're trying to use more gray water, to build one of those, what are they called, cistern systems. But until then, there's not much of a choice." These hundred goats, Sammypants among them, live off the grid. The ranch is entirely wind- and solar-powered; the closest power line is a mile away, farther than the snaking wall that defines the U.S.-Mexico border. They are off the grid but down in the ground, pumping water up from an underground reservoir, like every small farm and ranch scattered throughout these arid borderlands.

Lissa hands out a sample of goat feed for us to try, the group of six adults and a dozen children who have migrated inside. Goats eat just about everything—shirts, notebooks, hair—but these girls subsist on a feed mix of alfafa and bean chaff. "I think their feed makes a difference in the milk," Lissa tells us. "The bean chaff is sweet. When the girls finish eating, it makes their breath smell like peanut butter."

The children milk first. Lissa darts in and out, instructing them how to wrap their fingers around the udder to pull milk down into the teat. Cassie jostles about the middle position and kicks the milking bucket out from under her, eliciting a squeal from her eight-year-old milk maiden. When the children tire, Dave and I wash our hands and elbow in. Cassie twitches her right leg and shoos me away with the back of her hoof and I squeal like an eight-year-old. Finally, I reach my hand in and grab hold of her udder. It's soft and warm, heavy and shifting. The teat feels weirdly empty, like a deflated hose. I cup the udder with my palm and wrap my fingers tight around, peeling them shut from pinkie to thumb. It's less a pulling motion than a wrapping and squeezing, massaging and dodging the still-twitching leg. Finally, she calms, and finally—after three misfires—I pull on her udder, wrap around the small teat, and a thin stream of white milk hisses into the blue bucket.

After four or five minutes of pulling and wrapping, an inch worth of milk pools at the bottom of the blue bucket and the muscles in my fingers ache from the unaccustomed exertion. A new cluster of children has washed their hands and stand, queued at the ready, but I don't want to stop. I don't want to sever the connection of flesh on flesh, cold hand to warm teat. I want to linger and milk an inchoate understanding into something solid; I want to goad these goats and make them laugh. But children wait; so do tired boyfriends. I release my grip on the raw underbelly of this droll animal, we say our good-byes, and Dave and I drive back to Tucson.

THE PROBLEM OF MILK is not only that it comes from a living, breathing, resource-sucking animal; it is also the problem of people—that is, where we, most of the world's population, live in relation to those animals. It is essentially the same dilemma that plagued New York City in the nineteenth century. Breeding cows in the city presents the problem of production; cows thriving in the countryside make for challenging distribution when most people live in cities. It is hard to access small-scale dairies like Chiva Risa while remaining in Tucson, and it is hard to scale up small dairies without sucking up more groundwater and importing more feed. If the inefficiency of my individual salt production argued for centralized production, then dairy's difficulties are a case for scattered sourcing. Not only because dairy is best consumed fresh (while salt is not) but also because it would allow us to reclaim the diversity of dairy, fostering goats and sheep and buffalo and dismantling the unquestioned sovereignty of the omnipresent cow.

But today, small dairies don't stand a chance in a marketplace dominated by large dairies subsidized by the U.S. government both through antiquated price supports and direct financial support. In 2012, the *Washington Post* reported that if the U.S. government ended dairy subsidies, as it was threatening to do as we approached yet another "fiscal cliff," the price of a gallon of milk might hit $8. An unhappy development for consumers, surely, but one that also reveals how grossly underpriced a gallon of milk is when it costs $2.99.

This price is a choice, one that we as a country have made through priorities in our food policy. The system of subsidies that supports dairy is a complicated, sinuous one, but it is also one that mostly doesn't benefit organic dairies, especially small ones. Because organic cows graze on open pasture rather than an energy-dense mix of grain, corn, and soy, they simply don't produce as much milk as a Roxie, who enjoys a steady supply of cheap commodity crops. When organic farmers do need to supplement grass with feed, they find that organic feed is either cost prohibitive or simply unavailable, as higher-margin commodity crops, like corn, have lured struggling farmers away from growing organic grains for feed. And so, even though it requires fewer inputs and comes with a smaller environmental footprint, organic dairy is more expensive for consumers and less profitable for farmers.

One reason I started my year unprocessed was to see how possible it was to step outside our food system without stepping outside of urban society itself, without moving to a farm or otherwise dedicating my days to procuring and preparing food. With wheat, sugar, and tomatoes, I felt like I'd begun to reassert some small measure of ownership over my consumer choices. The system of milk production is an imperfect one, but what it reveals to me are my limits—the limits to what I can unprocess on my own. Food processing has always required certain compromises with the expectation that they provide greater gains. Pasteurize your milk, and it will be safer; centralize milk production and you will give more people access to more affordable protein.

But what if the cost of these compromises begins to outweigh their gains? What if the concentration of ten thousand animals on a thousand acres seems like a high price to pay for the cheap ubiquity of milk? The story of milk reveals to me the limits to my sovereignty as an individual consumer, the extent to which my dollars and decisions about food can't entirely forgo our industrial food system. If the cost of the compromises no longer justifies the gains, then the system itself must begin to renegotiate the relationship between the two.

Unprocessed is not a perfect framework to understand how to eat in a modern society, and so perhaps my struggle with milk is the struggle to find the right kind of compromise, the right bargain within the system. Just as compromises were made as we built up the infrastructure of a modern food distribution system, there are compromises to be made in its dismantling.

Unprocess Yourself: Dairy

Milk itself is not inherently processed. But once I began to consider the production of milk from an environmental standpoint, it became difficult to consume the same quantity as I had consumed before. I try to consume less, but better. By better, I mean whole—I eat eggs with all their yolks, milk with all its fat, cheese with all its curd. Not only do fat molecules help your body absorb the nutrients in milk, but also fat is delicious. Fat fills you up, so it's easier to eat less of it.

I *always* buy organic dairy, without exception. Environmental impact aside, organic milk has been shown both to be more nutritious than conventionally produced milk and also to contain fewer chemical and pesticide residues, and no leftover antibiotics or hormones. After organic, if I have an option, I try to buy milk from small dairies.

I continue to oscillate between plant- and animal-based milk. Some weeks, the additives in almond milk seem like a better deal than the environmental footprint in cow's milk. Some weeks, I really just want *cream*. I'm not lactose-intolerant, so I can flip-flop. When buying plant-based milks, check the ingredient label—many contain additives, such as emulsifiers like soy lecithin and xanthan gum, which are considered harmless but can affect sensitive stomachs; I always avoid products with carrageenan.

My sister just discovered WestSoy soymilk, sold by Westbrae Natural—we've both been looking for it for years; it's the only plant-based milk we've found that doesn't contain *any* additives. For $4.99, you get a half gallon of soymilk containing only filtered water and whole, organic soybeans. Since this discovery, I've settled on some sort of compromise between plant and cow. I buy half a gallon of Organic Valley half-and-half to put in my coffee—less packaging and it lasts me a month—and a weekly gallon of WestSoy soymilk for my smoothies.

I buy big blocks of cheese and shred it myself, not only because it's cheaper, but also because most shredded cheeses come coated with anticaking agents. Check the ingredient label regardless—usually, that bright orange cheddar didn't get so orange on its own. Although I occasionally make my own yogurt, I usually buy it in the store. Brown Cow and Straus Family Creamery are some of my favorite brands, but that's because they're based in California, which is about as local as we can do in Arizona. Nancy's Organics, based in Oregon, is another favorite. Skip flavored yogurts and add your own flavors—frozen blueberries turn plain yogurt the same bright blue, but don't require any food coloring to do so. And always check the label, as some companies add corn or tapioca starch or milk protein concentrate to thicken their yogurt.

In sum: If you're superconcerned about the environmental footprint of your dairy consumption, or if you're lactose-intolerant, buy plant-based milks with the fewest additives. If you like milk, if you don't want to give it up, buy organic and full-fat always, and local whenever possible.

If you have the time, making your own plant-based milk is pretty easy and very delicious. You'll need a blender or food processor and a good strainer—cheesecloth works best. To make almond milk, soak a cup of raw almonds in a bowl, covered by about an inch of water, at least overnight, but up to two days. The almonds will swell—they should feel slightly squishy. Discard any remaining water, and add the almonds to a blender or food processor, as well as two cups of fresh water. Blend for a few minutes, until the water turns white and creamy. Strain almond mixture through cheesecloth, making sure to press all the liquid from the meal. Add a dash of cinnamon, if you want, or a bit of sweetener, and refrigerate for up to two days. You can use the leftover almond meal in oatmeal or baked goods, or as a thickener in smoothies or soups. To make milk from oats, rice, or soybeans, follow basically the same steps: soak, rinse, blend, and strain.

11

MEAT

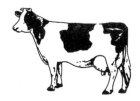

~~Meat is processed.~~ *Some meat is processed.*

Rain patters on the tin roof of the open-air ramada. We huddle in twelve chairs, a tight circle shivering against the damp wind. It is bone-cold—the words flash through my mind before I realize their aptness. My bones feel exposed, as if they are not wound in thick muscle, not padded by fat, and held together by tendons. I have no warm organs; no beating heart. I am just brittle skin and cracking bones, a tight skeleton clattering against thirty-degree rain. It's a good thing, too, with so many sharp knives around. I am not afraid of the other knives or of the people who wield them. I am afraid of my own—the piercing metal appendage that appeared on my belt loop this morning. It is brand new—purchased for this very event—and I am scared to slide it out of its flimsy plastic sheath.

But I will have to. My knife is one of the twelve eight-inch Craftsman-style knives that have convened at Bean Tree Farm at seven on a December morning to slaughter, butcher, and process a sheep.

Before we begin or remove our knives, the instructor of the workshop, a lanky midfifties farmer named Jeff, asks us to go around the circle and introduce ourselves. There is an implicit "why?" in this request—why wake up early in December's darkness to learn how to butcher a living animal?

Barbara begins. Welcome, she says, and her smile and the wave of long, loose hair relaxes us. Barbara and her partner, Bill, are hosting the two-day workshop at their permaculture farm located on twenty acres of saguaro forest in the mountains north of Tucson. Jeff and his wife, Ana, have driven back to Arizona from their home in tiny Boulder, Utah, to teach this animal processing workshop after a well-attended first class.

I'm surprised at how varied our group is—we are seven men and five women, the hands holding our knives aged across a span of sixty years. Uri, Clay, and Arlo are each handsome men in their midthirties, married with young children, and here for the same reason—to learn how to kill the animals they hope to raise. The five women in the group have a scattered set of reasons. Another Meghan, the director of a sustainable agriculture nonprofit whom I'd met before, wants to know more about where her food comes from. Nicole, who, wearing boots with two-inch heels and a stylish knit cardigan, seems vastly overdressed for this endeavor, has studied with Tohono O'odham healers and wants to be able to source ingredients for her bone broths—"Chicken feet are *so* hard to find," she says. Michelle, a mother of two teenagers, was diabetic before she rearranged her diet around fat and animal protein. Racheli sighs and uncrumples herself from a deep slouch before she begins. Her short, gray hair is matted and askew in the back; she's wearing baggy gray sweatpants, old running shoes, and a thick, oversize coat. "I'm nervous," she says, her voice accented from her Israeli upbringing. "I am very anxious for this. I do not know if this will be too much, but I am here, and we will see." Her voice cracks. "I want my children, these two, Uri and Tal," she says, gesturing at her two sons, "to understand this." Also, she says,

"My chicken hasn't laid an egg in four months and she laid one this morning! She must've known where I was going."

When it's my turn to speak, I offer a quick synopsis of the year I've nearly completed. "I stopped eating processed foods about a year ago and I'm trying to figure out how it is that we process foods from the wild," I say. "How we began, and how we've gotten to where we are today, when there is, I suppose, very little wild left to process." I look to my left, ready to pass the invisible talking baton to Tal, Racheli's youngest son, a nervous college student, and then I pause. I inhale sharply and add, "I've been a vegetarian on and off my whole life. I guess I just don't *know* how to eat meat." My voice cracks with frustration. "If there is a way to eat animals responsibly and intentionally . . . I guess I want to see what it really takes."

WHEN I WAS EIGHT YEARS OLD, my mom's parents visited us from Michigan and my grandfather announced he was treating us to a special night out. We drove down to Long Beach Harbor and boarded the *Queen Mary* for a three-hour cruise over dark, glassy waters, legs hidden under white linen tablecloths and hands clutching thick, cold silverware.

I was, somehow, my grandfather's last chance. My mom, his youngest daughter, had become a vegetarian when she went to college—if this was to be her only rebellion, he supposed he could handle a brief bout of it. But then she met a physicist and he didn't eat meat either! Meatless and married, they left the Midwest, moved to California, and now her daughters—*his* granddaughters, these writhing, skinny things who looked up at him with button-granddaughter eyes—were going to grow up without ever having tasted a proper steak!

My sister, with two years and two streaks of stubborn on me, refused to consider the possibility. I was, evidently, still malleable and just adventurous enough to be talked into ordering one of these proper steaks. I was swirling

Coca-Cola bubbles—another treat—around my mouth when a waiter's clean hand slid a wide plate onto an expanse of tablecloth before me. There must have been some mistake—this, *this* was what I had ordered? A slab of oozing brown flesh, splayed, unseemly, across a broad plate. I looked over at my dad, eyes wide. No way, José.

It was, my dad reassured me, like a hamburger. "It's just like a hamburger before it gets all ground up."

I looked left, at my grandfather. Seriously?

"Here, let's put some salt on it," he said, and reached over to switch my steak knife from my awkward left hand into my dominant right. I speared the chunk with my fork and examined the fibers that ran across it like hairs gathered in a ponytail. I glared at my dad. This was *not* a hamburger—not even close. But my grandfather was watching me and my sister was gagging—I'd show them. I sprinkled more salt on the chunk of meat and folded it in to my mouth.

The first time I tasted beer, I thought, *Meh.* The first time I sipped a martini, I dumped peanuts in my mouth to counteract the kick. Alcohol, like blue cheese, coffee, and oysters, is an acquired taste.

Steak, one might generalize, is not.

"You took one bite of that steak and you never went back," my dad would say later. "Your mom, sister, and I sat there looking at you like you were a cavewoman."

I still remember what that first bite tasted like—how it felt, as I chewed it through my mouth. First salt, then juice, then texture—a whole lot of texture, more than any vegetable I'd ever had. Feeling like a grown-up, a linen napkin that dabbed my mouth, a salty-skin rush of meat washed down by sweet Coca-Cola fizz. Unlike so many foods at that finicky age, I *liked* meat.

BEFORE WE CAN TRANSFORM OUR ANIMAL INTO MEAT, we must learn how to wield our knives safely. "A sharp knife is a safe knife," Jeff says. "You're more likely to get hurt with a dull knife because you'll have to exert more force." It is typical to cut oneself while butchering, Jeff says. "A nick on the finger is not critical." But we should try to avoid the danger zones, the spots on our bodies where an accidental swipe of a sharp blade will splice thin arteries. One swipe is all it takes—one short splice. "The neck is an obvious danger zone," he says. "Though if you manage to cut yourself there, you're doing some acrobatics that you really shouldn't be."

More likely, a careless cut will extend to an inner leg's arteries. Will slice a wrist or an ankle's tendon. Ana nods in agreement with Jeff. "We've had a few cut tendons before," she mutters, barely audible. A *few*? This casual count terrifies me. Petrified, I sit on my folding chair, unable to remove my knife for inspection, as every other member has done. Finally, I decide, with logic that unfreezes me, that allows me to move, to participate, that I will just lose a finger today. I will not cut a tendon, I will *not* slice an artery, but I might lose the tip of a finger, and that is just going to have to be okay.

So finally, I pull my knife out of its sheath. Bone fingers wrapped in dry skin grab the black rubber handle. The handle is black except for its top and bottom, beginning and ending with two rectangles of hard red rubber, wrapped around the black like signal flares.

"How do you know your knife is sharp?" asks Jeff.

"Try to cut a tomato?" I offer.

Jeff takes me seriously. "Sure, that works. But if you don't have a tomato handy, look at your edge in sunlight. If you can see a reflection, there's no edge." A knife with no edge is a knife that is not sharp.

The blade of my knife is made of carbon steel, a fact etched along a smooth side before the brand—Mora—and the words MADE IN SWEDEN. I pivot the handle to the right, like I'm turning a doorknob, and survey the edge of the thin blade that now faces me. The invisible edge slants imperceptibly toward thickness and then flares outward a fraction more at the abrupt end of the bevel—the narrowest part of the blade, the part we will have to sharpen, again and again, throughout the course of the workshop.

Jeff passes around wood blocks covered in six-hundred-grit sandpaper and shows us how to pin the bevel firmly against the grain and then stroke the knife up and down. For the stainless steel of kitchen knives, it takes the refined grit of a sharpening stone to grind down a knife's bevel to an invisible edge, the edge that will cleave two halves of a tomato. For our knives, sandpaper will do the trick; sandpaper will refine the edge that will slit the throat of a sheep. That will cut through its hide, crack apart its bones, saw off its haunches. The edge that will make meat out of an animal.

"WHAT IS IT THAT MAKES A CREATURE AN *ANIMAL*?" asks food writer Harold McGee. His answer draws on etymology—"The word comes from an Indo-European root meaning 'to breathe,' to move air in and out of the body." Animals breathe and animals *move*—they are beings with the self-contained power to travel through the world and shift pieces of that world around.

We'd have to go back two million years, to our primate ancestors scavenging the savannahs of Africa, to find a time when humans haven't eaten animals. Two million years ago, early humanoids fed themselves primarily on raw, foraged plants—fruits, leaves, tubers. It was a lot of work for these bodies to collect enough calories to sustain themselves and a lot of work for their guts to digest this high-fiber plant matter into accessible energy. It's not clear the cause—perhaps a shift in climate, making vegetation harder to find— but around the time that *Homo habilis* became *Homo erectus,* our ancestors began eating the animal carcasses that dotted their landscapes. Today, some evolutionary anthropologists suggest that it was this new diet of energy- and nutrient-dense animal flesh that catalyzed human evolution. You can, generally speaking, either have a big gut or a big brain, and energy-dense animal flesh provided the excess calories our ancestors needed to grow larger and more complex brains—calories that were previously unavailable on vegetarian diets. ("I know this will sound awful to vegetarians, but meat made us human," said Manuel Domínguez-Rodrigo, an archaeologist at Complutense University in Madrid.) Quite a bit later—1.9 million years, give or take—humans started hunting the meat for themselves. (Around that time, humans started painting hunting scenes on their cave walls—if meat made us human, it also made us artists.) It was only about ten thousand years ago that humans began intentionally raising animals for food, domesticating their first dogs, goats, and sheep, and then later, pigs, cattle, and horses.

Animals process the grains, grasses, and forbs of diverse landscapes into their muscles. Humans cultivate those muscles, care for that flesh, and then process these animals into meat. This relationship, the flow of energy from land to animal to meat to human, is primal, simple, and succinct. Or it should be.

JEFF ASKS US: "How does an animal die?"

There is a collective pause, a group inhale, a moment of silence.

He answers his own question: "Loss of blood to the brain. Our brains work for about four minutes after the blood supply is cut off." Animal brains, ours included, continue to work for four minutes after the body's heart stops beating.

The sheep will be lying down, head back and neck exposed. Someone's knife will be the knife that is pulled across the sheep's two carotid arteries. How will we know where to cut? Jeff asks us to feel our own arteries. "Put your fingers on your jaw," Jeff tells us. We obey. Run your fingers down your jaw to your trachea, the knobby column of calcium that protects your esophagus. Prod two fingers behind this column and feel the rubbery—imagined rubbery, imagined slippery—tubes.

Beat-beat. Beat-beat. Beat-beat.

"That's what you cut," Jeff says. "Those two arteries. If you don't cut them all the way through with one slice, you have to cut them again, or you prolong the sheep's death."

We consider this for a moment before Jeff sends us off on an explicitly solitary break. "Take a moment to reflect and decide if you want to be the one who makes that cut."

I unfold my cold, clenched body from the metal chair and begin walking on tight legs up into the prickly-pear-and-saguaro-dotted landscape. I weave down and up a ravine, and swerve to the east, away from the group; I duck under the hanging branches of a paloverde, and as I emerge, straighten my knees, and unbend my back, a two-step time lapse of human evolution, my right hand scrapes against an errant cluster of spines. Three distinct red scratches burst out of pale skin, three lines that touch in an alternating crisscross.

The rain has calmed to a light drizzle; the clouds have eased their tight grip along the red rock hills. I turn to my right, south, and survey Tucson's landscape spread across the flat plain below. I wipe my hand on the inside of my T-shirt and watch as beads of blood spring to the smooth surface like slow bubbles rising in soda pop. I lift my head to the cold clouds and once again poke two fingers behind my trachea to my throbbing arteries. Could I?

It is not a beat so much as it is as a push and retreat. It is matter then space, tick then tock, energy then rest. It is life, this pulse, and I had thought, really believed, until this moment, that I would volunteer my knife, my action, to slaughter the sheep. But I pulse—my hand bleeds. I pulse, I bleed; my skin is cold but my pulse is warm and my blood beats.

MY DAD GREW UP ON A FARM IN TEXAS. A farm with wheat and cotton, corn and vegetables, and forty head of cattle. My mom grew up eating midwestern meat, potatoes, and Velveeta cheese. They both grew up eating meat—summertime country-fried steak in Texas and Sunday-night pot roasts in Michigan—and then they both stopped eating meat.

"I was a sophomore in college, living in the dormitory at Michigan State," my mom says. We're sitting in our living room in California and my parents are answering my questions—why? And, how? My parents have been vegetarians as long as I've known them—they are vegetarians like they are my parents, prior lives unimaginable—and so I have never asked them so explicitly to explain themselves. "I read books about killing animals, how awful it is. I was eating pretty low-quality meat, so it was easy to give up," my mom says. "Then I got into the whole 'we shouldn't kill animals and eat them' thing." She pauses, remembering. "Oh yeah, around the same time, when I was a senior in college, there was a big scare in Michigan. They had fed fire retardant to cows and the meat got contaminated. Stuff like that comes out and you think, 'Oh no, I don't think so.'"

"Wait," I say. "They fed fire retardant to *cows?* Who is *they?*"

"Yup," she says. "I guess they got it mixed up with the cow feed."

As it turns out, "they" is the Michigan Chemical Corporation, and how they "got mixed up" is that illiterate workers accidentally swapped a bag of FireMaster, a flame retardant made from polybrominated biphenyl—a chemical that is now illegal—for a bag of Nutrimaster, a feed supplement made from magnesium oxide. (The bags had previously been color-coded.) According to Joyce Egginton, the author of *The Poisoning of Michigan,* when the poisoned cattle feed was distributed to farms throughout the state in the early 1970s, nine million residents consumed contaminated meat and milk. Nine million people, just about 85 percent of the state's population, unwittingly received some exposure to PBB, in what, three decades later, remains one of the most widespread chemical contaminations in U.S. history. I'd never heard of it.

"Come on"—my dad chimes in—"even if they hadn't put them in the wrong bags, how can you have a company that's making fire retardant *and* cow food on the same machinery?"

"Were you living in Michigan then?" I ask him.

"No, I was still in graduate school but I had gradually stopped eating meat. I'd always been a finicky meat eater. I'd eat a well-done hamburger, but when we moved onto the other cuts of the cow—bones and ribs—it was like, what is *that*? There's *blood* on my plate." He shakes his head and grimaces. "At first, it was, I don't want to eat that bloody stuff. Only later did I start to become concerned about the energy and water resources it took, the waste and health issues."

"So why'd you let us eat meat?" I ask. "When Katie and I were born, why weren't we vegetarians, too?"

My parents pause and look at each other. Finally, my dad says, "It seemed like a decision that should be your decision, not ours."

"When you and your sister were babies, we'd give you ground-up baby food with meat in it," my mom says. "We were worried about you missing some nutritional component."

"When you got older, your mom cooked meat probably once a week," my dad says.

"I'm sure it tasted horrible," my mom says. "I had no idea what I was doing."

"But really, you girls ate vegetarian," my dad says. "Meat was an occasional supplement so you'd acquire the taste and then make your own decision. Mostly, we ate vegetarian."

I STILL EAT MOSTLY VEGETARIAN—rather, I still haven't made that decision. When I left home and went to college, I was presented with an array of prepared meat, ready for the taking: pepperoni pizza, flat hamburgers, white chicken breast. Someone else cooked it for me, so it was all too easy to slide onto a plate and into my stomach. Once I started cooking for myself, I realized all of the recipes I had inherited from my mother were vegetarian and thus so were mine. Occasionally, once a month, I'd wonder if I needed more protein and so I'd pull a slimy palmful of Tyson chicken out of its plastic-wrapped

Styrofoam packaging and toss it on an electric George Forman grill with a grimace, slamming the lid shut and returning only when I knew the meat would be aggressively well done.

When I moved to Nicaragua, I learned to reckon with raw meat. Juan bought whole chickens at the supermarket and Isolina and I would pull apart their carcasses to drop wings, breasts, and thighs into pans of sputtering vegetable oil. We went fishing, trolling for miles out over the sparking blue Pacific in small, metal motorboats. I reeled in heavy mackerel and learned how to break their necks to stop their bodies from writhing. At daybreak on Thanksgiving morning, in preparation for our American-style celebration, I watched as Manuel, the hotel's groundskeeper, bound two flapping, feathered turkeys around a thick tree trunk and beheaded them with two quick swings of a machete. Before Juan and Manuel defeathered the birds, I poured hot water over their flesh to help loosen the skin; I watched while Isolina cleaned and gutted, seasoned and roasted. When, twelve hours later, the turkeys appeared at the end of the Thanksgiving buffet with our grateful grace, the meat felt earned.

When I moved back to Los Angeles, I read Michael Pollan's *The Omnivore's Dilemma* and realized the same thing my mom had three decades before—there's something wrong with the way we produce and consume meat in this country. But I earned minimum wage and decided that I couldn't afford to buy meat; at least, not the meat I thought I should be buying. I defaulted to a mostly meatless life. I wasn't a vegetarian. I just didn't happen to eat meat.

I didn't eat meat—except for when I did. When my brother-in-law made apple-bacon risotto—my sister is a finicky meat eater but decidedly a meat eater—or when carne asada tacos were a dollar each at happy hour. I ate meat when someone else cooked it for me, when I didn't have to consider raw flesh sourced from living animals.

When I moved from Los Angeles to Tucson and met new friends out for dinner, I'd order cheese enchiladas or stretch across the table for a slice of veggie pizza. When these new friends asked, "Oh, are you a vegetarian?" I said, "Sure." I forgot to buy meat at the supermarket and I preferred vegetables anyway, so sure, I could be a vegetarian. I went out of my way to eat one last In-N-Out cheeseburger and called my parents to tell them the news. I don't remember if I was embarrassed or proud; the prodigal meat eater returning to roost in the tofu tree.

"Oh," my mom said. "Okay."

"That's it?"

"Should there be more?"

"I guess not. I thought you'd have some reaction. Can I tell Dad?"

"Jeff, Megan's a vegetarian now," my mom called out, and I heard my dad's voice reply, deflected from around the corner: "Okay!"

WE HUDDLE QUIETLY, the carnivores and I, around the sputtering fire, in the accumulating mist. Uri drew the straw to make the cut, so he stands away from the group, away from the sheep's arrival. When we had returned from our solitary sojourns, Uri, Arlo, Clay, and Tal had all volunteered for the butchering. When the women of the group realized that none of us had stepped forward— only the men had—we looked at each other, embarrassed and unsure what to make of the gender divide. We sputtered excuses: not now, not ready, not yet. But the fact remains, and although it is discomfiting, it is also a comforting reminder of our specific culture, one distinctly human. A reminder that the words "male" and "female" do not simply refer to anatomy.

There is a soft bleat muted by fog, and then Jeff returns, carrying the sheep in his outstretched arms like a blinking bag of groceries. The sheep looks like a goat. It is a hair sheep—*he* is a hair sheep, bred for meat rather than wool. Coarse auburn hair wraps around a breathing body and fades into a thick stripe of black hair cutting across a soft stomach. Jeff lays the sheep on its side in the cold dirt, holding its body in place with a firm hand. The sheep is alive and warm. Frightened glassy eyes blink, roll, and stare.

As Jeff pulls the sheep's neck back, stretching it over the six-inch hole we've dug into hard dirt, the sheep offers one last twitch of resistance. But as we cluster around him, holding his hooves to the ground, weighing his haunches with our hands, he relaxes. Uri finds the sheep's arteries. Jeff nods. Uri exhales. He points the sharp end of his knife into the soft neck, pivots the knife by the handle, and pushes down four inches, a quick crunch through flesh.

The sheep's neck falls open. Blood falls into the ground. The neck stays open—a vacant V of space.

The sheep doesn't fight death. Blood falls from its open artery into the small hole in the earth, and the sheep waits. Or we wait. Four minutes, and suddenly I don't know how or when or why—I didn't expect this—tears stream down my cheeks.

MANY PEOPLE, ACROSS MANY CULTURES, believe that it is immoral to kill animals and eat them. Throughout history, many people, across many cultures, have also believed that it is moral to sacrifice animals in order to honor life. It is an interesting ethical argument, but at the end of the day, for me, it comes down to the fact that life takes life. Life requires the energy from other lives to sustain and thrive, to fold and unfold, and so the reason I cry when we kill the sheep is not that I believe it's wrong to kill animals, but that killing animals becomes right—to me—when I understand their measure. I cry when we kill the sheep because it is sentient; because it was alive and now it's not. I don't love this particular sheep, but I love many animals that are alive, and a quick, sturdy slit across a thick throat reminds me how fragile a beating body really is.

The sheep dies. We watch, silent. The sheep dies, and then it is no longer a sheep. The sheep dies and it becomes a carcass; it becomes potential energy, potential food for our human bodies. After four minutes, muscle becomes meat. Our knives' work begins.

Jeff lays the carcass on the ground under the ramada and then joins it, placing his leg parallel to the sheep's. "The anatomy is the same," he says. "The way you can dismantle an animal using only a knife is by finding the joints and popping them open." Slice the hide and find the ankle joint, wiggle it apart with the blade, crack it open with two clasped hands.

Hooves, then head. The head comes off—rather, we cut it off. Jeff pulls the hide open from neck to sternum, pulling out the trachea and esophagus, letting the stomach juices drizzle onto the ground before hoisting the carcass to hang by the cartilage of its heels.

We each work a bit at a time. Slow, so slow. Piece by piece. We step in and out of the work like subs in a basketball game; the game progresses, back and forth, and our team advances even as the players swap out. Jeff coaches us on. He calls a play and then steps aside for the blade of a volunteer. I am still scared of my knife, but finally, when he asks for someone to cut the hide from sternum to anus, I feel myself step forward. I hear myself say, "I can."

He maps the trajectory of my cut. I grasp the handle of my blade and slide it out with a careful hand. Two fingers pull the hide away from the muscle—it is a hard pull, a strong tug—and guide the knife blade, an inch at a time, along the sheep's body. The knife follows the crease between my fingers. The knife works—it cuts. It cuts, cleanly, and it is harder to pull the hide away from the muscle, to manually break the connective tissue, than it is to slice it with my knife. I don't know how long it takes to make the two-foot incision. But when I am done, my knife has blood on it and my fingers are sticky with the mucus that once held this sheep together.

IN MOST INDUSTRIAL MEAT PRODUCTION TODAY, spinning saws and colossal blades do the work of Craftsman knives. It simply takes too long to dismantle an animal by hand. One problem with butchering a carcass in a matter of minutes is that the process often sends bone shards into flesh. Bones fracture just like glass, and although many of these shards are too small to cause harm, bone fragments and "bone constituents" often show up in X-rays of commercial meat.

There are, of course, many other problems with industrial meat, apart from the occasional bone shard. Indeed, even if you have forgotten the specifics, by intent or accident, you might know that there is a lot to be said about meat. There is so much to be said about meat that it is a far cheerier choice to remain in bacon-adorned bliss—as I did for a very happy time—rather than consider the enormous, insurmountable complexity of what it means to be a meat eater in a modern society. Speaking of meat is a complex thing, but this is part of the industry's game. If feedlots and slaughterhouses were transparent, there might be a lot fewer of them.

If you wanted to know it, you'd know it by now—all of the reasons *not* to eat meat. You might know that today, 99 percent of all land animals eaten or milked in the United States come from a factory farm. If you are eating meat, as a rule, you are eating an animal born, bred, and slaughtered in a crowded, disease-ridden, resource-intensive feedlot. Animals in this system are not animals; they are commodities. Corn in, flesh out; if you are eating meat today, you're eating a commodity that was produced on a Concentrated Animal Feeding Operation—a CAFO. "The economic logic of gathering so many animals together to feed them cheap corn in CAFOs is hard to argue with; it has made meat, which used to be a special occasion in most American homes, so cheap and abundant that many of us now eat it three times a day," writes Michael Pollan in *The Omnivore's Dilemma*. "Not so compelling is the biological logic behind this cheap meat. Already in their short history CAFOs have produced more than their share of environmental and health problems: polluted water and air, toxic wastes, novel and deadly pathogens."

Again, there are a lot of ways to tell this story, but here's one: Livestock contributes over a third of the world's methane emissions. According to *National Geographic,* an average-size steer living on a feedlot sucks up two hundred gallons of fuel over its lifetime, fuel that is embedded in feed, fertilizers, and machinery, but not the price of beef at the supermarket. Remember wheat? Processed wheat? Forty percent of grain grown across the world is fed to animals; if it takes twenty-five gallons of water to grow a pound of wheat, it takes five thousand gallons of freshwater to produce a pound of steak. Put another way, it takes ten thousand pounds of grain (really, corn) to grow a thousand-pound cow.

Grain goes in, waste comes out. Farmed animals in the United States produce 130 times more waste than their human caretakers—three hundred million tons of it a year. Unlike cities, which have built sewage systems and treatment plants to deal with human waste, animal feces are flushed into waterways and otherwise dumped, literally, onto open swaths of land. Factory farming is so destructive to our soils, water, and air that Jonathan Safran Foer writes in *Eating Animals,* "Someone who regularly eats factory-farmed animal products cannot call himself an environmentalist without divorcing that word from its meaning."

Well then, screw the environment. What about *our* bodies? "The meat industry's big public relations problem," writes Marion Nestle in *What to Eat,* "is that vegetarians are demonstrably healthier than meat eaters." Every body is different, of course, as is every eater's relationship to the foods they eat, but Nestle writes in her landmark book *Food Politics* about how the meat industry has so successfully strong-armed the USDA's health guidelines that when, in 1977, the agency first offered the advice "decrease consumption of meat," it caused such an uproar that they've never done it again—even when studies published in respected medical journals show that significant meat consumption increases our risk for heart disease and certain cancers. (The fact that the

USDA is the federal agency publishing dietary guidelines is yet another quagmire, one that gets all the more complex when U.S. agricultural interests—beef and corn, namely—misalign with the advice of health professionals.)

So what if meat causes cancer—doesn't *everything* cause cancer these days? As it turns out, the risks inherent in eating industrial meat are more acute. Cattle aren't supposed to eat corn, just like humans haven't evolved to eat grass. When cattle eat corn, they get sick. And, with the exception of organic cattle, sick cattle get treated with drugs. According to the USDA, 80 percent of all the antibiotics sold in the United States are consumed by chickens, pigs, cows, and other food-producing animals. Because meat and poultry producers aren't required to disclose what they do with the drugs once they purchase them, it's tricky to prove that routine antibiotic use in animals causes antibiotic-resistant infections in the people who eat those animals. There is enough evidence, however, to suggest a correlation.

It doesn't stop there—although I'll stop soon. When cattle eat corn, a natural bacterium in their guts, *Escherichia coli,* mutates into a new, toxic strain. When that corn becomes waste, cows are left standing in it, so they then arrive to the slaughterhouse—there are now only *thirteen* major slaughterhouses in the United States, compared to the thousands that operated in the 1970s—covered in their own feces. A factory slaughtering four hundred cows an hour might not have the time to make sure every carcass is clean before they saw it in half, and so some fecal matter might get into flesh that is then ground up with hundreds of other slaughtered carcasses before it's shaped into hamburgers. The last count by the Centers for Disease Control estimated that every year, sixty-two thousand people are infected with E. coli O157:H7 traceable to the meat they eat. Every year, fifty-two of those people die. In 2007, twenty-two million pounds of beef were recalled—enough meat to make a hamburger for every American—as the result of a single E. coli outbreak.

We fret, we sigh, we gag at inhumane horror. And then what? It's not as if we actively decide to participate in the system, to endorse the companies like Tyson and ConAgra that have co-opted our food system and gambled with our health. Rather, we go out to lunch. We go to company picnics and to holiday dinner parties, and meat is wound so intricately into the fabric of our food that it seems we must either abstain altogether or give up the fight.

I declared myself a vegetarian. Except—that apple-bacon risotto? My brother-in-law cooked it only five months after my big pronouncement, when I went to visit him and my sister in Seattle before Christmas. And then I had broken the seal, so I ate three slices of translucent prosciutto at a holiday party, and then one piece of pepperoni pizza on New Year's Eve. They were exceptions to the rule. When I started my year unprocessed, I was a vegetarian—I just ate meat occasionally.

Meat was, theoretically, unprocessed. But of course I knew better. Of course I knew meat's truth. The meat we eat today is one of the most intensely processed foods available in our supermarkets—we have, after all, taken animals' lives and strung them on assembly lines.

AROUND NOON, after hide peels painstakingly away from muscle and the carcass hangs from the rafters looking more like food than animal, Barbara brings out a bowl of fresh salsa and corn chips. With its ankles spread across a short wood dowel, its belly still closed and full of organs, with skinny, truncated arms reaching out from muscle-wrapped shoulders, the carcass has acquired a certain anonymity. I can see the animal's white ribs surrounded by this fleshy red; its thick haunches marbled with white fat, hard like a bar of soap. Now that the sheep is not one sheep, but any—it could well be a goat or a dog now—I can start to see cuts of meat rather than bandages of muscle.

I am not hungry, but I have been on this farm, with this animal, for days—I cannot remember a time when I was not butchering a sheep—so I wash my hands and scoop heaps of cholla-bud salsa into my cold mouth. I step back into the rotation to begin slicing the belly open, exposing the stomach and organs, and then relinquish my incision to Tal's knife. I wash my hands. I scoop more salsa into my cold mouth. I return to the carcass. It is bizarre, this back-and-forth, animal then vegetable, carcass then corn chip.

Once we have opened the body cavity and the stomach billows out into the cold air—held in place, as our organs are, by a thick cord of connective tissue that runs from neck to anus—Jeff cuts off the sheep's penis. Unlike a human penis, this organ is a mostly subterranean appendage, a white, narrow vessel running from between the ram's legs nearly a foot up its stomach.

"Does anyone have a dog?" Jeff asks after he slices the organ loose.

It's silent for a beat, and Uri says, almost reluctantly, "I do."

Jeff hands him the penis. "Your dog will love it."

Again, it's quiet. Uri holds the penis in his right hand like a rubber ribbon and Jeff continues his work scraping out the sheep's interior. "Um," Uri says finally. "Do you have a bag or something?"

It feels amazing to laugh. My emotions have been limited to a taut range of fear and fatigue, and with one laugh, some of this knot relaxes. I have been afraid not only of cutting myself, but also of cutting the sheep incorrectly. Now that the sheep no longer feels pain, now that I have wielded my knife, my concern is less with inflicting harm and more, simply, with screwing up. I am terrified that I will accidentally puncture something that shouldn't be punctured, that I will miss a bone or cut a sloppy line across flesh. It is one thing to mess up baking a loaf of bread. It is quite another to screw up while processing an animal that has absorbed so many resources during its life, that has been reared and transported and killed with so much care. With a knife in my hand, my movements have consequences. Yet I have been so preoccupied with these consequences that I forgot to notice the humor—the life, really—in what we're doing here.

While the team laughs at Uri's request for a penis bag, Coach Jeff takes him seriously. "No, what you want to do is find a rock and lay it out to dry," he says, continuing to carve away at the carcass. "Once the penis gets hard, it's the best play toy."

I can't help it. I chortle. I catch Arlo's eye and he's holding in a grin, too, and then it escapes and then we're all chuckling, even Racheli, even, finally, Jeff.

WE EAT THE ORGANS FIRST. It is the only thing to do with the shiny bundles that Jeff scoops out of the body cavity. The iron-rich liver, smooth, shiny, and brown; the kidneys' thin disk that steams when it's exposed to the cold air; the small fist of a heart, the anatomy of a life. The testicles, white and buttery, slipping out of their sack with an easy squeeze by Racheli. They land in a bucket and it is not a question. What else would be done?

Ana warms up a two-burner camping stove while Arlo and Racheli dice up the meat into inch-size cubes. Two cutting boards fill with chunks of meat and a broad cast-iron griddle sizzles when the raw flesh tumbles onto the hot surface. Immediately, it smells like lamb. Flesh hits hissing heat and suddenly it is food. Suddenly it smells like meat. It smelled, before, of dirt and fur, of faint flesh and indistinct animal. Now the smell is inescapable. Animal becomes meat.

The smell makes me woozy. Woozy with hunger, faint with fatigue. I sit down on one of the cold folding chairs that remains from our tight morning circle. Ana sets a cast-iron skillet brimming with organ meat—one of the most iron-rich foods on the planet—sautéed and seasoned among carrots, cabbage, and celery, and I barely breathe as I scoop heaps of the steaming stir-fry into my ceramic bowl and then into my mouth. The meat itself is chewy, pungent, and flavorful; chunks of liver, kidney, and heart explore the corners of my mouth in strange, new ways, and although I don't fall as hard for my first organs as I did for my first steak, still I return for a second helping.

OF COURSE, there are many reasons *to* eat meat.

For as many China studies and vegan doctors as there are today, there are an equal number of thoughtful researchers and journalists who have suggested *more* meat as a solution to our failing health. Since the 1950s, when researcher Ancel Keys correlated saturated fat and cholesterol intake with higher instances of coronary heart disease—what's now known as the "lipid hypothesis"—hordes of nutritionists and dieticians have lined up to dispel this dictum. Journalists Gary Taubes and Michael Pollan are only the most notable among many who have blamed our expanding waistlines on all the "low-fat" processed sugars and carbohydrates we now inhale rather than their full-fat counterparts. Meat, of course, provides one of the largest sources of saturated and unsaturated fats in our diets, but "the belief that saturated fat clogs arteries by raising cholesterol is a hangover from the state of science thirty to forty years ago," writes Taubes in *Why We Get Fat.*

Today, if you've heard of the Paleo diet, you've heard of the work of Weston A. Price. Price was the dentist who traveled around the world in the 1930s documenting the teeth and mouth cavities of a dozen different indigenous groups. "While the primary quest was to find the cause of tooth decay," he writes in his seminal book *Nutrition and Physical Decay,* published in 1939, "[this] was established quite readily as being controlled directly by nutrition." Across the world, across a wide array of available foods, again and again Price documented how the introduction of modern processed foods such as refined wheat and sugar caused abrupt "degenerations" in total physical health, often within a single generation.

Price documented modern hunter-gatherers as surrogates for our hunter-gatherer ancestors, contrasting their diets to those of agriculture-based societies. Although there were significant differences, what all of the indigenous diets had in common was a high intake of animal fat—"namely, sea foods, organs of animals, or dairy products." And it was precisely these communities that showed the lowest incidences of tooth decay, diabetes, obesity, along with a host of other modern maladies. In other words, according to Price, meat begat health.

I BEGIN CARVING THE BACKSTRAP OFF THE ANIMAL, the thick, lean muscle that might be sliced and sold as a fillet. As Ana renders fat onto the griddle and fries chunks of testicle to a golden brown, I carefully slide my knife through sticky red muscle.

Nicole peers around my shoulders as I work. "God, that looks delicious."

Racheli ambles over from her chopping station. "Looks like dinner!" She turns to Jeff, who stands near the stove with Ana. "Can we try it?"

"Try what?" he asks.

"The meat!"

"Raw?"

"Of course," says Racheli, the commanding grandmother, matted hair askew.

We look at Jeff. He shrugs. "I suppose, why not?"

Racheli leans in with her knife and, with two deft slices, cuts off a small sliver of sticky red fillet and drops it into her mouth. "Yum!" she says, walking away, done with her project.

Nicole and I are left standing, staring at each other. "Well, shoot," she says. A small, sticky sliver lands in her mouth. Michelle and then Tal come over, and they, too, attempt the raw flesh.

"I guess I'll have to try some, too," Jeff says, laying his knife blade parallel to a rib and using it to remove a translucent sheet of meat.

And then, so do I. It occurs to me, as I'm chewing on the rubbery ball of flesh—it's not bloody or tangy; it doesn't taste like much, actually, more gelatin than animal—that *this* is meat unprocessed. The thought clatters around with some amusement, and then swallows itself back into my brain as my molars, long evolved and dulled by the work of steak knives, continue to work the flesh into smaller bits. When I finally swallow the meat into my own stomach, the memory of this raw texture rolls around, lingering as I carve away at the animal's ribs.

WE WORK UNDER THE HEAVY DRIZZLE of a cold afternoon until it gets dark. Almost twelve hours after we began, I fold my creaky limbs into my Civic and shift the car into gear. The car drives by muscle memory, winding along a dark dirt road until the road ends, suddenly, and I merge onto a bright six-lane cement street. There is, I realize after I turn left, no wine in my home. There is no wine, and I realize, as I am sitting at the stoplight at Silverbell and Twin Peaks Road, that I want wine, more than I've wanted anything. There is a Safeway on the corner on Silverbell and Twin Peaks Road. I don't think. I pull into the parking lot.

My muddy shoes are three steps in the door, backpack slung on one shoulder, knife still on my belt loop, when I am hit by the stupidity of this action. I stagger into a bright, brilliant *whoosh* of fluorescent prosperity and nearly stumble in shock.

Where could all this food have come from? How could it all be here, in one place, in one moment, when it takes so much effort—I am so tired—so much time—I am so tired—to pull apart just one animal? The transition from the quietly cold smell of sheep to this screaming smells-like-nothing place is unexpectedly violent. I feel like I've run against one of those pink-rimmed force fields that people collide into in sci-fi movies. I force my eyes to focus, ask them to lead me to the aisle labeled SPIRITS. On the way, I walk past a slanted glass case of sterile refrigeration. Columns of cuts, precise and similar—so perfectly square, so neatly arranged, so cleanly unblemished. MEAT. I sway over the section titled MEAT, suddenly so much more aware of my own skeleton. A right shoulder that slouches since I injured it in college; arms of skinny muscles and pull-apart bones. My thighs flex with the strength of a runner; my haunches curve with the fat of a female. I have seen what I am made of—I have touched and cut it, stretched and carved it.

I think about the night eleven months ago, when I went to Safeway and bought a DiGiorno pizza on the eve of my year unprocessed. I think about wandering through bright aisles laced with memory and nostalgia, considering mini pancakes and stacks of chocolate chip cookies—would that Megan even recognize this one, wandering around a different Safeway, looking for a bottle of wine after butchering a sheep? I feel a bit like an expat visiting home after a long sojourn. Just as one does not renounce citizenship overnight—it is a process, an untangling—I have not made it here, standing with a knife in my belt and sheep in my gut, by simply boarding a plane. I made the choice once but it has happened slowly, gradually; unprocess by accumulation rather than event.

If it is alive, it is muscle, Jeff had said. If it's dead, it's meat. The difference between muscle and meat is the difference between life and death, but what of the differences between muscles? How can this meat, here, be the same as that meat, there? Meat sizzling on a cast-iron grill—from a sheep from a farm—and meat puddled in a Styrofoam container—from an assembly line from a feedlot. How can this be described by the same word? I ate sheep today and here is lamb, but it is *not the same*. I start pacing in front of the clear case, suddenly angry that there isn't a better signifier, no casual way to convey the space between "vegetarian" and "omnivore," no word that offers different parameters of selectivity. Almost a decade after Michael Pollan offered us the modern omnivore's dilemma—it is not *meat* or *no meat* but rather *which* meat—there is *still* no socially acceptable way to articulate this difference. No way to express, without sounding like a high-maintenance eater or overzealous labeler, the difference between the two.

Meat. It is all just meat.

I DREAM ANIMAL DREAMS on Saturday night and return to Bean Tree Farm early on Sunday morning. We'll finish butchering the animal today, cut the meat off the bones and bake bread in the stomach, tan the hide, dismantle the hooves, and make rope from the intestines. We will make use of the whole animal—we will honor all of its parts, not just the ones our culture has deemed "valuable."

Before we begin our work anew, we cluster in a circle around a crackling campfire and reflect, once again, on the *why* and *how*. Before we slaughtered the animal, Michelle had said—many had said—"I want to know where my food comes from." But everyone who said this had put their words in implicit quotation marks, in the subtle tone reserved for clichés that we cannot help but lean on, and I wonder if we cannot *all* know where *all* of our food comes from, not if we want to order tacos from carts and travel to Mexico.

"I'm really glad I did this," I say. "But I don't know if I want to keep doing this—to have to kill every animal I eat. But that's the thing, that's why we formed communities, right? So people could specialize according to ability and interest. So that each homestead didn't have to fulfill every function themselves." After two days with a sheep, I know that I won't continue to process my own meat. But I can imagine it. Now that I have tried, just once, to experience how beating muscle becomes seasoned meat, I can imagine—I can understand—what meat is, and what it is not. I can still support this, this process of producing meat from animals that have been raised with care and killed with respect. But I can do it with my dollars, not my knife.

BARELY TWO WEEKS LATER, I wake up midmorning on a Sunday and drive myself to the St. Philip's Farmers' Market. The market bustles, bright in the unseasonably warm weather; the Catalina Mountains silhouette the sky above the Spanish-style plaza full of vendors. I'm walking toward the Chiva Risa booth—I see Lissa spearing samples of her goat cheese onto tiny toothpicks—

when I'm stopped by the blond ringlets of a wide-eyed girl. She's wearing a frilly yellow dress and white Sunday shoes, the kind you can only own when you're ten years old.

"Do you want one?" she says, and before I can respond, she hands me a glossy postcard adorned with a mountain panorama and the logo of the Double Check Ranch. The girl turns and prances away. I follow, weaving through the crowd until I see the brim of Paul Schwennesen's wide cowboy hat.

I'd been out to the Double Check Ranch the week before, still recovering from the animal processing workshop but still craving meat, still hoping to find someone to give my dollars to in exchange for flesh and iron. I drove an hour north from Tucson and into winding and windy grasslands. I got lost and arrived late, but Paul had smiled and ambled his cowboy boots around the pasture, showing me what was visible—twenty acres here, in the San Pedro River Valley—and telling me about what was not—ten thousand acres on the New Mexico state border. While he talked about native grass species and nitrogen-fixing legumes, about rainfall this year and last, I'd leaned over the wood-fenced coral to gaze at the cows, catching the eye of a brown steer. Big and beautiful, he'd blinked up at me with dark eyes and swished his tail back and forth across his soft, auburn coat. When I'd outstretched my hand to try to pet his broad forehead, he had backed away and, after a frowning moment, eased back toward me as I lowered my hand, palm up.

If it turns out that Weston Price is right and meat really is better for our bodies, the question remains—what about the environment?

"Ranchers are the best ecological stewards you'll find," Paul told me. "Hands down."

"Why's that?" I asked.

"We bear the burden. We benefit or lose from our decisions, how we treat our land."

If Paul doesn't take care of his soils so they can grow healthy stands of native grasses—grasses that require little water or fertilizer inputs—his cows won't have anything to eat. Anything to eat that's free, that is. Paul and his wife, Sarah, both have master's degrees in economics, training for their pre-ranching careers with the air force, and for a Harvard-trained economist, feed and fertilizer are unnecessary inputs that decrease the profit margins on his outputs. Which are, I reminded myself, hamburgers and briskets.

"I always say we're a business that converts growing plant matter into cash to support a family," said Paul. "The vehicle for that conversion is a cow."

Landscapes depend on animals to nourish them. Indeed, one of the reasons monoculture agriculture depends so heavily on chemical fertilizers is that without manure—without animal waste—soil degrades. A soil's fertility depends on the communities of microbes that thrive on the nutrient-rich waste produced by animals. Without manure, those degraded soils won't grow good grass to feed those animals—and they don't grow good vegetables either.

"Ranchers *have* to manage their land for long-term ecological sustainability," Paul said, yanking up a clump of grass to peer at its root structure. A ranch that resembles a natural ecosystem, one that has ebbed and flowed according to nature's will rather than a rancher's desire, will be a ranch that's been around for a long time. Ranchers like Paul quarrel with the idea that conservation happens *out there,* on parcels of land roped off from all economic activity. (Indeed, it's ranchers like Paul who have convinced groups like the Nature Conservancy to start buying and running ranches in the name of land stewardship; who have recognized the value of open land for migrating or endangered species and put some of their acres into conservation easements, thus protecting the land from future development.) For one, Paul's livelihood—and that of his family—depends on his ability as a steward of grass and water as much as of animals.

"Something is afoot," Paul said, "when people are willing to pay more for a product when they perceive it's also an investment in something they care about."

What we are buying, if we buy one of Double Check's eight-dollar-a-pound steaks, is not only quality meat, but also a certain quality of land. We understand that, in raising steers to sell for meat, Paul and his family are also raising grass on ten thousand acres of Arizona rangeland. Contained in the price of his beef is the cost of what are known as "ecosystem services." Ecosystem services used to simply be called externalities, those unfortunate by-products of industrial production that fell by the wayside in the great rush to sell cheap goods—by-products like clean air, healthy wildlife, or uncontaminated water. Although it's been diluted, the word "organic" began as a way to ask consumers to pay for ecosystem services, to monetize the value of pesticide-free ground.

And it turns out that we consumers are quite willing to pay for landscapes that do not look like feedlots. While Cargill makes pennies on the carcass, said Paul, he and Sarah earn over a thousand dollars, net return, on every animal.

Part of the reason they are profitable—although they are not all *that* profitable, earning only about $24,000 a year between the two of them—is that Double Check is one of only a handful of ranches in southern Arizona with a USDA-certified slaughtering house and packing plant on its premises. The story of the decline of local slaughterhouses—1,211 in 1992 compared to 809 in 2008—parallels the story of the decline of local food, a problem that's plagued farmers and ranchers trying to get back into the game. (It was, Paul said, "pure misery" to get the state of Arizona to certify their slaughterhouse.)

At Double Check, I got it—how an animal becomes meat. Rather, I got how enough animals became enough meat at a quick enough pace to be scalable, to feed a reasonable amount of people and make a reasonable-size profit.

(Though what constitutes a scalable amount of meat for a reasonable amount of people, Paul would say, is exactly the difference between Cargill and Double Check—the difference between $1.29 or $10 for a pound of beef.)

The cows come into the slaughterhouse one at a time—a stun gun to the head outside, a horizontal roll through the door, and a quick hook to the hind feet. Bleed-out, hide-off, organs-out. A carcass, split then quartered and hung in a walk-in freezer. Eight cows every Tuesday, and it all takes place feet from where they graze for the last few weeks of their lives, where they sleep and sway their tails, so they are not stressed when they go to die.

In the weeks since I butchered a sheep, I've asked at every restaurant I've patronized—feeling, it must be said, like a total asshole—where the kitchen buys their meat. I've gotten an array of answers, from "I dunno" to "a distributor in town." ("But where do *they* get *their* meat," I pressed, to which the cashier had said, "Why, you lookin' to buy a buncha meat?")

In addition to his weekly stand at the St. Philip's Farmers' Market, Paul sells bulk cuts of beef to La Cocina, my favorite twinkle-light-adorned restaurant in Tucson, to the Canyon Café in the UA Student Unions, to the Blue Willow Café and Time Market; to a handful of other restaurants in Tucson and a dozen more in Phoenix.

As we walked back over to the cows after leaving the slaughterhouse, Paul had said, rather out of the blue, "I'm not saying I'm better than everyone else. Shoot, I eat Wendy's when I'm starving."

I couldn't help it; a quick "hmm" spilled out of my mouth. Paul looked at me, questioning. "That's interesting," I said, lamely. "Um. Has your relationship to meat changed since you started ranching?"

"Don't get me wrong. We did not evolve to eat eighty-six pounds of meat per person per year, which is what we eat in the United States," he said. But sometimes he is in town and he is hungry. "I'm not going to tell you what to buy," he continued. "Prices are a market mechanism for conversation between consumer and supplier"—and, he implied, our continued dollar-based discussion with retailers that sell corn-fed beef reveals that we're fine with what's being said.

I told him it sounded like he was arguing against his own system.

"I do believe that we're producing full-bodied animals with lots of complexity. I believe they're better for you and better for the land. But if you're at the farmers' market or the supermarket, and it's cheaper to buy meat that hasn't been humanely raised and you're not particularly worried about animal welfare, by all means, go for it. I believe my animals improve the land, but if you don't much care about land health, then sure. Shop by your value systems."

And so I was—so I was going to buy meat, believing that eating animals wasn't always incompatible with a healthy environment. That, taken seriously and consumed infrequently, eating animals might actually help *restore* landscapes. I had come to the St. Philip's Farmers' Market to buy myself meat to cook at home, only the second time I'd done so all year. There's a Crock-Pot full of slow-cooked pulled brisket on the table and Paul scoops me a pinch into a paper cup.

"Yup," I say. "That. I want that." Paul paid attention in Marketing 101—people who taste are people who buy.

As Paul ducks back into the Double Check trailer—the very same trailer I had peered into, feet from his slaughterhouse, the week before—and stoops over an open cooler, I consider his revelation at the ranch. Even this eco-rancher eats burgers from Wendy's. Although it had frustrated me at first—if even *Paul* was eating fast-food burgers, what hope was there for the rest of us?—I realize as he emerges stooped from the trailer, holding on to his cowboy hat with his right hand, that Paul's eating at Wendy's was precisely the point of my year unprocessed. I had set out at the beginning of the year searching for a way to live in the world, full of its messy temptations and perverse consumptions, in a way that was ethical and sustainable. Knowing what we know today, how can we do both—know *and* live? I'd found, of course, that the answer lives in the messy middle.

Paul hands me a brick-size bundle wrapped in clean white paper and says, "Ten." I pull a crumpled bill from my skinny wallet and hand it to him. Ten dollars seems like a lot of money for a pound of brisket, but as I walk away with the heavy meat cradled in my skinny arms, the weariness of clutching a knife in cold, tense fear returns to me—my bones remember it—and suddenly, ten dollars for this cut of meat seems like an amazing bargain.

Unprocess Yourself: Meat

The easiest and cheapest way to unprocess your consumption of meat is simply to eat less of it. Take a vegetarian cooking class—or, if you have a friend who's a vegetarian, ask them to teach you how to cook their three favorite meals. As a matter of habit, I forget about meat. I don't usually cook meat, which means I forget to buy it at the market, which means I don't eat it at home. On the rare occasion when I do eat meat, often when I'm out to dinner with friends or at Sunday brunch, if the server doesn't know where the meat comes from, I consider it processed.

When I am eating meat as an unprocessed food, I buy it directly from a farmer or rancher at the farmers' market; at the Tucson Co-op, where it's labeled with its source; or at a restaurant where the menu or server tells me exactly where it came from. Wherever I am, I ask questions. Yes, believe me, I know: This is an easy thing to say and a very awkward thing to actually do. But keep in mind—if you don't ask, and if restaurants and markets don't have to answer for where their meat comes from, they will continue business as usual.

Even for me—raised by vegetarians, nearly a vegetarian myself—meat marks occasion. For our Christmas dinner, Tyler, Katie, and I bought pork chops at the farmers' market. On Valentine's Day, Dave and I made grass-fed steak from the 47 Ranch, near Tucson. Meat has weight—physically, emotionally, and financially—and it pairs well with occasions, with celebrations and commemorations. The trade-off is that meat might simply be too weighty for the everyday, in a passing sandwich or hurried salad.

When cooking meat, the best way to honor an animal is to use all of it, not just the best bits. I'm no expert in nose-to-tail cooking—I can barely sear a fillet—but chefs across the country are embracing the art of cooking with "other" parts, offering dishes like pig ear tacos or potted chicken liver. Fergus Henderson's cookbook *The Whole Beast: Nose to Tail Eating* instructs home cooks how to use every part of a pig; Jennifer McLagan's *Odd Bits* focuses on how to cook with offal. You could also just go to a farmers' market and ask what's for sale; many ranchers will set aside bones and offal, especially if you ask. The marrow inside bones makes amazing meat broths; and organ meat offers an incredible—and often delicious—nutritional bang for your buck.

12

HUNGER

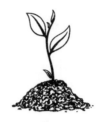

People unprocess.

At Food City, the produce is cheap. It seems too cheap, way cheaper than I remembered produce could be. Glossy yellow signs announce unfathomable prices—3AVOCADO/$1 and 2PINEAPPLE/$1 and 3LBSROMATOMATOES/$1. I know the reason for these prices is pesticides and semi trucks, but for my last official week of unprocessed eating, I am not trying to flee further from an anonymous food system; rather, I am jumping back in. This week will still be unprocessed—there will be no added sugars, no refined flours, no preservatives, food colors, or emulsifiers. I would eat fresh, whole, unprocessed foods, but I'd do it—I hoped—for twenty bucks.

Twenty dollars a week, $4 a day, $1.33 a meal—the amount that forty-six million people across the United States receive from SNAP, the federal government's Supplemental Nutrition Assistance Program (formerly known as the Federal Food Stamp Program).

It had first occurred to me to finish my year unprocessed with the SNAP Challenge—an official challenge sponsored by Community Food Banks across the country—sometime around the time my friend Cory had asked me to hold his half-eaten brownie. We had run into each other outside Bentley's Coffee & Tea; as Cory struggled to wrestle bike keys from bag and fasten helmet to head, he'd extended his brownie—folded in a loose pile of Saran Wrap, wafting sweet chocolate fumes through its seams—and said, "Hey, can you hold this?"

"Seriously?" I'd snapped back, before I could help it, before I'd realized how closely I teetered on the edge of intolerable. I was in the final stretch of my year unprocessed, but as my energy waned, the holidays brimmed, full of festive cookies and holiday-party pasta, end-of-the-year indulgences and cold-weather convenings. I watched my friends eat, hungry not simply to eat but to take part, to share in the sharing of food, and so I started focusing on all the things I couldn't have. I frowned when Dave ordered pizza, rolled my eyes when Sarah offered me a spoonful of ice cream. Christ—I was intolerable even to myself. I had *chosen* to do this, after all.

Before the brownie incident, it had crossed my mind to finish my year with one perfectly unprocessed week. A week in which I would take the knowledge I'd so painstakingly accumulated throughout my year and pull it together for one final heave-ho. Only eating bread I'd baked with White Sonora wheat, instead of the compromise sprouted whole-grain loaves I often bought at the co-op; drinking only home-fermented honey mead and homemade almond milk. I'd use only Malibu-sourced sea salt and chili powder ground from dried chilies. But as I thought about this week, I wondered: What would it prove? That with a great deal of time and energy, I could unprocess all my food all at once? If anything, my year had shown me that the opposite was true. I was still urban, broke, and busy; how I'd pulled off such a wide shift in my eating habits was by accumulating small movements, not jumping into grand gestures.

And after slaughtering a sheep—and in doing so, venturing as far out of my

Los Angeles–reared comfort zone as I'd ever been—I wanted to step back into the grocery store and contribute to a different conversation. This week, my quest was not to spend money better, to understand the reverberations of my food dollars, but to understand how I might live if I didn't have *enough* dollars to spend better.

IN FOOD CITY, my eyes skim across a profusion of colors: pyramids of red tomatoes, deep green avocados, and bright white onions; bins piled loosely with crisp green chilies and desiccated red ones. Oversize shopping carts pull along short families; women wearing heels, men in blue jeans. My ears pick up the cadences of family squabbles, rendered musical by Spanish, and then skip over to the actual music, a *bachata* beat that climbs up the white walls and slides across the linoleum floor, a song refusing to be consigned to the background. I linger in front of plastic-wrapped packages of *cacahuate dura* and *cocada horneada*—the treats I'd beg Juan to buy on his weekly grocery trips to Rivas—and walk past pyramids of dried hibiscus flowers, sticky cones of *piloncillo* sugar, and tan tamarind pods, the snacks I used to eat straight off the tree when I walked home from the beach. These reminders of my life in Nicaragua were the reason I sought out Food City when I first moved to Tucson, on a lonesome Sunday like this one, when I was missing Spanish and bursts of color. I drove south from my apartment, past peeling-paint corners and ladies sweeping their front stoops in house slippers, and I was reminded that I live only seventy miles north of the line where this particular America ends and the Latin one begins.

The Food City in South Tucson is a grocery store for this convergence. The fluorescent blue sign outside the store reads: FOOD CITY TORTILLERIA CHECK CASHING. Inside, the store is clean and bright, fresh and full. It's also disorganized and hodgepodge, Mexican Coke next to Rold Gold pretzels, colorful glass candles arranged above Pampers.

I force myself past a pile of mangoes—$0.79 a pop—and focus on another pile of color in this tropical display—bananas, nine of them for only $1.33. Three white onions for $0.72 and five pounds of potatoes for $1.69—too many potatoes for one week, but the price is too good to pass up. I plan to make soup with whatever vegetables I can find to accessorize the potatoes, and carrots are $0.49 a pound, so I grab two one-pound bags. Before I throw them in my cart, I hesitate, surveying the abundance of the produce section, suddenly stressed by the cheapness of it all. I remind myself that this week I am not asking where this food comes from; not requesting that it be locally grown or even be pesticide-free. I'd already done the math on organics—five pounds of locally sourced organic potatoes at the co-op would cost me twice as much as at Food City, and three times more on the carrots. This week, those seemingly small premiums would add up quickly.

I continue down the produce straightaway, stopping when I arrive at a green profusion of broccoli heads; they're on sale, a pound for $1.69. I pick up one head and then another, but before I place them in my cart, I wonder: How much broccoli is a pound of a broccoli? I've been duped by the heaviness of tomatoes before, and indeed, when I place my broccoli in the metal bowl of the produce scale, it sinks more exuberantly than I expected; the hand of the scale leaps and then jiggles between the two- and three-pound markers. I consider the math, and then the broccoli, carrots, onions, and potatoes—a week's worth of hearty, healthy soup for seven bucks.

Conventional wisdom claims that fresh foods are pricey, that fresh fruits and vegetables cost too much to be accessible to everyone, all the time. But if I learned anything wandering through a freezing warehouse full of a hundred thousand Mexican melons, it is that even though this far-flung network is built on hidden frailties and delayed costs, its benefits are undeniable. If you have four dollars a day to spend on food, this system brings you fresh produce in exchange for very little money.

In 2010, researchers at the USDA's Economic Research Service tallied the cost of fifty-nine fresh and processed fruits (frozen or canned) and ninety-four fresh and processed vegetables, and found that Americans could buy the variety and quantity of produce suggested for a two-thousand-calorie-a-day diet for between $2.00 and $2.50. Although the USDA certainly has some vested interest in finding that "A Wide Variety of Fruit and Vegetables Are Affordable for SNAP Recipients"—one study's title—the fact remains: Fresh produce is a bargain. And contrary to the dictum perpetuated by ninety-nine-cent menus, it is a bargain even when compared to its competitors. According to the USDA, on average, fruits and vegetables cost thirty-one cents per portion, while less healthy—more processed—snack foods cost thirty-three cents per portion.

This may be so, but as I wander up and down the aisles at Food City, I start to pay attention to the foods that had been invisible to me all year long, their cheapness too glaring to ignore. Eight Pop-Tarts for $2.39; a jumbo box of Fruit Loops, a full twelve cups, for $2.99. A box of mini pancakes, forty-eight of them, for only $3.19—how ridiculous, how amazing. My oatmeal-for-breakfast plan is soon derailed when I realize that although a pound of Food Club brand oatmeal costs $3.29, if I want it to be even slightly sweet, I will also have to buy a plastic bear full of maybe-honey for $3.99. A toast-and-peanut-butter plan B proves similarly untenable when I look at the ingredients on Bimbo Whole Wheat Bread—surely twenty-three ingredients is too many. Nature's Own 100% Whole Grain fares no better—what does that "100%" even *refer* to, since more than 2 percent of the loaf is made up of sugar.

I walk back to the oatmeal, muttering as I tally up the accumulation in my cart. I'm leaning over, reaching for the cheapest canister, when I hear a man's voice mutter behind me: *"Ay, qué guapa, la alta."* I turn around to find a man beaming at me. I don't think it through; I shoot back a quick, accented *"bueno, gracias,"* offering my smile as a challenge. Back off buddy, *te entiendo.*

The man nearly stumbles backward. *"Hablas español?"* he exclaims, clearly delighted.

"Sí."

He leans forward, beside himself. *"Qué bueno! Donde aprendiste?"*

"Yo vivía en Nicaragua hace uno año."

"Hablas bien," he says. I nod and turn down the aisle. I'm pleased to realize that he's right—I can still speak Spanish, at least at this basic level, and I haven't totally lost the Nicaraguan accent I worked so hard to acquire. But the wheels on my cart have barely budged when the man calls, *"Espera! Como te llamas?"* I turn around and hesitate. It would not be outrageously rude to smile and roll onward, but there is something about this man's demeanor, the enthusiasm of his stance—he reminds me of Juan a little bit, the way Juan leaned through life belly first—that yanks me back on the strings of nostalgia. "Megan," I say, and then *"Y tú?"*

José is an electrician from El Salvador who lives across the street from Santa Rita Park, where he sometimes plays baseball; José learns that I am a writer from Los Angeles who lives "nearby." When José asks what I write about and I tell him "food," he nods in a thoughtful way. He gestures at my cart. "So you're shopping for food, then," he says, deadpan. I cannot help but laugh. José's confidence is buoyed. "How about I cook you dinner?" he asks.

I smile and shake my head. "No thanks."

"Why not?"

I pause, fishing for an answer. *Porque no quiero*—I don't want to—seems a bit blunt, but really, what other reason is there? And then I remember. I *do* have a boyfriend, a real, live one, not one of the made-up, stop-hitting-on-me-variety. I tell José as much.

"I don't mind," he says. I'm trying to assemble a response to this when José turns to greet a teenage girl who approaches with a box of Frosted Cheerios. Her age and build suggest she's his daughter; their rapid-fire negotiation about the price of cereal offers a quick glimpse into another kind of life, one I am not privy to. I am at Food City attempting to understand this life's contours, but, of course, a week of SNAP simulation does not give me access to its nuances.

"Bueno, adios, José," I say. *"Mucho gusto."* I arrive at the end of the aisle, suddenly flooded with an unexpected burst of energy that has nothing to do with this odd offer of dinner. Rather, speaking Spanish reminds me of the vigor I had applied to my life in Nicaragua, the verve I'd found navigating that strange country on my own. Speaking Spanish reminds me of my last night in Nicaragua, when Juan, Isolina, and I had sat on the hotel's porch, drinking Toña cervezas, listening to *bachata,* and letting the Pacific's breeze lap our necks. When Juan and I had ventured into the kitchen for a snack, he asked me, "What are you going to do next?"

Juan was the big brother of my Nicaragua adventure, friend and protector against scary students and scorpions, and on that last night, when we stood in the kitchen and I folded the morning's leftover *gallo pinto* into a frying pan, I didn't have an answer for him. I stirred the *gallo pinto* around the pan, folding beans and rice together with Isolina's even pace.

"Isolina and I have this joke," I told him. "We never eat all the *gallo pinto* in the morning. There's always leftover after breakfast. So we put it in a Tupperware, store it in the fridge, and the next morning, when Isolina makes a new batch, she just dumps the old in with the new and stirs it all around. So we say that there's one bean that's been in there forever, going from Tupper to pan to Tupper. The leftover *gallo pinto* bean, always being stirred around."

Now, thinking of that moment, I am struck by the remembrance of how I had felt then, how full of energy, of possibility. I am also struck by the most obvious takeaway of this scene. *Gallo pinto!* The dish I ate every day in Nicaragua, the dish central to so many diets around the world: rice and beans. I loved *gallo pinto,* even more when Isolina would offer it up along with two oily scrambled eggs. I grab a one-pound bag of brown rice—$1.93—and a two-pound bag of black beans—$2.79. I return to the dairy and pluck a carton of *huevos grandes* for $2.49, and, while I'm there, a half gallon of whole milk for $2.07. Back in the produce section, I fill a bag with cheap tomatoes and grab a bunch of spinach, an easy $0.69.

I've got this. Twenty dollars, *sin problemas*. And then I remember—coffee. A yellow tin canister of Café Bustelo costs $4.99 for ten ounces; without knowing exactly how much my produce weighs, I estimate my cart has already hit $18. Maybe I've overestimated—maybe my little bits of rounding up will accumulate into the price of coffee. I head to the cash register, hopeful for the magic of math.

The woman in front of me holds her solitary purchase, a loaf of white Food City–brand bread. She's younger than me, wears tight jeans with bleach-whiskered pockets and a stretchy yellow T-shirt; she stares at her cell-phone screen as the customer before her completes his transaction. Finally, when it is her turn, she swipes a debit card through the small PIN-pad machine. When it replies with the cranky beep of rejection, she tries again. The cashier, a thick woman in a blue apron, looks at the young woman and then back at the screen. My eyes flicker toward it and I see the small, automated words: *SNAP purchase denied*.

After the woman asks, "Wait, how much is it?" and then runs out to the parking lot to grab more money, I start unloading my own cart, feeling humbled by this reminder that living on SNAP benefits is not a hypothetical proposition. As my tally grows, beep after beep, I begin to feel like an interloper in a land more foreign to me than Nicaragua had ever felt. Although I lived in a town where a family's monthly income might fluctuate between one and two hundred dollars, where houses were four walls of cinder block that flooded with mud every October, my students had never complained of hunger—or rather, I realize now with a start, they'd never complained to *me*.

My food trundles forward. The tally grows, beep after beep. Fourteen dollars by the time all the produce has passed, but then a quick leap with the milk and eggs, a slight rise with the rice and beans, and then an all-out lurch, straight from $20.37 to $25.36 with the pass of the coffee canister. I should tell the cashier that I'll skip the coffee. But I want coffee, I think stubbornly, and a line stretches behind me. Of course, I can go over the limit. I will not be denied; my debit card is tied to my bank account, not a government-issued SNAP account. With only seconds to make up my mind, I decide to just slide my debit card through the machine.

WHAT DOES IT MEAN TO BE HUNGRY? Rather, what is hunger? The difference between the adjective and the noun is the difference between a casual word for the day-to-day and the abstraction of a statistic. Hunger affects one out of five Arizonans. One in six American adults—four of every ten children—struggle with hunger. Hunger is, according to the 2010 Census, on the rise.

To distinguish between the two, we now speak of "food security"—or insecurity. To be food insecure is to be uncertain how you will next feed yourself. The "U.S. Household Food Security Survey Module" administered by government officials reads like the worst kind of choose-your-own-adventure novel. "Did you ever worry your food would run out before you got money to buy more?" Often, sometimes, never. If you answer "often" to enough questions, you may continue. "How often was this true: I couldn't afford to eat a balanced meal?" Often, sometimes, never. "In the last 12 months, did you ever not eat for a whole day because there wasn't enough money for food?" To this last question, 8 percent of adults in the United States will respond with "often." It is "often" that accumulates into hunger.

If you are often uncertain about how you will feed yourself or your family, the U.S. government tries to offer some certainty. You can walk in the door of a food bank and walk out with a box full of food through what's known as The Emergency Food Assistance Program, or TEFAP. In Arizona, for a single-person household, if you earn less than $1,265 a month, you can apply for continued relief through SNAP or WIC, the Special Supplemental Nutrition Program for Women, Infants and Children.

I earn $1,387 a month, so I don't qualify for SNAP benefits—I take the online screening questionnaire. I'm a slim—or large, depending on who's counting—$200 over the $1,211 threshold. But the margin by which I do *not* qualify for SNAP benefits is much larger than this $200 would reflect—the screening questionnaire rightly does not ask about upbringing or education.

"I don't think it matters as much if you're educated or not educated," says Bill Carnegie, the CEO of the Community Food Bank of Southern Arizona. "Maybe it is your social upbringing in relation to food." He's trying to answer my question about what it is that determines whether you rely on a dollar menu or a dollar bag of beans to get through a week on SNAP benefits. He's stumbling his way to an answer, just as I stumbled my way through the question. It's hard to know what's relevant, what bears on the parameters of our food choices.

Bill Carnegie is the CEO of one of the country's largest food banks—they distributed thirty million pounds of food last year alone—but he's happy to talk to me about the items in my small shopping cart. Bill tells me that when he took the challenge, he went $1.25 over budget, and still ran out of food. "It was eye-opening to realize how expensive food really is."

Eye-opening. The stated purpose of the SNAP Challenge is to raise awareness, not only of the relative power of a dollar, but also the power of nine billion—the amount the federal government will cut the SNAP program over the next decade, even as the number of people in need has more than doubled over the last ten years. Five years ago, the Community Food Bank of Southern Arizona was serving 98,000 people a month; today, that number is closer to 225,000.

Cans of creamed corn and Chef Boyardee Ravioli, plastic jars of peanut butter, squashed bags of Sunbeam Bread, blocks of bright orange "government cheese." Thousands of pounds of food arrives and departs the Food Bank's fourteen-thousand-square-foot warehouse every day.

"But for us," says Bill, "it is not just about providing food for people *today*. We know that we cannot solve hunger just by giving away boxes. I tend to focus more on poverty these days than hunger. Hunger is just a symptom of poverty."

Although I do not qualify for SNAP benefits, my annual income places me well below the federal poverty line. I earn $16,780 annually, well short of the $20,665 yearly income that defines a single-person household as "poor." But I am not poor. I earn $16,000 a year *by choice*. Because I am a graduate student, working for my education, working for some next step, a step unknown but assumed to be up. I have a savings account and an education, but there is something else, too, something that cannot be quantified. My mom asks me every so often, every other month, if I have enough money, and although I always say yes, the support is assumed. My safety net stretches, strong and invisible.

I am not poor. I am broke. The difference between poor and broke is a difference contained within all the other challenges that come along with a life that requires government-supported benefits just to make ends meet—hunger, as Bill Carnegie said, is a symptom of poverty. The difference between poor and broke is the difference between every week and this week. It might be a challenge, but it will only be a week that I will have to depend on twenty dollars.

OF COURSE, I have just spent twenty-*five* dollars. I have not even started and already I have failed. But as I am unloading groceries into my casita's kitchen, it occurs to me: If this is a challenge to raise awareness, the only way to fail is to fail to learn. I went over the limit, so I will just start sooner—I will eat this food for six days rather than five. I scramble two eggs, shred a potato, and fry up some hash browns in olive oil. (Technically, we are allowed to cook with preexisting condiments. "Is a tablespoon of olive oil a condiment?" is not a question answered in the SNAP Challenge FAQs.)

On Sunday evening, I load my Crock-Pot—a Christmas present from my mother, further evidence of that invisible support—with the bag of rice and dump my two-pound bag of dried black beans into a glass bowl to sort. I'm annoyed that I have to sort the beans, that there is no shortcut to removing shattered slivers and occasional bits of nonbean matter, that this has not been done *for* me. But sort I shall, and soon enough I relax into the methodic quiet of the task, of fingers caressing and plucking flecks of white from a sea of black, so different from the metallic crank of splitting open a can of precooked beans and sliding them, slimy, into a bowl.

On Monday morning, when I lift the lid of my Crock-Pot, I find a bundle of sticky brown starch. When I try to fluff some life into the rice with my fork, the kernels do not separate in discrete granules, but instead stick to the fork, more clay than sand. Did I add too much water? Turn the heat on too high? Any other week, I'd fume over this phenomenal loss of food and my $1.93 and then throw the whole mess into the compost bin. But today, it is this rice or no rice, so I scoop out the mostly mushy middle section, give the rest a vigorous tear-through with my fork, and adjust my breakfast strategy to accommodate the rice's insolence. More hash browns, this time with spinach and eggs. It is a good strategy, one that keeps me full until well past 2 P.M., when I finally get up from my desk and use our office microwave to heat up a glass Tupperware full of rice and beans and two bright diced tomatoes. I arrive home on Monday evening, frigid from a dark bike ride and tired from my night class, to the wafting smell of simmering salt. Two diced potatoes, a head of broccoli, four carrots, and half of a diced onion spent the day in the Crock-Pot; when I lift the lid, an exhale of sweet steam bathes my face. I add a dash of garlic powder—the week is also open-spice—and a bit more salt, and then puree the whole thing into a creamy, delicious green.

Spinach-scrambled eggs and potatoes, *gallo pinto* and tomatoes, broccoli-potato-carrot soup. Monday slides into Tuesday into Wednesday, and my belly is warm and full.

But when I arrive home on Wednesday night, well after dark on a day that started at eight, I'm cold, tired, and cranky. All I want to do is futz around in my kitchen, to unwind some of the stress of my day into stirring or sautéing. But there is nothing to futz *with*. My broccoli-potato-carrot soup is made and awaiting new heat from the stovetop. Though a microwave-free home makes leftovers less alluring, the real reason I cook anew every night is that I like my nightly fifteen minutes in the kitchen, a time that transitions me from day to night. Just as my fifteen-minute bike ride from home to work offers me a much-needed transition from here to there, standing in my kitchen when it is dark outside, chopping carrots or sautéing greens, suggests a slip and shift from there to here. While I occasionally love burrowing into the kitchen without regard for time—kneading dough, tempering chocolate, canning tomatoes—fifteen minutes is my weeknight sweet spot. Enough time to maneuver a hand-ful of whole veggies into something edible by way of dice, puree, or sauté, but not so much that I fatigue or fret over the looming to-dos. My Wednesday-night dinners are not masterpieces—they often employ precooked grains or beans, store-bought corn tortillas or whole-grain pasta—but they are quick and cheap, whole and fresh.

As the pureed soup reheats in a saucepan on the stovetop, I mope around my little house. I am moping not only because I had a long day and there is nothing to do tonight except reheat my soup and watch *The Daily Show*, but also because all of my friends are at this moment sitting together around a table, eating cheap tacos and drinking cheap beer, as we do every Wednesday night. "Just 'cause she's on food stamps doesn't mean a gentleman can't buy a pretty lady a drink," Dave had offered, and I was tempted, but it was, after all, a slippery slope. Not only can't SNAP dollars be used to buy alcohol, but

SNAP Challenge rules also explicitly request that we challengers "avoid accepting free food from friends, family or work." Once I had a beer in front of me, why not let this generous gentleman buy his pretty lady two veggie tacos and a side of properly prepared rice?

JUST SOUTH OF SILVERLAKE ROAD, down the straight and gray Cottonwood Lane, past small, boxlike houses, quiet cars, and knobby speed bumps, beyond a gate adorned with a block-letter sign, I catch a glimpse of green.

Three years ago, Las Milpitas—which means "little fields" in Spanish—was an abandoned plot of land—long, dusty, shadeless. Today, ninety-four garden plots brim with vegetation. Broad mesquite trees spread shade. Thick foliage emerges out from dark soil, wide leaves that hide heads of cauliflower or bunches of broccoli. There is kale: curly, lacinato, purple. Spicy arugula and perky heads of lettuce. The beginnings of basil; the promise of sweet summer corn. Some plots are adorned with yellow sticks, a signal to other gardeners that the produce in this plot is for the picking—for the sharing.

The sum of these small impressions is striking: This is a *lot* of food.

"Las Milpitas is an example of a process that really captures the essence of what we want to do," says Robert Ojeda, the director of the Community Food Resource Center, or CFRC, a branch of the Community Food Bank that focuses on long-term food security and sustainability. The CFRC began thirteen years ago when a few food-bank employees, focused on access to healthy food and nutrition, built a small demonstration garden next to the food bank. Since then, they've offered free, bilingual training on home food production, youth farm training apprenticeships, and support of fifty school gardens and four farmers' markets that accept SNAP and WIC vouchers.

And then they built a farm. When City High School approached the Community Food Bank and asked to partner in developing the space that would become Las Milpitas, "We first went out to the neighborhood, before we did anything," Robert says. "We said, 'There's this space next door. What would you like to see happen in that space?'"

The community consensus was clear: They wanted the capacity to grow their own food.

Anna Pain was one community member who dug in right away. "My neighbor saw me trying to fill some pots in my backyard and she said, 'You know, they're giving away plots of land next door for free,'" she says. "I didn't have a green thumb in my body. I really didn't think I could do this, but here I am!"

It's a sunny winter's day at Las Milpitas and Anna has work to do. Aphids have been munching on her broccoli. She pulls out a spray bottle filled with soapy water and starts her assault. When she pulls back a beefy leaf on the edge of the plot, she comes face-to-face with a bright white sphere of cauliflower and exclaims an ecstatic "Oh!"

I've been wandering around the garden for twenty minutes, watching bees bump into sunflowers and chickens cluck around their coop. I'm here at Robert's suggestion; it is refreshing—it is hopeful—to see all this potential energy sprouting from the ground instead of piled on crates and stamped with price tags at Food City. After sitting on my couch, slurping up the same soup night after night, the bright, cold wind of a winter's garden is needed—it is perspective.

Anna spent nearly a decade working as a cashier at Safeway until 2011, when she was diagnosed with fibromyalgia, a condition characterized by chronic fatigue and pain. She believes it was a series of unlucky car accidents that damaged her nerves and catalyzed the fibromyalgia; in any case, she could no longer bear the physical strain of cashier work—standing on her feet for eight-hour shifts, lifting fifty-pound bags of cat food or twenty packs of water bottles. "My thumbs were giving out on me. I'd get home and I wouldn't be able to move them," she says. "But working in the garden helps me. It keeps my joints limber. It's grounding. Especially in the summer, when the ground is hot—it's healing for my hands."

She's been receiving SNAP benefits for the past year and a half. Before she started gardening, she says that she and her daughter didn't eat nearly as many fresh vegetables as they do now. "We're eating much healthier," Anna says—and they're spending less money. "I used to spend maybe fifty dollars a week at the store. Now I go maybe every two to three weeks and just buy canned foods and herbs. I'll get a few pieces of meat and stick them in the freezer—and they sometimes stay there a long time," she says.

"I don't know how long food stamps will be around. I hope I can grow enough stuff so that I don't have to worry about going to the grocery and so I don't have to rely on food stamps."

Later, Robert tells me that the Food Bank is trying to quantify the value of a place like Las Milpitas. "Traditional food banks tend to look at pounds that are brought in and the pounds that are distributed to what number of people. We're a food bank that distributes millions of pounds of food. But what is the true value of a home garden? If you had to buy the thirty to forty monthly pounds of organic produce that a home garden yields, how much would it cost? What is its nutritional value?"

ON SATURDAY, my kitchen contains a surplus: two extra bananas, eight potatoes, half a can of coffee, some increasingly goopy rice, and enough black beans to make another month's worth of *gallo pinto*. I'd eaten unprocessed for six days (fine, five and two-thirds) and spent $25.69. But I wasn't sure what, exactly, I had proved. That eating unprocessed on roughly $4 a day could be done? Sure, I'd done that. My week had been frustrating and solitary, but I'd had plenty of fresh, whole foods at my disposal. I had, after all, been practicing, by necessity, the art of eating unprocessed on a budget for a full year.

It's true that I had eaten no processed food, but I'd eaten no local or organic food either. I certainly could have split my CSA share in half for the week and used the other ten dollars to buy rice, beans, and potatoes, but that had felt like cheating somehow. My CSA is a spectacular bargain—twenty dollars for an excess of locally grown, organic produce—and although I think this proves that organic and local are not synonymous with expensive and elite, the problem is again one of awareness. More often than not, those who take the SNAP Challenge have access to CSA programs, farmers' markets, and gardens, while most of those who eat on SNAP benefits do not.

Although the USDA has shown otherwise, the fact of the matter remains that, per calorie, subsidized foods are cheaper for the consumer than those that are not, and the United States does not subsidize farmers who grow organic broccoli. (Or grass-fed beef. A ten-dollar brisket, a mere two meals' worth of meat? Not this week.) According to a study published in the *American Journal of Clinical Nutrition,* at an average American supermarket, one dollar buys either 1,200 calories' worth of potato chips or 250 calories' worth of carrots; 875 calories of soda or 170 calories' worth of fruit juice. Studies like this are thrown around a lot, and the way they are often summarized is: If you had only four dollars to feed yourself for a day, what would *you* buy?

But the idea of a food calorie—which is the energy needed to raise the temperature of one kilogram of water by one degree Celsius—is as abstract to the sensory experience of eating warm soup as studying internal combustion is to the experience of driving a car. Calories are discrete units that power our bodies to go out and interact with the world. But we do not go to supermarkets explicitly seeking calories. All of us, rich or poor, under or overweight, want to buy and eat—or grow and eat—*food,* and the food we buy is determined by much more complex considerations than calorie per dollar.

"Until we change people's perspective on what they are eating and how self-sufficient they're being about what they're putting in their bodies, things aren't really going to change," Bill Carnegie said, and indeed, the great irony of hunger today is that it now most often appears alongside obesity. If nearly 20 percent of Arizonans struggle with hunger, and 63 percent of the state is either obese or overweight, logic dictates that these statistics might even refer to the same people. (In 2009, a study at Ohio State University found that the longer a person relied on SNAP benefits, the higher the likelihood that they would become overweight or obese.)

What is at stake here is not just hunger, but health. Nine percent of Arizonans have diabetes, costing the state $3.3 billion a year in medical costs. Four dollars a day does not cause diabetes, but when you consider this $3.3 billion against the $9 billion of proposed cuts to the SNAP program—cuts that will make it harder for low-income families to afford healthy, whole foods—some measure of cause and effect seems overlooked.

Just as we travel on shared roads, send our kids to learn at public schools, and pay taxes to build dams and bridges, we eat through our food system, and this is an infrastructure that has been outsourced to the highest bidder. Although we now have a national mandate for public health coverage, we still assume: For better care, go private. The same is now happening to our food system—if you want good food for your body and the environment, it is assumed: Don't go to the supermarket. After a year of traveling on privately built back roads—roads built by enterprising and hardworking individuals and communities—I'd taken the SNAP Challenge to better understand this public food system, to inhabit the food superhighways of our national infrastructure.

I wanted to prove that eating fresh, whole foods—unprocessed and unpackaged—could be done on a budget. But the economics of food and the politics of hunger are two very different challenges, and while they are intertwined, the issue of hunger in our society has as much to do with how much aid we give to hungry people as how much food costs for everyone.

And how much food costs is determined almost entirely by an omnibus piece of legislation known as the Farm Bill. The Farm Bill has inertia—seven hundred pages of it—and a legacy that supports commodity growers and large agribusinesses. Renewed every five years, the Farm Bill provides income and price supports for commodity crops; funds food stamp and nutrition programs; supports trade and foreign food aid; and provides funding for research in forestry, food safety, energy, and very recently, organic agriculture. In other words, there is little the Farm Bill does not touch; it's very size and scope help perpetuate the idea that it is impenetrable, accessible only by those interests whose scale matches its own.

When the first Farm Bill was passed in 1933, as a cornerstone of Franklin Delano Roosevelt's New Deal agenda, it was sorely needed. Farm profits had plummeted, partly because, after years of overplanting and poor land management by desperate farmers, a million tons of topsoil had vacated the Great Plains. With the first Farm Bill, the government promised to buy up grain surpluses to prevent the market from being flooded, offer crop insurance for farmers to safeguard against risk, and subsidize conservation practices like leaving land fallow. And so it did, with reasonable success, for two decades.

But in the era after World War II, as farming became mechanized, soils fertilized, and plants hybridized, the Farm Bill facilitated our transformation from a nation that depended on small, diversified farms to one beholden to consolidated "megafarms" and agribusinesses. By the 1970s, under the leadership of Secretary of Agriculture Earl Butz, "American farmers assumed a manufacturing mentality," writes Daniel Imhoff in *Food Fight: The Citizen's Guide to the Next Farm Bill*. "They become low-cost producers of the industrial ingredients of modern food."

Indeed, the Farm Bill is *the* reason we have so many cheap, processed foods made from corn and soybeans. "If the government removes all financial risk from growing corn, offers generous tax breaks to ethanol producers and writes six-figure checks to feedlot operators . . . then farmers will plant corn and lots of it," writes Imhoff. "Even when the real winners are the agribusinesses and food manufacturers that buy it."

Ironically, fresh fruits and vegetables, so heartily recommended by the nutrition programs of the USDA, are largely ignored by its agricultural objective. Corn, cotton, wheat, rice, and soybeans—these are the foods we support, to the tune of 70 percent of total commodity subsidies. Of California's eighty thousand farms—which produce nearly half of our fruits, vegetables, and nuts—only 10 percent receive some form of governmental support. In 2002, research in organic agriculture received $78 million in funding, less than 1 percent of the USDA's annual research budget. (Investment in local and organic agriculture *is* growing, albeit slowly, with programs like the Farmers Market Promotion Program and the Beginning Farmer and Rancher Development Program.)

Today, more than 70 percent of the bill's funding goes to supplemental nutrition programs like SNAP. That this number has more than tripled in the past decade reveals the spectacular failure of decades of food policy designed to produce a lot of cheap food. Our food may be cheap, but we're still hungry.

But, of course, no one eats in a vacuum, just as no one spends money strictly by the budget. Life swirls in and things come up. Cars break down, employers cut hours, rent goes up. But life also swirls in with unexpected dignity. If hunger is a symptom of poverty, just because you are poor doesn't mean you are hungry. No one makes two pounds of beans just for themselves; the point of making a big batch of food is not to hoard it for a week's rations but to share it among a community's members. This is where my week failed—I'd attempted to do it alone. Hadn't I learned this by now? Single-serving packaging and seaside salt making; goat's milk and butchered sheep. Again and again, the lesson was: There is a reason humans clustered into communities. Social endeavors turn out better than solo ones.

The dysfunction of our food system is not simply that it has removed us from our food; it is has removed us from each other.

Unprocess Yourself: Hunger

The easiest way to save money on food is to buy in bulk and cook at home. Make beans—they are cheap, full of nutrients, and taste *so much better* home-cooked than out of a can. (And they're *so much cheaper*—a pound of dried beans makes about the equivalent of three cans of beans, and it usually costs half as much. Too many beans for you? They freeze well.) I'm terribly imprecise about beans—I tend to forget to pre-soak them, although they cook quicker if you do. In a large saucepot or Crock-Pot, submerge beans in water, plus about an inch; add salt now, or later. On the stove, bring the beans to a boil and then reduce heat to a simmer; cook from three to eight hours, sampling every hour or so— beans should be tender, but not mushy. I often put a pound of beans in my Crock-Pot on low heat just before I go to bed; when I wake up, eight hours later, I've made enough for a week's worth of lunches.

Donate healthy foods to food drives—canned tomatoes instead of canned ravioli; whole-grain bread instead of squishy white Wonder Bread—or volunteer to help fill and distribute emergency food boxes at your local food bank, especially around the holiday season. If you're a gardener, ask if your food bank has a program in which you can help people in low-income neighborhoods install or maintain gardens.

Consider donating to or volunteering with Wholesome Wave, a nonprofit organization working to improve the accessibility and affordability of locally grown fresh fruits and vegetables. In some cities, Wholesome Wave's Double Value Coupon Program doubles the amount of money SNAP recipients receive if they buy fresh fruits and vegetables at farmers' markets. They're also launching a fruit and vegetable prescription program, where doctors can write "prescriptions" for qualifying patients, which can then be exchanged for fresh produce at farmers' markets.

That said, we're not going to be able to address hunger and the cost of fresh, healthy foods unless we get political. In 2010, agribusiness spent $140 million lobbying members of Congress; the only way to combat this influence is by exerting our power as voters. Visit Food Fight2012.org for ideas on how to get involved. Check to see if your senator or representative sits on any of the important food or agricultural committees that influence the Farm Bill; if they do, tell them how you think our agricultural policy should change. Tell your city council that investing in local food will help stimulate your city's economy. Ask them to adopt a local food charter or a list of Farm Bill principles, as Seattle did in 2010. As cities and counties take on the Farm Bill at a local level, we can diminish some of its impenetrable power and communicate a new set of priorities to the USDA.

We need big change in our food system—but while that's happening, we can still do little things. We can eat together—as families, friends, and communities—share our foods, and spread whatever small resources we have as wide as we possibly can.

Receipts accumulate.

If Tex-Mex is what happened when Texas took over the tortilla, then the Sonoran hot dog is what happened when Arizona conquered the frank. A hot dog becomes Sonoran after it is bacon-wrapped, smothered in pinto beans, and stuffed into a Mexican *bolillo* roll, and although it is incredibly messy, doused with tomatoes, onions, jalapeño sauce, mustard, and mayo, the Sonoran dog is the grab-and-go food of Tucson. Among all the possibilities—and I'd considered *all* of them in these past few months—I chose a Sonoran dog for my first processed meal not because of the dog but because of its spontaneity. No one gets up on a Saturday and says, "I think I'll have a Sonoran dog for dinner tonight"; it is, sometimes, just what happens. I missed being able to be an unplanned eater out in the world, a world that was, like it or not, full of processed foods. What I hunger after the most—what had been making me so cranky in these final months—is the ability to eat a food not because it is healthy, whole, or ethical. I missed the satisfaction of eating something simply because it is there and so are you.

So, finally, $4.39 buys me my first processed meal—a fizzy can of Diet Coke and a Sonoran hot dog from RobDogs, a sort-of stationary food truck parked just off Fourth Avenue. I'd never eaten the food before, but I'd stood in front of the truck countless times, waiting as one friend or another completed their purchase and we continued our mosey along the bar-filled avenue.

Of course, tonight, this is not a spontaneous purchase. I have asked the friends who supported and humored me through my long year to celebrate its closure with a hot dog and ice cream, and they have come out in force. Sarah and Hilary, of course, and new additions, Kati and Brenna, Mike, Tommy, and Chris. They're there, waiting for me when Dave and I walk up, three minutes after seven.

"Thanks for coming!" I say. "Hurray!" Everyone smiles and there is no line in front of the small window, but surely we should talk this over some more— surely it is not already time to finish unprocessed, not yet? But a group of college students turns the corner into the corral and so quickly we line up and I, the unprocessed eater, am rushed to the front. "One Sonoran dog, all the toppings, please!" I chirp, feeling like an eighteen-year-old ordering a drink on the authority of a fake ID. I pay for the dog and grab a Diet Coke from a white Styrofoam cooler. I'm nervous, so I don't open the cold can right away. I am not nervous for my stomach, although this seems to be the question on everyone's mind—will process cause Megan to explode? Rather, my nerves contain the ambivalence I feel about this year's end. I am excited, of course, for hot dogs and ice cream, but I'm anxious about the unwinding of all my parameters—the uncertain answer to the question I keep getting asked: "What next?"

I feel both like I put myself through so much—enough, already—and also like I've barely begun. I learned the processes that brought food to me, but more than that, I'd found their places and connected with their people. And so much had changed since I began my year. New wineries were popping up like weeds across Sonoita—and so were locally sourced restaurants in Tucson. The Tucson Co-op had completed its expansion and planted an urban farm in an adjacent parking lot. A CSA program in Denver, where Kara still lived, started selling canned-produce shares as winter rations for home-canning-averse. Jeff and Ana were coming back to Tucson to teach another animal processing workshop, and Dave—wonderful, absentminded Dave—tried a week of unprocessed eating with me *and* bought a home soda maker (no more tiny plastic water bottles!). My sister and her husband were getting ready to move back to Texas, where we both began—Katie had been offered a job teaching environmental economics at Southwestern University. Closer to Tucson, but still, we were so apart. And still there were so many more processes to unravel, networks to track, things I'd missed.

Maybe the goal of my year unprocessed was not only understanding the process of food, but also cultivating a different way to see the world. The curtain had been cast back on so many things, food and object alike, and I wanted to continue this process of peeling back layers, burrowing into unruly problems.

After a year of fighting to make my unprocessed choices my routine, I wasn't about to jump feetfirst back into the supermarket. It was a lot of work to get here, for one, and this work wasn't about this year in particular—the year had only been a frame in which to catalyze change, to test its tenability. And for the most part, eating unprocessed was tenable. It was doable and, in many regards, better—not only because of the food eaten, but also because of how it had felt to eat in accordance with what I believed.

Even if I missed chocolate chips and pizza, even if I now relaxed my grip on wheat and refined sugar, my attempt to unprocess my way of life and way of spending dollars would continue to build and exert its influence on my choices. I didn't know what was next, but I knew it wasn't going to stop here.

Finally, I crack open the can of Diet Coke and take a sip. The liquid bubbles into my mouth, cold and fizzy. It tastes sweeter than I remember it. A lot sweeter, but the sweetness doesn't linger. It sort of slides in with a fake hello, the kind you offer an aunt at Christmas; it waves hello and then saunters its way on through. It is a shrug at sweetness, an attempt at bubbles, but mostly, it tastes like an aluminum can. This . . . *this* was what I had been missing all these months?

But when a hot dog slides through a small window with a call of "Megan!"—when I grab the narrow cardboard boat holding the piled-high hot dog—when my friends pivot toward me, cameras at the ready, and when I finally, intentionally, take a bite, I am not disappointed. The bun of the Sonoran dog is fluffy sweet, the condiments are cloying and complementary, and the hot-dog meat crunches with the salty juiciness of bacon. Even after I finish the whole sticky dog, finish the rest of the tinny-tasting Diet Coke, and we all walk to the Hub and spoonful after spoonful of red velvet ice cream, flecked with thick chocolate cake, melts in my mouth—it all tastes *so good*—still, I know that my year unprocessed isn't over. It is simply reprieved. Although I still believe more than ever before that our choices have consequences, I've also learned that sometimes, the experience of eating is less about the eating than about the experience.

IF AT THE BEGINNING OF MY YEAR, everyone asked, "What's processed?" then at the end, they asked, "How do you feel?" Did I feel different after a year unprocessed? I felt in control, focused, and aware. I felt stronger in mind and body, but mostly how I felt after eating unprocessed foods for a year was *full*. While this may seem trivial, before my year began, I'd been, in one form or another, dieting for over a decade. During my year unprocessed, I was rarely hungry—or if I was, it was because it was simply time to eat. The satiety of this year surprised me. After I'd restricted myself to unprocessed, I could eat whatever I wanted, and as much as filled me up. By allowing myself this freedom within restrictions, I learned how to listen to my stomach, to a body's cravings—and to discern their difference from a mind's.

As the end of my year had approached, I'd wondered: Should I step back on the scale? I was nervous and I was curious. Although I'd had many friends who started eating unprocessed to lose weight, that had never been my goal. But still, I wondered about weight. And wondered: Did it matter, if I didn't already feel it?

An unintended lesson I'd learned this year is that a number does not reveal a body or inform its shape. My body still fit into all its clothes—although, upon reflection, perhaps it did exercise with more vigor, stood with more strength. On the morning of January 15, when the number on the scale is the same, I wonder if the answer to the question "how do you feel?" is one of arrangement rather than quality. I feel mostly the same—I feel fuller, stronger, healthier, but mostly I feel like my body fits together more seamlessly and coherently than it ever has before.

My body is not just mine to mess with, to add and subtract from like debits and credits in a checking account. My body connects me to my family, to my sister, mother-father, grandmother-grandfather; to my friends, tight hugs, and flailed dancing; to that one person I'd chosen to love, kisses and caresses. Food had connected me to my body, and how did I feel? I felt unwound, unbound— and tethered. Solidly, to people and place, to food and friends. Megan to her body.

ON SUNDAY MORNING, after the Sonoran dog settles in my stomach with unexpected ease, when I have bought all the food I will buy for my year unpro- cessed, I confront the growing pile of grocery receipts that I'd been collecting all year. There must be two hundred of them, evidence of the kind of run-in, run-out trips that had become my norm. Once contained in a cup on the top of my spice cabinet, the receipts had expanded outward like unruly vines, covering the top surface of the cabinet and crawling up the back wall in curls of white paper.

Slowly, the jumble becomes a flat stack as I enter total after total into an Excel spreadsheet, the marks of my purchases becoming strange portals into the past year.

There is a receipt for cacao powder and honey from when Katie had visited and we'd accidentally made chocolate butter; cheese and apples from Kara's midsummer visit to go with all the white wine we drank on my hot porch in hot June. Buried in a long list of Trader Joe's items, the first sack of Humpty-Dumpty whole-wheat flour that had started my year. One receipt with one item: $180 for a co-op membership. A receipt for nothing but vegetable broth and onions, presumably from one of the Friday nights I'd made soup for Sarah and Hilary and forgotten two critical ingredients; there's another solitary purchase, a receipt for organic cherries, the bag I'd bought on my way to Dave's for the first nondate-that-became-a-date. The receipts are crumpled and crinkled, printed on thin paper with smudged ink, and mostly they document mundane items that blur together into a year's food habits—onions and bananas, yogurt and milk, coffee and baking cacao. I exclude extras like dish soap and wine, the former because I didn't eat it, the later because the relative sobriety of my year didn't seem particularly pertinent.

During this year, I'd earned just over $18,000; in addition to my graduate assistant salary, I'd sold several freelance articles and essays. Although I enjoyed the freedom to allocate more of these earnings to groceries, to hand-crank wheat grinders, mini food processors, and mead-brewing buckets, this allocation also revealed my priorities—groceries before shoes.

Eaters in the United States spend a smaller fraction of their disposable income on food than eaters in any other country in the world. In 2013, just 6.1 percent of our disposable personal income went toward buying food for consumption at home. Compare this to the 19.3 percent of our income we spent to feed ourselves at home in 1929, the year the USDA's Economic Research Service first began keeping track—compare it to *any* year before, and you'll see that in spite of inflation and rising fuel and feed costs, year after year, we are spending a smaller fraction of our income on food. It is true that Americans have more disposable income than many other people in the world, but to make this point is simply to argue that we *could* spend more money on food. That we could, down the line, spend less on health care or treatments for diet-related diseases like obesity, diabetes, and hypertension. My pile of receipts was an investment in health that I hoped would pay me back in years to come. Compare the United States' 6.7 percent of consumer expenditures on food with the United Kingdom's 9.3 percent, with China's 26.1 or Russia's 30.5, and then compare those nation's health-care costs with ours. Proudly we soar above the rest.

Why have we as a society decided that food must first be cheap, and *then* be healthy?

At its core, the purpose of my year unprocessed was about a pile of receipts that represented a different way to live an urban life. Through January, February, and March, the slippery pieces of paper were stamped by Trader Joe's. Gradually, though, they shifted. There was payment after payment to the Tucson CSA, a smattering of Whole Foods purchases that document a year's worth of cacao butter, and a great pile of accounts owed to the Food Conspiracy Co-op. It is nearly a cliché to advocate shopping at a co-op, but how could I not when $100 spent in a national chain store sends $43 back into your community, compared to the $73 that sticks around when that $100 is spent at a locally owned business.

But of course, the $73 of my $100 doesn't cycle very far. It's only when $100 is spent again and again by person after person that our communities begin to fill out their emaciated figures. The figure I heard in June that struck me dumb is worth repeating: If a community the size of Tucson shifted 10 percent of its spending to local businesses, in one year, we would create $140 million in new revenue for the city and 1,600 new jobs.

"We are eliminating our own jobs and creating poorer jobs through the money we're spending," says Kimber Lanning, the founder of Local First Arizona. I finally get the nerve to call her only after the official end of my year unprocessed, after I have filled myself with Safeway chocolate chip cookies and cheddar Chex Mix and marveled, in a marvelously disembodied way, at the fact that I had ever savored them as treats. I am nervous when I call Kimber because she was the first person I'd heard say: Spend Money Better. What if I'd heard her wrong? What if the frame for my year came unglued?

"If I had to choose one word for what Local First Arizona is about, it would be empowerment," she says. "Empowering the American public so that they can see that *we* are the economy." Six months later, after meat and sheep, hunger and cows, it is uncanny to hear the same voice advocating the same message. Kimber reminds me of a story I'd heard before—one I'd participated in. In September of 2011, Bank of America announced it would charge debit-card customers with less than $20,000 in total holdings a $5 monthly ATM fee. Five dollars for the delight of withdrawing cash. We cried back, we of the lower $20,000—nope. When I got an e-mail from Bank of America informing me of this change—a quiet e-mail that arrived almost unseen—I had $44.76 in my account. Nope, not for me. We called, e-mailed, posted on Facebook, and hash-tagged on Twitter. Within twenty-four hours, Bank of America quietly rescinded the announcement with a sheepish "oh, you noticed that?" "The American public claimed its power for about twenty-four hours, and so one of the biggest corporations in the world changed direction," says Kimber. "We act like we are a nation of victims when in fact we are the ones pulling the strings. We just haven't claimed that power."

Of course, the problem with this reasoning is the oh-so-slippery "we." *We* don't do anything—you do things and I do things. If the things I do and the things you do are the same, *you* and *I* become *we*. I had just spent a year trying to spend money better, but as it drew to its close, I wondered: Did it matter? My dollars do not reverberate—*ours* do. But the collective cannot exist without the individual—maybe it is why "we" is always conjugated after "I" in the litany of learning a foreign language, and maybe the same order of operations holds for another kind of habit forming. *Yo compro, tu compras, él compra, nosotros compramos*—I buy, you buy, he buys, we buy. It's only when you and I decide to make small changes in our own lives that big "we" changes begin to happen.

I stumble my way through Excel's sum function and then finally, so quickly, there it is. Stuck in a little box, the total of my year unprocessed: $4,981.13. It seems like a large sum, larger than I was prepared for—27 percent of my income. I'm not sure how to contextualize it, so I divide my annual grocery bill by fifty-two weeks to arrive at $95.79 a week. It's only when I divide by seven that I realize what I've accomplished. I fed myself three mostly organic, largely local, totally unprocessed meals every day for a year and spent, on average, $13.60 a day—$4.50 a meal.

This total contains the various hobbies I'd explored throughout the year— home chocolate making, an endeavor more entertaining than economical; my adventures in canning and pickling; all my bread baking, all flat and lifted loaves. It includes all of the jars of honey I purchased, raw, rich honey that I ate by the spoonful; it includes all the lunches I'd packed in the morning, all the almonds I'd munched through the day, and the fifteen-minute meals I'd pre-pared in the evening. I'd wanted to spend money better when it was *my* choice, when it came down to just me and my dollars, and so there it is—$4.50 a meal.

In January, I hadn't thought to keep track of the dollars I spent in restau-rants. I didn't figure my unprocessed parameters would allow me to eat out much—my salary certainly hadn't before I started my year, when the mainstay of my social life had been dinners cooked at home with Sarah and Hilary. We went out, of course, but mostly it was to meet friends for a beer. But as my year progressed, I found myself eating out more and more. I'd gone out maybe once in January and February, a few more times in March and April, several rapid-fire dates in May, and then, in July, Dave had arrived. We didn't eat out very much, a couple times a month, but I stopped suggesting that we huddle in my small kitchen when I realized that if the point of my year was to find a way to sustain myself with unprocessed food, then I also had to heed my relationships. Dave and I may have started our relationship in the kitchen—or rather, on a breezy porch—but we sustained it over shared entrées and split checks. The meals I'd eaten out, while they had adhered as best they could to my unprocessed parameters, represented a different sort of unprocessing. That of my solitude, perhaps, in building an intimacy with people as much as with food. When I returned to my checking account to tally up the totals of meals eaten in the world—like most my age, I rarely have cash on hand—I find that, over the course of my year, I'd spent somewhere in the range of $500 at restaurants around town (supporting the local economy in yet another form).

If I started the year alone in my kitchen, I had ended it out in the world. Not literally, at the hot-dog stand, but in small connections that wound together. The lines began to blur between knowledge gathered and connections forged, sources for information and friends for socializing. When Sandor Katz visited Patagonia, I'd ended up eating sourdough pizza made with White Sonora wheat with Jeff Zimmerman on our lunch break. I ran into Jaime de Zubeldia at potluck dinners, sat next to Barbara Rose and sipped her prickly-pear lemonade. Now when I go to the farmers' market, I see J.C. and Lissa of Chiva Risa; I nod to Paul Schwennesen's wide cowboy hat.

That, really, seems to be the point of buying local. Dollars circulating through a community are important, but what they mean for my day-to-day is that I cannot move through the world anonymously. The realization of my CSA, where cranky hurriedness is taboo, became true for all my food purchases. I am not anonymous—*they* are not anonymous, these people who are willing to dedicate their life's energies to processing food from nature—and so we can't ignore the transfer of dollars from one to another. While it's true that dollars spent in your community are dollars withheld from the balance sheets of unaccountable corporations, it's also true that sometimes spending money better makes for a more lovely Sunday morning.

WHEN I STOPPED EATING PROCESSED FOODS back in January, I can't say I understood why. All I knew was that something needed to be done—that *I* needed to do something. I'd learned in Nicaragua that it is easy to get fired up about change, and much harder to figure out what you want to change—and how you want to do it. Some challenges feel so insurmountable that it seems as though nothing can be done. But we live in a world full of insurmountable obstacles. And we do things. Without small gestures, without localness and precision of place, it is hard to ask and harder to answer: How do we begin?

When I started unprocessed, I didn't have it totally figured out, couldn't have imagined all the complications I'd stumble into along the way—issues of health and money, time and family, community and independence. But after my year began, I'd tried to show, purchase by purchase, food by food, that even if you have very few, if you pay attention, your dollars have more purchasing power than you might believe.

We stir the proverbial frying pan of *gallo pinto,* turning and moving and working toward what comes next—hoping that we can summon the luck or energy to pluck out that last leftover bean and start something fresh.

Because, really, all you can do is begin.

ACKNOWLEDGMENTS

The support I've received in writing and researching this book is years long and dozens of people deep. I am so profoundly grateful that I get to do the only thing I've ever wanted to do.

Thank you first and foremost to my amazing agent, Mackenzie Brady, who is tirelessly enthusiastic and eminently talented. With Mackenzie at my side, nothing seemed quite so daunting. Thanks to my thoughtful, careful, considerate editor, Trish Daly. Trish got it—and then she went ahead and made it *so much* better.

This book took shape during the two life-changing years I spent in the MFA program at the University of Arizona. Thank you to my nonfiction cohort, who toiled on draft after draft, chapter after chapter, with patience, humor, and encouragement. Thanks to Fenton Johnson and Ander Monson for line edits and office hours. I'm humbled by the bundle of spirit that is Alison Deming, who provided much-needed inspiration, perspective, and balance.

Thank you, again and again, to Chris Cokinos, who challenged and focused me, who ignited latent energy, who made me rewrite paragraphs and reimagine chapters—and then reminded me to take it one word at a time. Thank you, Chris, for sitting across from me at lunch one January, and saying, "Yes. Write a book about *that*."

I humbly follow in the footsteps of Gary Nabhan, the food systems dreamer who has become, amazingly, a mentor, friend, and fellow adventurer. Thank you, Gary, for taking a chance on me—and for reminding me, always, why we write about food. Thank you for your optimism, resilience, and faith in our collective future.

Doug Biggers gave me my most favorite job and continues to support my life as a writer, in ways big and small. I love what I do and I get to do it because of Doug, who inhabits the wonderful space between brazen entrepreneur and fervent idealist. Thanks to his brother, Jeff Biggers, who nudged me along the path toward publication. Thanks to Steven Meckler, for my lovely author photo.

Before there was a year unprocessed—before there was graduate school or college—there was Bill Plaschke, who once told me how to be a writer over hamburgers at Magpie's Grill. It's all still true. Be hungry, ask questions, and everyone gets nervous. Thanks to Chris Erskine, for Zeli's Coffee and for believing in a young, hungry, nervous writer.

Thanks also to all those who welcomed me into the daily processes of their farms, kitchens, ranches, dairies, bakeries, offices, and homes: Jeff and Emma Zimmerman at Hayden Flour Mills; Jaime de Zubeldia at ReZoNation Farm; Prescott and Brian Vandervoet at Vandervoet & Associates; Frank Martin at Crooked Sky Farm and Philippe Waterinckx at the Tucson CSA—my favorite Wednesday evening activity. Thanks to Perry Dunson at Los Reales Landfill. Thanks to Tristan White at Dragoon Brewing; Marc Moeller at Flying Leap Vineyards; Todd and Kelly Bostock at Dos Cabezas Wineworks; and Stephen Paul at Hamilton Distillers—you all do amazing work. Thanks to Lissa Howe and J. C. Mutchler at Chiva Risa. Thanks to Barbara Rose at Bean Tree Farm and Jeff and Ana Sanders at Desert Dawn for a life-changing two days; thanks to Paul Schwennesen, for steak and conversation. To the wonderful, generous staff at the Community Food Bank of Southern Arizona, for letting me come in and peek around—Nick Henry, Robert Ojeda, Michael McDonald, and Bill Carnegie.

Thanks to Joe Abraham, for teaching me what a *murf* is. Thanks to Rob Dull, for a year at Hotel Brio, and Juan Delgado—*gracias, Juancho.* A quiet thanks, from afar, to Kimber Lanning, for the vision.

Thanks to my amazing friends, for tolerating my diet, supporting my frustrations, and finding the humor in unprocessed. Thanks to Sarah Minor, for dancing and baking and dating with me. Hilary Gan helped start my year; Heather Hamilton taught me the difference between a cow and a heifer; Jessica Langan-Peck made soup; Cory Aaland made the adventures more fun. Thanks to Dave Mondy, for coming along. Thanks to Courtney Trine and Kara Lyons, for their love and continuing support.

This book is for my family. For Joyce Kimble, the bravest woman who ever took on Texas—and Joel Kimble, who left his own courageous legacy. Thank you, Tyler, for your unprocessed inquiries and astute observations. To my big sister, Katie—my first reader, best critic, and unfailing cheerleader. You are the voice in my head; the first person I tell; my other half. I owe you a hundred big borrows. To my parents, Midge and Jeff Kimble. You are the foundation, the frame, and the roof. You are the start and the finish. You are home.

NOTES

INTRODUCTION

9   *Spend money better*—Loft Film Fest, Frances Causey and Kimber Lanning discuss Causey's new documentary, *Heist: Who Stole the American Dream?*
    shifted 10 percent—Local First, "Local Works! Examining the Impact of Local Business on the West Michigan Economy," *Civic Economics* (September 2008).

10   *a dollar distributed to the center*—Raj Patel, *Stuffed and Starved: The Hidden Battle for the World Food System* (New York: Melville House Publishing, 2007).

11   *three-fourths of food consumed*—Carlos Monteiro, "The Big Issue Is Ultra-processing," *World Nutrition* (November 2010).

12   *today, the goal of processing*—Ibid.

CHAPTER 1: SUPERMARKET

17   *the site of the first Safeway*—Olive Gray, "Seelig's Chain Is Now Safeway: Pioneer Grocery Business in New Hands," *Los Angeles Times,* March 15, 1925.
    But in 1916, when Clarence Saunders—Time, "Business & Finance: Piggly Wiggly Man," *Time* (February 25, 1929).

18   *M. M. Zimmerman marveled*—Max Mandell Zimmerman, *The Super Market: A Revolution in Distribution* (New York: McGraw-Hill, 1955).
    In 1929, an Irish immigrant—Tracie McMillan, *The American Way of Eating: Undercover at Walmart, Applebee's, Farm Fields, and the Dinner Table* (New York: Scribner, 2012).

19   *Today, aggressive food marketing*—Vance Packard, *The Hidden Persuaders* (New York: Ig Publishing, 2007).
    an intricate framework of slotting fees—Luis Therrien, "Want Shelf Space at the Supermarket? Ante Up," *BusinessWeek* (August 7, 1989).

21   *dissertations about supermarket layout*—Theodore Leed and Gene Garman, *Food Merchandising: Principles and Practices* (New York: Lebhar-Friedman Books, 1979).

22   *some foods are so irrationally irresistible*—David A. Kessler, *The Eat of Overeating: Taking Control of the Insatiable American Appetite* (Emmaus, PA: Rodale Books, 2010).

23   *We've processed foods*—Evelyn Kim, "Processed Food: A 2 Million Year History," *Scientific American* (August 20, 2013).

      Entrepreneurs bounded into—Diane Toops, "Food Processing: A History," *Food Processing* (October 5, 2010).

24   *In 1958, the FDA updated*—FDA: Generally Recognized as Safe (GRAS).

      According to a 2010 study—The PEW Charitable Trusts: Food Additives Project.

25   *the supermarket's "hypnoidal trance"*—Packard, *The Hidden Persuaders.*

26   *the "thousands of items offered"*—Mabian Manners, "Cornucopia of Foods Fills Market Baskets: Thousands of Items Offered," *Los Angeles Times,* September 16, 1961.

      By 2007, the average supermarket—Marion Nestle, *What to Eat* (New York: North Point Press, 2006).

CHAPTER 2: WHEAT

29   *as opposed to refined white flour*—Harold McGee, *On Food and Cooking: The Science and Lore of the Kitchen* (New York: Scribner, 2004).

32   *But then, ten thousand years ago*—Jared Diamond, *Guns, Germs, and Steel: The Fates of Human Societies* (New York: W. W. Norton, 1999).

33   *dated emmer cultivation*—Ibid.

35   *U.S. law required millers*—FDA, "Code of Federal Regulations Title 21: Food and Drugs."

      Archestratus, a contemporary—McGee, *On Food and Cooking.*

      chlorinated flour is illegal—United Kingdom Food Standards Agency, "The Bread and Flour Recommendations 1998."

40   *Weight Watchers calls a "trigger food"*—Weight Watchers Research Department, "Eating Triggers."

41   *Ancient grains are categorically*—Johan E. Hoff and Jules Janick, eds., "Wheat," *Food: Readings from Scientific American* (New York: W. H. Freeman & Company, 1973).

43   *a cohort of gastroenterologists*—Alberto Rubio-Tapia et al., "Increased Prevalence and Mortality in Undiagnosed Celiac Disease," *Gastroenterology* (April 2009).

44   *The word "foodshed"*—Jack Kloppenburg et al., "Coming into the Foodshed," *Agriculture and Human Values* (1996).

45   *the world's seed stocks*—ETC Group, "Who Will Control the Green Economy?" (November 2011).

46   *The decline of small mills*—USDA Economic Research Service, "Economic Analysis of the Changing Structure of the U.S. Flour Milling Industry" (2001).

50   *Price documented teeth*—Weston Price, *Nutrition and Physical Degeneration* (New York: Paul B. Hoeber, 1939).
      "All grains contain phytic acid"—Sally Fallon, *Nourishing Traditions: The Cookbook That Challenges Politically Correct Nutrition and the Diet Dictocrats* (Washington, D.C.: New Trends Publishing, 2001).

51   *They want fluffy flour*—Jeff Zimmerman, personal interview, October 20, 2012.

52   *White Sonora wheat is one of the oldest*—Slow Food USA, Ark of Taste, "White Sonora Wheat."

53   *In 1874, Charles Trumbull Hayden*—Richard Ruelas, "Tempe Man Revives Hayden Flour Mill Name," *Arizona Republic*, July 21, 2012.

57   *"The word* dough *comes*—McGee, *On Food and Cooking.*

CHAPTER 3: SWEET

63   *chocolate was consumed*—John S. Henderson et al., "Chemical and Archeological Evidence for the Earliest Cacao Beverages," proceedings of the National Academy of Sciences, October 8, 2007.

64   Xocolatl *became chocolate*—Harold McGee, *On Food and Cooking: The Science and Lore of the Kitchen* (New York: Scribner, 2004).

66   *an affinity for sweetness*—Sidney W. Mintz, *Sweetness and Power: The Place of Sugar in Modern History* (New York: Penguin Books, 1986).
      something that is sweet—*Oxford English Dictionary* definition of "sugar."

68   *All sugars are some combination*—McGee, *On Food and Cooking.*

69   *it's essentially irrelevant*—Gary Taubes, *Why We Get Fat: And What to Do About It* (New York: Anchor Books, 2011).

70   *By quantity, sugarcane is*—Food and Agricultural Organization of the United Nations, "Crop Production."
      the knobby reed contained—Mintz, *Sweetness and Power.*
      A fellow named Dioscorides—Andrew Dalby, *Food in the Ancient World from A to Z* (New York: Routledge, 2003).

71   *Sugar remained on the periphery*—Ibid.

      granulated sugar was a rarity—Mintz, *Sweetness and Power.*

      But it was in the Americas—Ibid.

72   *Making sugar from sugarcane*—Andrew Wilder, "What is the healthiest sugar?"
      EatingRules.com.

73   *bone char from cattle*—Jeanne Yacoubou, "Is Your Sugar Vegan? An Update on
      Sugar Processing Practices," *Vegetarian Journal* (2007).

      Initially, the incentive to process—Mintz, *Sweetness and Power.*

74   *sugar is "defined as any*—Robert J. Lustig, "The Toxic Truth About Sugar," *Nature*
      (February 2, 2012).

      sugar consumption has tripled—Ibid.

      how your body responds to sugar—Taubes, *Why We Get Fat.*

75   *"If the stars should appear*—Ralph Waldo Emerson, *Nature and Selected Essays* (New
      York: Penguin Classics, 2003).

      "The bees are cranky today,"—Jaime de Zubeldia, personal interview, March 19,
      2013.

76   *honey was the sweetener*—Dalby, *Food in the Ancient World.*

      That space is in fact called "bee space"—Tammy Horn, *Bees in America: How the
      Honey Bee Shaped a Nation* (Lexington: University Press of Kentucky, 2005).

78   *honey without pollen isn't honey*—Andrew Schneider, "Tests Show Most Store
      Honey Isn't Honey," *Food Safety News* (November 7, 2011).

80   *the Trader Joe's demographic*—Beth Kowitt, "Inside the Secret World of Trader Joe's,"
      Fortune (August 23, 2010).

83   *On the Vivapura blog*—"The Best Raw Chocolate Ever," http://blog.vivpura.com.

CHAPTER 4: PRODUCE

92   *The food that catalyzes this transformation*—Frank Martin, personal interview,
      January 4, 2013.

96   *In the past thirty years, many farmers*—Peter Pringle, *Food, Inc.: Mendel to
      Monsanto—The Promises and Perils of the Biotech Harvest* (New York: Simon &
      Schuster, 2003).

97   *the precedent of substantial equivalence*—Ibid.

98   *California tried to legislate*—"Who's Funding Prop 37, Labeling for Genetically
      Modified Foods?" KCET Election 2012.

100   *roughly 75 percent of farmworkers*—National Farmer Worker Ministry, "Farm
      Worker Issues."

101   *It is a well-worn story*—USDA 2012 *Census of Agriculture,* Tom Vilsack, Secretary.
      thirteen million acres of prime farmland—"Summary Report: 2010 National
      Resources Inventory," Natural Resources Conservation Service, 2013.
      it is not work that pays—Ken Meter, "Finding Food in the Border Counties," *Hungry
      For Change: Borderlands Food and Water in the Balance* (Southwest Center's Kellogg
      Program in Sustainable Food Systems: 2012).

102   *the average age of the American farmer*—USDA 2012 *Census of Agriculture,* Tom
      Vilsack, Secretary.
      In the winter, 60 percent—Prescott and Brian Vandervoet, personal interview,
      October 2011–February 2013.

103   *food has flowed across this region*—Gary Paul Nabhan, "A Brief History of Cross-
      Border Food Trade," *Hungry for Change: Borderlands Food and Water in the Balance*
      (Southwest Center's Kellogg Program in Sustainable Food Systems: 2012).

106   *Every mango eaten*—Robert R. Alvarez, "The Transnational State and Empire:
      U.S. Certification in the Mexican Mango and Persian Lime Industries," *Human
      Organization* (2006).

110   *Legally, a food is organic*—USDA Agricultural Marketing Service: National Organic
      Program.

111   *The problem of Big Organic*—Stephanie Strom, "Has Organic Been Oversized?"
      New York Times, July 7, 2012.
      While there are a few brokers—Phil Ostram, personal interview, February 1, 2012.

112   *"The landscape of any farm*—Aldo Leopold, "The Farmer as Conservationist," *The
      River of the Mother of God: And Other Essays by Aldo Leopold* (Madison: University
      of Wisconsin Press, 1992).

113   *65 percent of conventionally grown*—Environmental Working Group, "EWG's 2014
      Shopper's Guide to Pesticides In Produce."

114   *one in four strawberry samples*—EPA, "Technology Transfer Network Air Toxics Web
      Site: Captan."

115   *Most are grown in the Central Valley*—Eric Schlosser, "In the Strawberry Fields,"
      The Atlantic Monthly (November 1995).

116   *ninety-one cents of every dollar*—Steven Gorelick and Helena Norberg-Hodge,
      "Think Global . . . Eat Local," *The Ecologist* (September 2002).

116   *shifted just five dollars each week*—Meter, "Finding Food in the Border Counties."

117   *twenty thousand acres of farmland*—Julie Murphree, "Arizona Agriculture in High Cotton!" Arizona Farm Bureau, September 25, 2013.

CHAPTER 5: SALT

123   *In June of 1862, John Commins*—Mark Kurlansky, *Salt: A World History* (New York: Penguin , 2002).

    Facing severe salt shortages—Ibid.

124   *the 10,000 chemicals added*—Center for Science in the Public Interest, "Food Additives."

    to pull salt from the earth—Harold McGee, *On Food and Cooking: The Science and Lore of the Kitchen* (New York: Scribner, 2004).

126   *Salt keeps our electrolytes*—Ibid.

    "Salt is perfect—Marion Nestle, *What to Eat* (New York: North Point Press, 2006).

130   *"We say food ingredients*—Steve Ettlinger, *Twinkie, Deconstructed: My Journey to Discover How the Ingredients Found in Processed Foods Are Grown, Mined (Yes, Mined), and Manipulated into What America Eats* (New York: Hudson Street Press, 2007).

    Only 8 percent of the salt—U.S. Geological Survey, "2010 Minerals Yearbook: Salt."

CHAPTER 6: STUFF

137   *this fragility is no mistake*—Bernard London, "Ending the Depression Through Planned Obsolescence" (Madison: University of Wisconsin, 1932; digitized 2009).

139   *one of the first "unrepairable products"*—Giles Slade, *Made to Break: Technology and Obsolescence in America* (Cambridge, MA.: Harvard University Press, 2006).

    Repair or replace it? *asks an article*—Consumer Reports, "Repair or Replace It? CR's Guide to Having Products Fixed—or Not," *Consumer Reports* (November 2008).

140   *During World War II*—Raytheon Company, "Our Company History," www.raytheon.com.

    "Basically, you dig a big hole—Perry Dunson, personal interview, February 7, 2013.

141   *In 1976, the EPA mandated*—EPA, "Resource Conservation and Recovery Act," 1976.

142   *cause climate change by releasing*—EPA, "Overview of Greenhouse Gases: Methane Emissions."

143 *These UA folks are a group*—William Rathje and Cullen Murphy, *Rubbish!: The Archeology of Garbage* (New York: HarperCollins, 1992).

144 *40 percent of our food*—Jonathan Bloom, *American Wasteland: How America Throws Away Nearly Half of Its Food* (Boston: De Capo Lifelong Books, 2010).

145 *The first public garbage management*—Rathje and Murphy, *Rubbish!*
more than nine thousand municipalities—EPA, "Municipal Solid Waste Generation, Recycling, and Disposal in the United States: Facts and Figures for 2010."
Tucson's Materials Recovery Facility—Augie, personal interview, February 11, 2013.

149 *According to a study by Local First*—Local First, "Local Works! Examining the Impact of Local Business on the West Michigan Economy," *Civic Economics* (September 2008).
Cooperatives purchase 20 percent—National Cooperative Grocers Association, "Healthy Foods Healthy Communities: Measuring the Social and Economic Impact of Food Co-ops," 2012.

150 *Case in point: A study of a food*—"Waste Reduction in Food Retail: Case Study Report of the People's Food Co-op," Solid Waste Research Group (Lansing: University of Michigan, 1991).
the "skin of commerce"—Daniel Imhoff, *Paper or Plastic: Searching for Solutions to an Overpackaged World* (San Francisco: Sierra Club Books, 2005).
containers and packaging make up—EPA, "Municipal Solid Waste Generation, Recycling, and Disposal in the United States: Facts and Figures for 2010."

151 *RISE Equipment Recycling Center*—Ruben Vejar, personal interview, March 28, 2013.

155 *the new food processor promised*—Cuisinart Marketing Pamphlet, Cookery Ephemera Index, Los Angeles Public Library Archives (accessed May 14, 2012).

158 *I spent a frantic two weeks*—Beth Terry, *Plastic-Free: How I Kicked the Plastic Habit and How You Can Too* (New York: Skyhorse, 2012).
so is the documentary Bag It—*Bag It! Is Your Life Too Plastic?* dir. Suzan Beraza, Paramount Classics, 2011.

CHAPTER 7: OUT

161 *Hugh Grant plays*—*Notting Hill*, dir. Roger Michell, Polygram, 1999.

165 *either abstainers or moderators*—Gretchen Rubin, *The Happiness Project: Or, Why I Spent a Year Trying to Sing in the Morning, Clean My Closets, Fight Right, Read Aristotle, and Generally Have More Fun* (New York: HarperCollins, 2009).

172   *"Monocultures of the mind make*—Vandana Shiva, *Monocultures of the Mind: Perspectives on Biodiversity and Biotechnology* (London: Zed Books, 1993).

174   *the minute we include*—Deborah Madison, *What We Eat When We Eat Alone: Stories and 100 Recipes* (New York: Gibbs Smith, 2009).

CHAPTER 8: DRINK

179   *the early process of alcohol making*—Elias Lönnrot, *The Kalevala: An Epic Poem after Oral Tradition* (London: Oxford University Press, 2009).

184   *"From the start, it seems that beer*—Tom Standage, *A History of the World in Six Glasses* (New York: Bloomsbury, 2006).

185   *"A lot of people ask us*—Tristan White, personal interview, August 12, 2014.

186   *Indeed, there are no laws*—FDA, "Guidance for Industry: Labeling of Certain Beers Subject to the Labeling Jurisdiction of the Food and Drug Administration."

187   *"I think the coolest thing*—Stephen Paul, personal interview, August 24, 2014.

192   *"I am tempted to place the craving*—Jean-Anthelme Brillat-Savarin, *The Physiology of Taste* (New York: Penguin Classics, 1970).
        Temperature and time are finicky—Harold McGee, *On Food and Cooking: The Science and Lore of the Kitchen* (New York: Scribner, 2004).

193   *I found an article online*—Gary Miller, "A Cheap and Easy Homemade Wine Recipe," *Mother Earth News* (September/October, 1970).
        A few weeks before, we'd both—Sandor Ellix Katz, Fermentation Workshop, October 23, 2012.

194   *Sulfites are any sulfur-based*—McGee, *On Food and Cooking.*
        more than seventy other additives—Code of Federal Regulations, Title 27: Alcohol, Tobacco Products and Firearms, "Materials Authorized for the Treatment of Wine and Juice."
        These additives might include enzymes—Christopher Null, "How to Make Mass Produced Wine Taste Great," *Wired* (April 24, 2014).

196   *On the first day of the grape harvest*—Marc Moeller, personal interview, August 9, 2014.

200   *"We have a lot of history here"*—Todd Bostock, personal interview, August 9, 2014.

203   *if you want to make mead*—Sandor Ellix Katz, *The Art of Fermentation: An In-depth Exploration of Essential Concepts and Processes from Around the World* (White River Junction, VT: Chelsea Green, 2012).

CHAPTER 9: REFRIGERATION

207   *the French military offered*—Encyclopædia Britannica, "Nicolas Appert," *Encyclopædia Britannica.*

Fifty years before Appert—Encyclopædia Britannica, "Refrigeration," *Encyclopædia Britannica.*

208   *the U.S. Office of Education*—Federal Security Agency, U.S. Office of Education Division of Visual Aids, "Principles of Refrigeration."

The chemicals we've used—Barbara Krasner-Khait, "The Impact of Refrigeration," *History Magazine* (2013).

a team at General Motors synthesized—DuPont Heritage Timeline, "1930: Freon."

In the 1920s, relatively few homes—Krasner-Khait, "The Impact of Refrigeration."

Within two decades, a General Electric—General Electric Consumers Institute, "Frozen Foods: How to Prepare, Package, Freeze, and Cook," Cookery Ephemera Index, Los Angeles Public Library Archives (accessed May 14, 2012).

209   *Freezers captivated a generation*—Borg-Warner Corporation, "Cooking with Cold" (1937), Cookery Ephemera Index, Los Angeles Public Library Archives (accessed May 14, 2012).

210   *Why can my own food*—U.S. Bureau of Human Nutrition and Home Economics, "Wartime Canning of Fruits and Vegetables" (1943), Los Angeles Public Library Archives (accessed May 14, 2012).

213   *the average time we spend*—USDA Economic Research Service, "How Much Time Do Americans Spend on Food?" November 2011.

about three hours a day in the 1920s—Lindsey Smith, "Trends in US Home Food Preparation and Consumption:Analysis of National Nutrition Surveys and Time Use Studies from 1965–1966 to 2007–2008," *Nutritional Journal* (April 11, 2013).

While in 1926, women were spending—Laura Shapiro, *Something from the Oven: Reinventing Dinner in 1950s America* (New York: Penguin, 2004).

this new culture of convenience—American Can Company, Marketing Pamphlet, Cookery Ephemera Index, Los Angeles Public Library Archives (accessed May 14, 2012).

214   *"I do not believe that 'employment*—Wendell Berry, *What Are People For?* (Berkeley, CA: Counterpoint, 2010).

219   *tells an anecdote to prove his point*—Mark Albion, *More Than Money: Questions Every MBA Needs to Answer* (San Francisco: BK Life, 2008).

CHAPTER 10: DAIRY

230   *"Roxie is funny, sweet, sassy*—Shamrock Farms Farm Tour, October 20, 2012.

232   *the 6 billion gallons we guzzle up*—"U.S. Fluid Milk Demand: A Disaggregated Approach." *International Food and Agribusiness Management Review,* 2012.

234   *a controversial additive*—Andrew Weil, "Is Carrageenan Safe?" DrWeil.com, October 1, 2012.

235   *Nine or ten thousand years ago*—Harold McGee, *On Food and Cooking: The Science and Lore of the Kitchen* (New York: Scribner, 2004).
    For this reason, fluid milk—Ibid.

236   *"Sweet, fresh cow's milk*—Melanie DuPris, *Nature's Perfect Food: How Milk Became America's Drink* (New York: New York University Press, 2002).

237   *In March of 2012, a Wisconsin farmer*—"Farmer Accused of Selling Raw Milk Stays Free," Channel3000.com, March 2, 2012.
    Modern historian P. J. Atkins—"White Poison? The Social Consequences of Milk Consumption, 1850–1930," *Social History of Medicine* (1992).
    infected with cholera infantum—DuPris, *Nature's Perfect Food.*

238   *Americans clamored for reform*—Ibid.
    the reason to drink raw milk—Sandor Ellix Katz, *The Revolution Will Not Be Microwaved: Inside America's Underground Food Movements* (New York: Chelsea Green, 2006).

239   *"this mixed community*—Jennifer Ackerman,"How Bacteria in Our Bodies Protect Our Health," *Scientific American* (May 15, 2012).

241   *Although the milk from cows*—Marion Nestle, *What to Eat* (New York: North Point Press, 2006).

242   *two companies—Horizon Organic*—Ye Su, Scott Brown, and Michael Cook, "Stability in Organic Milk Farm Prices: A Comparative Study," University of Missouri, 2013.
    two "mega-dairy" farms—DuPris, *Nature's Perfect Food.*
    Is milk healthy?—U.S. Department of Agriculture, "Dietary Guidelines for Americans, 2010."

243   *"the dairy industry is large*—Nestle, *What to Eat.*
    The American Institute for Cancer Research—"Independent Researchers Issue New Assessment of Possible Milk-Prostate Cancer Link," American Institute for Cancer Research, February 26, 2002.

243   *The most compelling evidence*—T. Colin Campbell, *The China Study: The Most Comprehensive Study of Nutrition Ever Conducted* (Dallas: BenBella Books, 2006).

244   *The Weston A. Price Foundation*—Denise Minger, "The China Study Myth," Weston A. Price Foundation, March 24, 2012.

      New research shows that eating—Allison Aubrey, "The Full-Fat Paradox: Whole Milk May Keep Us Lean," National Public Radio, February 12, 2014.

      Other studies show that the fats—Sally Fallon, *Nourishing Traditions: The Cookbook That Challenges Politically Correct Nutrition and the Diet Dictocrats* (Washington, D.C.: New Trends, 2001).

247   *the total footprint of a pint of milk*—Mike Berners-Lee, *How Bad Are Bananas: The Carbon Footprint of Everything* (Vancouver: Greystone Books, 2011).

249   *make oat milk at home*—"How to Milk an Oat," *Chocolate Covered Katie: The Healthy Dessert Blog,* September 2, 2010.

      where 80 percent of the world's—Eric Holthaus, "The Thirsty West: 10 Percent of California's Water Goes to Almond Farming," *Slate* (May 14, 2014).

      more than a gallon of water—Julia Lurie and Alex Park, "It Takes How Much Water to Grow an Almond?" *Mother Jones* (February 4, 2014).

252   *"Saturday. Goat day!"*—Lissa Howe and J. C. Mutchler, personal interview, November 3, 2012.

256   *In 2012, the* Washington Post *reported*—Editorial Board, "The 'Milk Cliff,'" *Washington Post,* December 22, 2012.

CHAPTER 11: MEAT

261   *Rain patters on the tin roof*—Animal Processing Workshop, Bean Tree Farm, December 15–16, 2012.

266   *"What is it that makes a creature*—Harold McGee, *On Food and Cooking: The Science and Lore of the Kitchen* (New York: Scribner, 2004).

      Two million years ago—Katharine Milton, "A Hypothesis to Explain the Role of Meat-eating in Human Evolution," *Evolutionary Anthropology* (1999).

      our ancestors began eating the animal—"Earliest Porotic Hyperostosis on a 1.5-Million-Year-Old Hominin, Olduvai Gorge, Tanzania," *PLOS ONE* (2012).

      it was this new diet—Charles Q. Choi, "Eating Meat Made Us Human, Suggests New Skull Fossil," LiveScience.com, October 3, 2012.

267   *Quite a bit later—1.9 million years*—Jared Diamond, *Guns, Germs, and Steel: The Fates of Human Societies* (New York: W. W. Norton, 1999).

269   *there was a big scare in Michigan*—Science, "Michigan's PBB Incident: Chemical Mix-Up Leads to Disaster," *Science* (April 16, 1976).

        They had fed fire retardant—G. F. Fries, "The PBB Episode in Michigan: An Overall Appraisal," *Critical Reviews in Toxicology* 16, no. 2 (1985): 105–56.

        According to Joyce Egginton—Joyce Egginton, *The Poisoning of Michigan* (East Lansing: Michigan State University Press, 2009).

275   *the process often sends*—N.J.B. McFarlane et al., "Detection of Bone Fragments in Chicken Meat Using X-ray Backscatter," *Biosystems Engineering* (June 2003).

        all of the reasons not *to eat meat*—Food and Agriculture Organization of the United Nations, "Livestock's Long Shadow: Environmental Issues and Options," 2006.

        Corn in, flesh out—Michael Pollan, *The Omnivore's Dilemma: A Natural History of Four Meals* (New York: Penguin, 2007).

276   *Livestock contributes over a third*—Food and Agriculture Organization of the United Nations, "Livestock's Long Shadow."

        an average-size steer—Tim Appenzeller, "The End of Cheap Oil," *National Geographic* (June 2004).

        Forty percent of grain grown—Michael Pollan, "Farmer in Chief," *New York Times Magazine* (October 9, 2008).

        Grain goes in, waste comes out—Jonathan Safran Foer, *Eating Animals* (New York: Back Bay Books, 2010).

        What about our *bodies?*—Marion Nestle, *What to Eat* (New York: North Point Press, 2006).

        "The meat industry's big—Marion Nestle, *Food Politics* (Berkeley: University of California Press, 2003).

277   *sick cattle get treated with drugs*—Sabrina Tavernise, "Farm Use of Antibiotics Defies Scrutiny," *New York Times,* September 3, 2012.

        thirteen *major slaughterhouses*—*Food, Inc.* dir. Robert Kenner, Magnolia Pictures, 2010.

        sixty-two thousand people—Denise Eblen, "E. Coli O157:H7 in Ground Beef," USDA's Food Safety and Inspection Service podcast, September 16, 2009.

281   *many reasons* to eat *meat*—Gary Taubes, *Why We Get Fat: And What to Do About It* (New York: Alfred A. Knopf, 2011).

        heard of the Paleo diet—Weston Price, *Nutrition and Physical Degeneration* (New York: Paul B. Hoeber, 1939).

286 *what about the environment?*—Paul Schwennesen, personal interview, January 8, 2012.

288 *known as "ecosystem services*—Daniel Imhoff, *Farming with the Wild: Enhancing Biodiversity of Farms and Ranches* (San Francisco: Sierra Club Books, 2003).
The story of the decline of local—Kate Zezima, "Push to Eat Local Food Is Hampered by Shortage," *New York Times,* March 27, 2010.

CHAPTER 12: HUNGER

294 *Twenty dollars a week*—USDA, Supplemental Nutrition Assistance Program, Eligibility.

295 *SNAP Challenge—an official challenge*—Community Food Bank of Southern Arizona, "About the SNAP Challenge."

298 *the cost of fifty-nine fresh*—Hayden Stewart, Jeffrey Hyman, Jean Buzby, Elizabeth Frazao, and Andrea Carlson, "How Much Do Fruits and Vegetables Cost?" USDA, Economic Research Service, February 2011.
some vested interest—Andrea Carlson and Hayden Stewart, "A Wide Variety of Fruits and Vegetables Are Affordable for SNAP Recipients," USDA, Economic Research Service, December 2011.
on average, fruits and vegetables—Andrea Carlson and Elizabeth Frazao, "Are Health Foods Really More Expensive? It Depends on How You Measure the Price," USDA, Economic Research Service, May 2012.

302 *Hunger affects one out of five*—USDA, A. Coleman-Jensen, M. Nord, M. Andrews, and S. Carlson, "Household Food Security in the United States in 2011," 2012.
One in six American adults—James Mabli, Rhoda Cohen, Frank Potter, and Zhanyun Zhao, "Hunger in America 2010: Local Report Prepared for the Community Food Bank of Tucson," Mathematica Policy Research, 2010.
The "U.S. Household Food—USDA, Economic Research Service, "U.S. Adult Food Security Survey Module: Three-Stage Design, with Screeners," September 2012.

303 *if you earn less than $1,265*—USDA, SNAP eligibility.
"I don't think it matters—Bill Carnegie, personal interview, February 1, 2013.

307 *"Las Milpitas is an example*—Robert Ojeda, personal interview, January 22, 2014.

310 *one dollar buys either*—Adam Drewnowski and S. E. Specter, "Poverty and Obesity: The Role of Energy Density and Energy Costs," *American Journal of Clinical Nutrition* (January 2004).

310   *63 percent of the state*—Trust for America's Health, "F as in Fat: How Obesity Threatens America's Future," July 2011.

311   *relied on SNAP benefits*—Melanie Mason, "Food Stamps for Good Food," *The Nation,* March 10, 2011.

Nine percent of Arizonans—Arizona Department of Health Services, "Arizona Diabetes Burden Report: 2011."

The Farm Bill has inertia—Daniel Imhoff, *Food Fight: The Citizen's Guide to the Next Food and Farm Bill* (Healdsburg, CA: Watershed Media, 2012).

313   *these are the foods we support*—Ibid.

Today, more than 70 percent—Ibid.

EPILOGUE

321   *Eaters in the United States*—USDA Economic Research Service, "Percent of Household Final Consumption Expenditures Spent on Food, Alcoholic Beverages, and Tobacco That Were Consumed at Home, by Selected Countries," 2013.

In 2013, just 6.1 percent—USDA Economic Research Service, "Food Expenditures by Families and Individuals as a Share of Disposable Personal Income," 2012.

322   *to advocate shopping at a co-op*—National Cooperative Grocers Association, "Healthy Foods Healthy Communities: Measuring the Social and Economic Impact of Food Co-ops," 2012.

323   *"We are eliminating our own jobs*—Kimber Lanning, personal interview, April 1, 2013.